Development and Prevention of Behaviour Problems

T0383756

Development and Prevention of Behaviour Problems: From Genes to Social Policy brings together world leading researchers from diverse fields to explore the potential causes of the development of behaviour problems. The book presents theories that hope to influence public health, education and social policy in the prevention of the costly social troubles that behaviour problems can cause.

Featuring contributions from researchers whose backgrounds range from the social and behavioural sciences to economics, the varied chapters assess the potential role of gene–environment interactions, biological factors and gender differences in the development of behaviour problems. The book includes a review of studies that attempt to understand why antisocial behaviour is concentrated in families, and concludes with three chapters that link developmental research directly with policy issues. It provides a framework for students, scientists, educators and care givers to understand where frontier research on behaviour problems is going and how it can be applied in the social, educational and health services.

This collection will interest all students of behavioural psychology and the behavioural sciences as well as those with an interest in public policy, sociology, abnormal psychology, psychopathology and personality disorders.

Richard E. Tremblay is Professor of Paediatrics, Psychiatry and Psychology at the University of Montréal, Professor of Child Development in the School of Public Health at University College Dublin, and co-director of the International Laboratory for Child and Adolescent Mental Health Development (INSERM U669, Paris).

Marcel A. G. van Aken is full professor and chair of the Department of Developmental Psychology at Utrecht University. His research focuses on transactional relations between personality and social relationships.

Willem Koops is distinguished professor in Foundations and History of Developmental Psychology and Education at Utrecht University, The Netherlands. He is Dean of the Faculty of Social and Behavioural Sciences and Editor of the *European Journal of Developmental Psychology*.

Development and Prevention of Behaviour Problems

From Genes to Social Policy

**Edited by Richard E. Tremblay,
Marcel A. G. van Aken and Willem Koops**

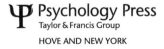

Ψ Psychology Press
Taylor & Francis Group

HOVE AND NEW YORK

First published 2009
by Psychology Press
27 Church Road, Hove, East Sussex BN3 2FA

Simultaneously published in the USA and Canada
by Psychology Press
711 Third Avenue, New York, NY 10017

Psychology Press is an imprint of the Taylor & Francis Group, an Informa business

First issued in paperback 2012

Typeset in Times by RefineCatch Limited, Bungay, Suffolk

Cover design by Andy Ward

This publication has been produced with paper manufactured to strict environmental standards and with pulp derived from sustainable forests.

British Library Cataloguing in Publication Data
A catalogue record for this book is available from the British Library

Library of Congress Cataloging-in-Publication Data
Development and prevention of behaviour problems : from genes to social policy / edited by Richard E. Tremblay, Marcel A.G. van Aken and Willem Koops.
    p. cm.
Includes bibliographical references and index.
ISBN 978-1-84872-007-7 (hb)
    1. Conduct disorders in children—Prevention. I. Tremblay, Richard Ernest. II. Aken, Marcel A. G. van, 1958– III. Koops, W. (Willem)
RJ506.C65D48 2009
618.92'89–dc22

                                                            2008044652

ISBN: 978-1-84872-007-7 (hbk)

ISBN: 978-0-415-64720-5 (pbk)

Contents

Figures

viii   *Figures*

Contributors

Michal Abrahamowicz Centre de Recherche, Centre Hospitalier de l'Université de Montréal, Montréal, Quebec, Canada

Jason Almerigi Child Development Department, Tufts University, Medford, MA, USA

Nadine Arbour Groupe ECOBES, CEGEP Jonquiere, Jonquiere, Quebec, Canada

Manon Bernard Brain & Body Centre, University of Nottingham, Nottingham, UK

Sylvana M. Côté Social and Preventive Medicine, Montréal University, Montréal, Canada and Utrecht University, Utrecht, The Netherlands

Alan C. Evans Montréal Neurological Institute, McGill University, Montréal, Quebec, Canada

Lynette Feder College of Liberal Arts & Sciences, Portland State University, Portland, OR, USA

Daniel Gaudet Complex Hospitalier de la Sagamie, Chicoutimi, Quebec, Canada

Pavel Hamet Centre de Recherche, Centre Hospitalier de l'Université de Montréal, Montréal, Quebec, Canada

Petr Hanzalek Brain & Body Centre, University of Nottingham, Nottingham, UK

Sara Jaffee Institute of Psychiatry, King's College, London, UK

Marianne Junger IPIT Institute for Social Safety Studies, School of Management & Governance, University of Twente, Enschede, The Netherlands

Willem Koops Department of Developmental Psychology, Utrecht University, The Netherlands

Michael Kramer Montréal Children's Hospital, McGill University, Montréal, Quebec, Canada

Luc Laberge   Groupe ECOBES, CEGEP Jonquiere, Jonquiere, Quebec, Canada

Susan Leal   Baylor College of Medicine, Houston, TX, USA

Gabriel Leonard   Montréal Neurological Institute, McGill University, Montréal, Quebec, Canada

Jackie Lerner   Child Development Department, Tufts University, Medford, MA, USA

Richard M. Lerner   Child Development Department, Tufts University, Medford, MA, USA

Jean Mathieu   Complex Hospitalier de la Sagamie, Chicoutimi, Quebec, Canada

Patrick O. McGowan   Douglas Hospital Research Center, and McGill Program for the Study of Behaviour, Genes and Environment, 6875 LaSalle Blvd, Montréal, Quebec, Canada

Michael J. Meaney   Douglas Hospital Research Center, and McGill Program for the Study of Behaviour, Genes and Environment, 6875 LaSalle Blvd, Montréal, Quebec, Canada

Tomáš Paus   Brain & Body Centre, University of Nottingham, Nottingham, UK and the Montréal Neurological Institute, McGill University, Montréal, Quebec, Canada

Zdenka Pausova   Brain & Body Centre, University of Nottingham, Nottingham, UK and the Centre de Recherche, Centre Hospitalier de l'Université de Montréal, Montréal, Quebec, Canada

Michael Perron   Groupe ECOBES, CEGEP Jonquiere, Jonquiere, Quebec, Canada

Anne C. Petersen   Center for Advanced Study in the Behavioral Sciences, Stanford University, Stanford, CA, USA

Nadine Provencal   Department of Pharmacology and Therapeutics, McGill University, Montréal, Quebec, Canada

Bruce Pike   Montréal Neurological Institute, McGill University, Montréal, Quebec, Canada

Alain Pitiot   Brain & Body Centre, University of Nottingham, Nottingham, UK

Louis Richer   Department of Psychology, University of Quebec in Chicoutimi, Chicoutimi, Quebec, Canada

Jean R. Séguin   Research Unit on Children's Psychosocial Maladjustment (GRIP), University of Montréal, Montréal, Quebec, Canada

Stephen J. Suomi Laboratory of Comparative Ethology, Eunice Kennedy Shriver National Institute of Child Health and Human Development, Poolesville, MD, USA

Catriona Syme Brain & Body Centre, University of Nottingham, Nottingham, UK

Moshe Szyf Department of Pharmacology and Therapeutics, McGill University, and McGill Program for the Study of Behaviour, Genes and Environment, 6875 LaSalle Blvd, Montréal, Quebec, Canada

Richard E. Tremblay International Laboratory for Child and Adolescent Mental Health Development, INSERM U669, Paris, France; University of Montréal, Quebec, Canada; School of Public Health and Population Sciences, University College, Dublin, Ireland; and Utrecht University, Utrecht, The Netherlands

Marcel A. G. van Aken Department of Developmental Psychology, Utrecht University, Utrecht, The Netherlands

Jacques van der Gaag Depertment of Economics, University of Amsterdam, The Netherlands

Suzanne Veillette Groupe ECOBES, CEGEP Jonquiere, Jonquiere, Quebec, Canada

Kate Watkins Department of Experimental Psychology, University of Oxford, Oxford, UK

Ian Weaver Douglas Hospital Research Center, and McGill Program for the Study of Behaviour, Genes and Environment, 6875 LaSalle Blvd, Montréal, Quebec, Canada

Preface

This book is the product of important developments at Utrecht University's Department of Developmental Psychology (Utrecht, The Netherlands). The Department has been especially fortunate in receiving several resources to invite eminent scholars from abroad who study the development and prevention of behaviour problems from an interdisciplinary perspective.

First, a generous award was given by the Joannes Juda Groen Foundation for Interdisciplinary Behavioural Research (in Dutch: the Joannes Juda Groen Stichting voor Interdisciplinair Gedragsonderzoek, or SIGO), to offer Richard Tremblay a chair during the years 2004–2007. He presented his inaugural lecture on 9 June 2006 with Marcel van Aken, who became professor of Developmental Psychology following the nomination of Willem Koops as Dean of the Faculty of Social and Behavioural Sciences. In connection with these two inaugural lectures an international symposium on the Development and Prevention of Behaviour Problems was organized with the aim of offering an overview of the interdisciplinary frontier work being done on this topic.

Second, in 2005 the "Belle van Zuylen" chair was offered by the Department of Developmental Psychology to Sylvana Côté. The chair is offered annually by Utrecht University to an internationally renowned scholar on a topic related to the work of Belle van Zuylen, a writer born near Utrecht in 1740, who died 65 years later in Switzerland where she lived with her Swiss husband. Writing in French under the name Isabelle de Charrière, Belle published novels, pamphlets, plays and a voluminous correspondence with famous intellectuals such as James Boswell and Benjamin Constant. Sylvana Côté creatively built on the work of Belle van Zuylen by concentrating on gender differences, in this case in aggressive behaviour, the topic of her inaugural lecture (7 June 2007) and her chapter in this book. We are grateful for the award from Utrecht University and grateful to Sylvana Côté for her stimulating and motivating collaboration with the Department of Developmental Psychology.

Richard Tremblay was the main "auctor intellectualis" of the symposium and book, heavily supported by Marcel van Aken, who also took care of much of the logistics of the symposium. Willem Koops, in his capacity of

Dean, obtained the financial support from the foundations. We are grateful to Mrs Madelon Pieper who took care of the desk editing process and contacts with the authors.

Finally, we want to express our gratitude towards the SIGO foundation who financed the professorial chair of Richard Tremblay and also subsidized the publication of this book. SIGO is the guardian of the intellectual heritage of the Dutch physician Joannes Juda Groen (1903–1990), a scientist with a passion for interdisciplinary research (Van Daal & De Knecht-van Eekelen, 1994). The aim of the colloquium and the book was to highlight fundamental changes in research on behaviour problems that are still hard to grasp by most investigators. Dr J. J. Groen would most certainly be thrilled to see the incredible advancements made since he died. Thanks to his foresight the Groen Foundation contributes to widening the horizons.

Reference

Van Daal, M. J. G. W., & De Knecht-van Eekelen, A. (1994). *Joannes Juda Groen (1903–1990). Een arts op zoek naar het ware welzijn* [A doctor looking for the real well-being]. Rotterdam: Erasmus Publishing.

1 Research on the development and prevention of behaviour problems

A fundamental change still hard to grasp for most investigators

Richard E. Tremblay, Marcel A. G. van Aken and Willem Koops

This book brings together world leading investigators to illustrate how different fields of expertise are coming together to unravel the development of behaviour problems and, hopefully, influence public health, education and social policies in preventing costly health and social problems.

There was a time, not so long ago, when social, cognitive, psychodynamic, behavioural and biological investigators were each working in their own small corner of the world trying to find "The Cause" and "The Cure" of behaviour problems. We vividly remember the freshly minted PhD from one of the top child development research institutes in the USA proudly telling, in a job interview, that he specialized in emotional development rather than cognitive development because it was the "real" basis of behaviour problems, and the candidate for a postdoctoral position claiming that her knowledge of multi-level analyses was essential and foundational for the future of research of behavioural problems, if not for any behavioural research.

Students were not the only naïve members of the academic and public policy environment. In the years leading to the last decade of the 20th century, the McArthur Foundation joined forces with the National Institute of Justice, investing very large amounts of money to plan a longitudinal study aimed at understanding the development of antisocial behaviour from an interdisciplinary perspective (Farrington et al., 1990; Tonry et al., 1991). The genetic-biological component that the first author of this chapter worked on with Felton Earls and David Rowe was not the most popular during the planning phase and, eventually, had to go "underground" because the project was finally targeted at an African-American community in Chicago (Sampson, Raudenbusch, & Earls, 1997). This was all before the worldwide collaborative-competitive effort launched by geneticists succeeded in giving us the tools to use genetic information in our behavioural studies (Roberts, 2001), and before neuroscientists acquired effective brain imaging tools (Albright, Jessell, Kandel, & Posner, 2001; Raichle, 1998) to help understand the brain mechanisms involved in cognitive, emotional and social behaviour.

However, not all of the prejudices disappeared with the advent of the new millennium and the new technologies. University departments still breed millions of young professionals blind to most of the other disciplines studying their object of interest. Research on the development of behaviour problems is still done mostly from a behavioural, cognitive, genetic, hormonal or social perspective, to name only a few of the multitude of angles that can be taken.

If most investigators are still trained with tightly fitting blinkers, it is easy to imagine the resistances new interdisciplinary research results are meeting in the public arena. For example, in 2004 the first author was invited by the French national research institute of health (INSERM) to be a member of an expert panel charged with reviewing the state of knowledge on conduct disorder. The 428-page report appeared one year later (INSERM, 2005) and included chapters on development, prevention, treatment and risk factors such as perinatal events, family characteristics, parenting, attachment, neuro-cognitive deficits and genetics. On the day the report was released an editorial appeared in one of the main French daily newspapers accusing the report, among other things, of proposals that would stigmatize children and promote the use of medication to "cure" a "social" problem (Le Monde, 2005). A group of university professors and professionals working in the child protection area created a web site denouncing the report and asking the public to sign a petition against its recommendations. Within a few months 200,000 people had signed the petition, dozens of newspaper articles, radio, and television programmes were debating whether conduct disorder existed or not, whether it was a medical or social problem, whether there were clear long-term risk factors, and whether we should try to prevent these social problems by intervention programmes before adolescence. The "revolt" against the national research institute was clearly led by professionals trained within university departments where biological and behavioural research was depicted as a threat to human dignity (Tremblay, 2008a). Demonization of a biological approach to "social" problems is not limited to French psychoanalysts. A good example can be found in a recent New York Times Bestseller, *The Lucifer Effect* (Zimbardo, 2007). The book presents in detail social psychology experiments which try to explain "how good people turn evil". In the book's Foreword the author writes that he challenges "the traditional focus on the individual's inner nature". However, the only reference to research on "individual inner nature" was to the eugenics movement more than a century ago (p. 313)!

The chances that the present book will be a bestseller among professionals who have made up their minds concerning the "causes" of behaviour problems are perilously close to zero. Our aim is not to convert those who have long adhered to the idea that the human mind and human behaviour escape the laws of nature. Our hope is that the chapters of this book will help a new generation of students, scientists, educators and care givers to understand where frontier research on behaviour problems is going and how it can be applied in the social, educational, and health services.

This being said, it will be easy to understand that we start with non-human animal studies. Chapter 2 describes fascinating work with rhesus monkeys, relatives that are close enough to accept that the mechanisms that explain their behaviour should be a good approximation of the mechanisms underlying human behaviour. Steve Suomi has published on rhesus monkey behaviour for close to 40 years and has been extremely successful in answering questions that help investigators working with human subjects to go beyond the traditional frontiers. For example, the work on gene–environment interactions he presented at an International Society for the Study of Behavioural Development (ISSBD) symposium in Beijing (Suomi, 2000) sparked the work of Caspi et al. (2002) on gene–environment interactions for violent behaviour in humans. In this book he shows how both genetic and experiential mechanisms are implicated not only in the expression of behaviour patterns but also in their transmission across successive generations of monkeys.

Chapter 3 takes over from where Chapter 2 ends by investigating the mechanisms that could explain the statistical gene–environment interactions. The chapter was written as an introduction to the new and vibrant version of a relatively old concept, epigenetics (Tremblay, 2005, 2008b). The first author, Moshe Szyf, spent most of his career applying epigenetics (environmental programming of gene expression) to cancer research before turning to the effects of the environment on non-human and human behaviour through gene expression. The chapter starts with a detailed discussion of epigenetics (i.e., how the environment has an impact on gene expression) and then summarizes groundbreaking work that explains the long-term epigenetic effects of maternal care on the behaviour of rats. It ends with an incursion in no less groundbreaking work on human aggression.

Chapter 4 is an excellent introduction to human studies of gene–environment interactions aiming to understand numerous long-term outcomes of maternal behaviour during pregnancy. Tomas Paus, a brain imaging specialist, and Zdenka Pausova, a hypertension geneticist, initiated this retrospective study to understand the extent to which maternal smoking during pregnancy has an impact on brain and behaviour development as well as on cardiovascular and metabolic health in adolescence. The study is a good illustration of the broad interdisciplinary work needed to link complex interrelated causal factors such as genes and environment with a host of interrelated outcomes such as brain development, cardiovascular functioning and behaviour. Too often we forget that "mental" health is based on health of a physical organ, the brain!

With Chapter 5 we turn to prospective longitudinal studies of behaviour development to highlight the importance of long-term descriptions of the phenotypes we want to "explain". The mechanisms that control the development of a phenotype can be understood only if we have a good description of that specific phenotype's development. Richard Tremblay describes a series of longitudinal studies that showed we had been asking the wrong question when, for decades, we tried to find "how children learn to physically aggress".

The chapter also summarizes a series of studies that tested the genetic and environmental contributions to the development of a chronic physical aggression trajectory. The story about the long-term follow-up of thousands of children maps well on the rhesus monkey results in Chapter 2, on the maternal smoking during pregnancy issues of Chapter 4, and extends the last part of Chapter 3 on epigenetic differences between boys on a chronic trajectory of physical aggression and boys on a "normal" trajectory.

The focus of Chapter 6 is on individual differences in temperament and personality among children. The debate over the genetic and environmental origins of temperament and personality is as old as research in psychology. Marcel van Aken summarizes studies on the stability of personality from childhood to adulthood, which also highlight how personality, together with environmental factors, influences children's social adjustment and mental health. Several possible connections between personality and psychopathology in children are illustrated. The chapter ends by showing how temperament and personality are useful concepts for thinking about interventions with children.

Chapters 7 and 8 review research on two very well known facts that have led to numerous hypotheses and studies: males physically aggress more than females and antisocial behaviour (disruptive behaviour, rule breaking, delinquency, criminality) runs in families. In Chapter 7 Sylvana Côté takes a developmental perspective to sex differences in aggression showing that although males generally use aggression more often than females, the magnitude of the difference between the sexes varies widely according to the type of aggression that is considered (physical versus indirect), and according to the developmental period studied. She also reviews biology and social learning hypotheses that attempt to explain these complex differences between males and females who are essentially brought up by the same parents in the same environments. In Chapter 8 Sara Jaffee reviews the large body of studies that attempted to understand why antisocial behaviour is concentrated in families. She first reviews the studies that took a psychosocial perspective aiming to show that children learn from their environment to behave in an antisocial way (e.g., antisocial parents and deviant friends) and concludes that the studies provide at best inconclusive results. She then summarizes recent studies that take into account genetic and environmental factors and concludes that they need replications but hold promise of providing more useful results for predictive purposes and hopefully for preventive purposes.

The last three chapters link developmental research with policy issues. In Chapter 9 Marianne Junger and colleagues address policy issues from the perspective of violence prevention. They first summarize research on the development of physical aggression, followed by research on the early prevention of chronic physical aggression. Subsequently, they discuss a series of policy options based on supporting evidence from experimental research. Finally they describe social policy choices that have been made by different countries.

Chapter 10 by Jacques van der Gaag links with the early childhood story developed in Chapter 9, but marks an important change of perspective and language. Jacques worked for a long time at the World Bank as an economist. We invited him to contribute a chapter that would help take a broad social view of efforts to prevent children's behaviour problems. In this chapter he shows how programmes that foster early childhood development are a first step in a global human development perspective. He argues that four pathways link early childhood development to human development: education, health, social capital, and equality. He concludes that each of the four pathways to human development leads to economic growth. We must admit that economic issues have rarely been on the mind of behaviour problem investigators, let alone their research projects. However, the times are changing. As can be seen from Jacques' chapter, economists are starting to pay attention to developmental work (see also Heckman, 2006).

In the final chapter Anne Petersen makes use of her dual experience as a social scientist and her close collaborations with social policy makers. Her ultimate aim is to get policy makers to use research results, but here she writes for investigators to help them get their message across to policy makers. She does this by exploring the relationships between research and social policy and by describing some promising examples of research that managed to influence policy.

References

Albright, T. D., Jessell, T. M., Kandel, E. R., & Posner, M. I. (2001). Progress in the neural sciences in the century after Cajal (and the mysteries that remain). *Annals of the New York Academy of Sciences, 929*, 11–40.

Caspi, A., McClay, J., Moffitt, T., Mill, J., Martin, J., Craig, I. W., et al. (2002). Role of genotype in the cycle of violence in maltreated children. *Science, 297*, 851–854.

Farrington, D. P., Loeber, R., Elliott, D. S., Hawkins, J. D., Kandel, D. B., Klein, M. W., et al. (1990). Advancing knowledge about the onset of delinquency and crime. In B. B. Lahey & A. E. Kazdin (Eds.), *Advances in clinical child psychology* (Vol. 13, pp. 283–342). New York: Plenum Press.

Heckman, J. J. (2006). Skill formation and the economics of investing in disadvantaged children. *Science, 312*, 1900–1902.

INSERM (Institut National de Santé et de Recherche Médicale) (2005). *Trouble des conduites chez l'enfant et l'adolescent* [Conduct disorder in children and adolescents]. Paris: INSERM.

Le Monde (2005, September 23). Zeros de conduite [Zero tolerance of conduct problems]. *Le Monde*, p. 3.

Raichle, M. E. (1998). Behind the scenes of functional brain imaging: a historical and physiological perspective. *Proceedings of the National Academy of Sciences of the USA, 95*(3), 765–772.

Roberts, L. (2001). Controversial from the start. *Science, 291*, 1182–1188.

Sampson, R. J., Raudenbusch, S. W., & Earls, F. (1997). Neighborhoods and violent crime: A multilevel study of collective efficacy. *Science, 277*, 918–924.

Suomi, S. (2000). *Physical and indirect aggression: Their development and consequences.*

Paper presented at the XVIth biennial meetings of the International Society for the Study of Behavioural Development, Beijing, China.

Tonry, M., Ohlin, L., Farrington, D., Adams, K., Earls, F., Rowe, D., et al. (1991). *Human development and criminal behavior: New ways of advancing knowledge*. New York: Springer-Verlag.

Tremblay, R. E. (2005). Is there a World beyond genetics? *Bulletin of the Centre of Excellence on Early Childhood Development, 4*(2), 1.

Tremblay, R. E. (2008a). *Prévenir la violence dès la petite enfance* [Preventing violence from early childhood]. Paris: Odile Jacob.

Tremblay, R. E. (2008b). Understanding development and prevention of chronic physical aggression: Towards experimental epigenetic studies. *Philosophical Transactions of the Royal Society of London, Series B: Biological Sciences, 363*, 2613–2622.

Zimbardo, P. (2007). *The Lucifer Effect*. New York: Random House.

2 How gene–environment interactions shape biobehavioural development[1]

Lessons from studies with rhesus monkeys

Stephen J. Suomi

Introduction

The question of whether the features that make us unique as individuals are largely determined by our genetic heritage or shaped by our personal experiences has been argued since at least the time of Aristotle – clearly the "nature–nurture" debate is not exactly new. What has been relatively new among those who study development is the realization that the basic question underlying this debate over the years may have been largely misdirected. Instead of arguing whether behavioural and biological characteristics that emerge during development are genetic in origin or are the product of specific experiences, these researchers now acknowledge that *both* genetic *and* environmental factors can play crucial roles in shaping individual developmental trajectories (Collins, Maccoby, Steinburg, Hetherington, & Bornstein, 2000). For example, behavioural geneticists (e.g., Plomin, 1990) have sought to determine the relative contributions of specific genetic and environmental factors to a variety of physical, physiological, behavioural, cognitive, and socio-emotional features. Other investigators (e.g., Rutter, 2001) have focused on possible *interactions* between genetic and environmental factors.

Unfortunately, direct study of potential gene–environment interactions and their possible influence on human development poses numerous methodological, practical, and even ethical problems. Demonstrations of specific gene–environment interactions are arguably most convincing when a range of predetermined genotypes can be studied prospectively across a range of systematically varied environments, yet that is almost never ethically proper and seldom practically feasible with human studies. Instead, such interactions must be largely inferred, typically after the fact. Specific genetic factors often tend to co-vary with particular rearing environments, such that the resulting gene–environment *correlations* can obscure actual gene–environment interactions (Reiss, Neiderhiser, Hetherington, & Plomin, 2000). Even when specific genes can be characterized in different individuals who are then followed prospectively in different environments, the actual basis for any emerging gene–environment interactions may be difficult to discern.

For example, Caspi et al. (2003) recently reported that the likelihood that individuals would experience episodes of depression was significantly related to the number of stressful life events they had experienced in the previous 5 years, but only if they possessed either the "LS" or "SS" variant of the serotonin transporter (5-HTT) gene; if they had the "LL" variant of the 5-HTT gene there was no relationship between recent depressive episodes and previous stressful life events. They also reported that individuals who had been maltreated as children were similarly more likely to experience depressive episodes in young adulthood than if they had not been maltreated, but again only if they possessed either the LS or SS (but not the LL) 5-HTT allele. However, the researchers were unable to specify exactly what aspects of the stressful life events or childhood maltreatment might be responsible for these apparent gene–environment interactions. In addition, they acknowledged that:

> This evidence that 5-HTTPR variation moderates the effect of life events on depression does not constitute unambiguous evidence of a G × E interaction, because exposure to life events may be influenced by genetic factors; if individuals have a heritable tendency to enter situations where they encounter stressful life events, these events may simply be a genetically saturated marker.
>
> (Caspi et al., 2003, p. 387)

Thus, even in this groundbreaking epidemiological study the lack of direct experimental control over environmental factors somewhat clouded precise interpretation of the extant findings.

Developmental researchers who study animals in captive environments are not faced with the same set of ethical and practical restrictions regarding manipulations of rearing environments characteristic of virtually all human studies. Instead, they can selectively breed or otherwise choose subjects with particular genetic pedigrees and rear them in different standardized environments in which various aspects of those environments can be systematically altered at various points throughout development. Such a research design readily permits the identification and characterization of specific gene–environment interactions. Of course, the degree to which any findings from studies with animals can answer questions or address issues concerning human developmental phenomena is largely dependent on the degree to which the phenomena of interest generalize from the human case to the animal under study (Harlow, Suomi, & Gluck, 1972). In the case of many basic aspects of biological, behavioural, and socio-emotional development, a growing body of evidence suggests considerable generality between humans and advanced non-human primate species.

This report summarizes findings from a series of studies investigating genetic and environmental factors – and their interactions – that can shape individual differences in biobehavioural developmental trajectories in rhesus monkeys, especially with respect to the development of excessively fearful behaviour, on the one hand, and overly aggressive behaviour on the other. It begins with a description of the complex social contexts that rhesus monkeys growing up in the wild normally encounter throughout development. Next, developmental trajectories for two subgroups of rhesus monkeys (*Macaca mulatta*) – one who consistently exhibit unusually fearful and anxious-like behavioural reactions to novel mildly stressful situations, and the other who are likely to exhibit impulsive and/or inappropriately aggressive responses in similar situations – will be described in terms of their distinctive behavioural and biological features and propensities. Although many of these characteristics appear to be highly heritable, evidence will be presented demonstrating that they are also subject to considerable modification by environmental factors, especially those involving early social attachment relationships. Finally, the results of studies investigating possible gene–environment interactions involving polymorphisms in the rhesus monkey 5-HTT gene that are structurally similar and functionally identical to the polymorphisms in the human 5-HTT gene cited above will be described, and their relevance for considerations of human development will be discussed.

Species-normative development in rhesus monkeys

Humans are not the only beings who grow up in a variety of complex social contexts. Most monkeys and apes living in natural settings spend their lives as active members of distinctive social communities, each typically characterized by elaborate kinship- and status-defined social relationships. These primate communities often encompass three or more generations within individual family units and usually retain their basic identity long beyond the life span of any single community member or generation of members. Moreover, in most primate species the relationships between individual family members, between families within a given community, and even between different communities are dynamic in nature, and changes in each type of relationship often can have long-term consequences for all individuals involved.

An illustrative example of the complex and dynamic nature of social contexts within primate communities has been provided by extensive studies of rhesus monkeys in both captive and field settings over the past half-century. Rhesus monkeys inhabit a wider geographic range, encompassing a broader mix of climate and habitat variation, than any other non-human primate species, with perhaps one or two exceptions. In contrast to many primate species currently classified as endangered or threatened, rhesus monkeys are actually expanding their local populations in certain parts of their extensive range. They have also consistently demonstrated an impressive ability to adapt to and indeed thrive in a wide variety of captive environments (Novak & Suomi, 1991).

In nature, rhesus monkeys reside in large social groups (troops), each comprised of several different female-headed families (matrilines) spanning several generations of kin, plus numerous immigrant males. This pattern of social organization derives from the fact that rhesus monkey females stay in their natal troop for their entire lives whereas virtually all rhesus monkey males emigrate from their natal troop around the time of puberty, usually in their fourth or fifth year, and then join other troops (Lindburg, 1971). These troops are also characterized by multiple social dominance relationships, including distinctive hierarchies both between and within families, as well as a hierarchy among the immigrant adult males, whose relative status seems to be largely a function of their ability to join and maintain coalitions, especially with high-ranking females. Indeed, the dominance status of any particular rhesus monkey within its troop depends not so much on how big and strong it is but rather who its family and friends are – and the latter is clearly dependent on the development of complex social skills during ontogeny.

Given the multiple social relationships and the variety of social networks embedded within each rhesus monkey troop, how do infants born to troop members become integrated into the overall social fabric of that troop? An impressive body of both laboratory and field data suggests that such integration is an emergent consequence of the species-normative pattern of socialization that rhesus monkey infants experience as they grow up (Sameroff & Suomi, 1996). In particular, the social networks of rhesus monkey infants initially are largely limited to members of their immediate families but expand dramatically in both scope and complexity as these infants mature.

Rhesus monkey infants begin life completely dependent on their mother for all their essential needs. They spend virtually all of their first month of life in physical contact with or within arm's reach of their mother, and mothers typically limit any other social contact of their infants to female members of their immediate family (Harlow, Harlow, & Hansen, 1963; Hinde & Spencer-Booth, 1967). During this time a strong and enduring social bond inevitably develops between mother and infant, recognized by Bowlby (1969) to be basically homologous with the mother–infant attachment relationship universally seen in all human cultures.

Once infants have established an attachment bond with their mother they quickly learn to use her as a secure base from which to start exploring their environment, beginning as early as their second month of life. Shortly thereafter, they spend increasing amounts of time engaging in social interactions with other troop members, especially peers. Although mothers show considerable variability in the degree to which they permit, if not encourage, these interactions with peers, by 6 months of age most youngsters typically are spending many hours each week in peer-directed activities. Interactions with peers continue to increase in both frequency and complexity throughout the rest of the young monkeys' first year of life. In contrast, the amount of time they spend interacting with their mother declines substantially after weaning, and this decline typically accelerates if the mother becomes pregnant again (Berman, Rasmussen, & Suomi, 1993).

Peer-directed activities continue at high and essentially stable rates through-out the second and third year of life (Ruppenthal, Harlow, Eisele, Harlow, & Suomi, 1974). During this time peer play becomes increasingly gender-specific, sex-segregated (i.e., males tend to play more with males and females with females), and involves behavioural sequences that appear to simulate virtually all adult social activities, including courtship and reproductive behaviours as well as dominant–aggressive interactions. However, both male and female juveniles still retain unique social ties with their mother even as she becomes increasingly involved with their younger siblings. They continue to use her as a secure base, they routinely seek physical contact with her under stressful circumstances, and they actively solicit her participation (and respond to her solicitations) in agonistic exchanges with other monkeys both inside and outside their troop (Suomi, 1998).

The social activities of and contexts for male and female juveniles change dramatically and differentially with puberty, which usually begins at the end of the third year for females and the start of the fourth year for males. Although females remain in their natal troop throughout adolescence and thereafter, their interactions with peers decline substantially from prepubertal levels as they redirect many of their social activities toward matrilineal kin, including both their mothers and the offspring they subsequently bear and rear. Nevertheless, females do retain some aspects of previous relationships with female peers throughout adult life, although their mutual activities tend to be greatly diminished in frequency and are largely limited to grooming bouts and (paradoxically) agonistic encounters rather than play. Much more time is instead invested in family-directed activities; indeed, females remain actively involved in family affairs for the rest of their lives, even after they stop having babies themselves.

Pubertal males, by contrast, leave both their family and their natal troop permanently, typically joining all-male "gangs" for varying periods before attempting to enter a different troop. In doing so, these young males effect-ively terminate their relationship with their mother and all other female relatives, inasmuch as they are not permitted to re-enter their natal troop once they have emigrated. They also end their relationships with most of their natal group peers (Suomi, 1998). Once a male has joined a new troop he must not only establish new relationships with the various members but also learn about the specific kinship relationships and multiple dominance hierarchies in order to become successfully integrated within that troop. Not surprisingly, this period of transition represents a time of major stress and potential danger for adolescent and young adult males – the mortality rate for males during the process of natal troop emigration and subsequent immigration approaches 50% in some wild monkey populations (Dittus, 1979). Some surviving males remain in their new troop for the rest of their lives, whereas other males may transfer from one troop to another several times during their adult years, but they never return to their natal troop (Berard, 1989).

Individual differences in the regulation of fear and aggression

Although virtually all rhesus monkeys growing up both in the wild and in social groups maintained in captivity go through the same basic developmental sequences described above, the specific social experiences that any individual accrues and the specific contexts in which they occur throughout development can vary considerably both within and between families. For example, numerous studies have demonstrated that most rhesus monkey mothers are acutely sensitive to those aspects of their immediate physical and social environment that pose potential threats to their infant's well-being, and they appear to adjust their maternal behaviour accordingly. Both laboratory and field studies have consistently shown that low-ranking mothers tend to be much more restrictive of their infant's exploratory efforts than are high-ranking mothers, whose own maternal style has been termed "laissez-faire" (Altmann, 1980). The standard interpretation of these findings is that low-ranking mothers risk reprisal from others if they try to intervene whenever their infant is threatened, so they minimize such risk by restricting their infant's exploration. High-ranking mothers have no such problem; hence, they can afford to let their infant explore as it pleases.

Other studies have found that mothers generally become more restrictive and increase their levels of infant monitoring when their immediate social environment becomes less stable, such as when major changes in inter-family dominance hierarchies take place or when alien males try to join the troop. Changes in various aspects of the physical environment, such as the food supply becoming less predictable, have also been associated with increases in maternal restriction of early infant environmental exploration (Andrews & Rosenblum, 1991), as have increases in the population of any one troop (Berman, Rasmussen, & Suomi, 1997). For infants whose opportunities to explore are chronically limited during their first few months of life, development of species-normative relationships with others in their social group, especially peers, can be compromised, often with long-term consequences for both the infants and their social group (Suomi, 1997).

There are also substantial differences among individual troop members in the precise timing and relative ease with which they make major developmental transitions, as well as how they manage the day-to-day challenges and stresses that are an inevitable consequence of complex social group life. In particular, recent research has identified two subgroups of monkeys who exhibit specific problems in their socio-emotional regulation that can result in increased long-term risk for behavioural pathology and even mortality. Members of one subgroup, comprising approximately 15–20% of both wild and captive populations, seem excessively fearful. These monkeys consistently respond to novel and/or mildly challenging situations with extreme behavioural disruption and pronounced physiological arousal (Suomi, 1986).

Highly fearful monkeys can usually be identified during their initial weeks and months of life. Most begin leaving their mothers later chronologically and explore their physical and social environment less than other infants in their birth cohort. Highly fearful youngsters also tend to be shy and withdrawn in their initial encounters with peers – laboratory studies have shown that they exhibit significantly higher and more stable heart rates and greater secretion of cortisol in such interactions than do their less reactive age-mates. However, when these fearful monkeys are in familiar and stable social settings they are virtually indistinguishable, both behaviourally and physiologically, from their peers (Suomi, 1991b). In contrast, when fearful monkeys encounter extreme and/or prolonged stress, their behavioural and physiological reaction differs from others in their social group.

For example, young rhesus monkeys typically experience functional maternal separations during the 2-month-long annual breeding season when their mothers repeatedly leave the troop for brief periods to consort with selected males (Berman, Rasmussen, & Suomi, 1994). The sudden loss of access to its mother is a major social stressor for any young monkey and, not surprisingly, virtually all youngsters initially react to their mother's departure with short-term behavioural agitation and physiological arousal, much as Bowlby (1973) described for human infants experiencing involuntary maternal separation. However, whereas most youngsters soon begin to adapt to the separation and readily seek out the company of others in their social group until their mother returns, highly fearful individuals typically lapse into a behavioural depression characterized by increasing lethargy, lack of apparent interest in social stimuli, eating and sleeping difficulties, and a characteristic hunched-over, foetal-like posture (Suomi, 1991a).

Laboratory studies simulating these naturalistic maternal separations have shown that, relative to their like-reared peers, highly fearful monkeys not only are more likely to exhibit depressive-like behavioural reactions to short-term social separation but also tend to show greater and more prolonged hypothalamic-pituitary-adrenal (HPA) activation, more dramatic sympathetic arousal, more rapid central noradrenergic turnover, and greater immunosuppression (Suomi, 1991b). These differential patterns of biobehavioural response to separation tend to remain remarkably stable throughout prepubertal development and may be maintained during adolescence and even into adulthood (Suomi, 1995). Moreover, individual differences in infant biobehavioural response to separation are predictive of differential responses to other situations experienced later in life (e.g., Fahlke, Lorenz, Long, Champoux, Suomi, & Higley, 2000). An increasing body of evidence has demonstrated significant heritability for at least some components of these differential responses to stress (Higley et al., 1993; Williamson et al., 2003).

Highly fearful males usually emigrate from their natal troop at significantly older ages than the rest of their male birth cohort and, when they do finally leave, they typically employ much more conservative strategies for entering a new troop than do their less fearful peers. This pattern of delayed emigration may actually be adaptive, in that the physically larger and heavier a male is at the time he emigrates from his natal troop, the greater the likelihood that he will survive and successfully join another troop (Rasmussen, Fellows, & Suomi, 1990). Therefore, if a male is able to postpone emigration until he has largely finished his adolescent growth spurt, he appears to be better able to make the transition to adult male life than if he leaves home prior to or during the growth spurt. Because fearful adolescent males pose little apparent threat to adult females and their offspring, they tend to be tolerated by other troop members at ages when the other males in their birth cohort have either left voluntarily or been forcibly driven away. Thus, even though excessive fearfulness apparently puts an individual male at increased risk for adverse biobehavioural reactions to stress throughout development, there may be some circumstances where this characteristic can actually be adaptive (Suomi, 2000b).

A parallel situation exists for females: Highly fearful young mothers in the wild tend to reject and punish their infants at higher rates around the time of weaning than do other mothers in their troop (Rasmussen, Timme, & Suomi, 1997), and in the absence of social support they appear to be at increased risk for infant neglect and/or abuse (Suomi & Ripp, 1983). Yet, under stable social circumstances these fearful females may not only turn out to be highly competent mothers but also often achieve relatively high positions of social dominance (Rasmussen et al., 1997). In sum, excessive fearfulness in infancy appears to be associated with increased risk for developing anxious- and depressive-like symptoms and potential problems in parenting in response to stressful circumstances later in life, but such long-term outcomes are far from inevitable.

Other rhesus monkeys appear to have problems regulating aggression. These monkeys, comprising approximately 5–10% of the population, seem unusually impulsive, insensitive, and overly aggressive in their interactions with other troop members. Impulsive young males seem unable to moderate their responses to rough-and-tumble play initiations from peers, frequently escalating initially benign play bouts into full-blown aggressive exchanges that may result in actual wounding (Higley et al., 1992). Not surprisingly, most of these individuals tend to be avoided by peers, and as a result they become increasingly isolated socially. In addition, many of these juvenile males often appear unwilling (or unable) to follow the "rules" inherent in rhesus monkey social dominance hierarchies. For example, they may directly challenge a dominant adult male, a foolhardy act that can result in serious injury, especially when the juvenile refuses to back away or exhibit submissive behaviour once defeat becomes obvious. Impulsive males also show a propensity for making dangerous leaps from treetop to treetop, sometimes with injurious or even fatal outcomes (Mehlman et al., 1994).

Overly impulsive monkeys of both genders consistently exhibit chronic deficits in central serotonin metabolism, as reflected by unusually low cerebrospinal fluid (CSF) concentrations of the primary central serotonin metabolite 5-hydroxyindoleacetic acid (5-HIAA). Laboratory studies have shown that these deficits in serotonin metabolism appear early in life and tend to persist throughout development, as was the case for HPA responsiveness among highly fearful monkeys. Monkeys who exhibit such deficits are also likely to show poor state control and visual orienting capabilities during early infancy (Champoux, Suomi, & Schneider, 1994), poor performance on delay-of-gratification tasks as juveniles (Bennett et al., 1999), and sleep disturbances as adults (Zajicek, Higley, Suomi, & Linnoila, 1997). Moreover, individual differences in 5-HIAA concentrations appear to be highly heritable among monkeys of similar age and comparable rearing background (Higley et al., 1993).

Recent field studies have found that the timing of natal troop emigration typical for impulsive males is seemingly the reverse of that for fearful males, often with deadly consequences. Ostracized by their peers and frequently attacked by adults of both sexes, most of these excessively aggressive young males are physically driven out of their natal troop prior to 3 years of age, well before the onset of puberty and long before most of their male cohort begins the normal emigration process (Mehlman et al., 1995). These males tend to be grossly incompetent socially and, lacking the requisite social skills necessary for successful entrance into another troop or even into an all-male gang, most of them become solitary and typically perish within a year (Higley et al., 1996b).

Young females who have chronically low CSF levels of 5-HIAA also tend to be impulsive, aggressive, and generally rather incompetent socially. However, unlike the males, they are not expelled from their natal troop but instead remain with their family throughout their lifetime, although studies of captive rhesus monkey groups suggest that these females will likely remain at the bottom of their respective dominance hierarchies (Higley, King, Hasert, Champoux, Suomi, & Linnoila, 1996a). While most become mothers, their maternal behaviour is often inadequate or even abusive, such that the attachment relationships they develop with their offspring tend to be avoidant, if not disorganized (Suomi, 2000a). In sum, rhesus monkeys who exhibit poor regulation of impulsive and aggressive behaviour and low central serotonin metabolism early in life tend to follow developmental trajectories that often result in premature death for males and chronically low social dominance and poor parenting for females.

Effects of peer-rearing on rhesus monkey biobehavioural development

Although the findings from both the field and laboratory studies cited above have shown that individual differences in expressions of fear and aggression tend to be quite stable from infancy to adulthood and are at least in part heritable, this does not mean that they are necessarily fixed at birth, immune to subsequent environmental influence. To the contrary, an increasing body of evidence from laboratory studies has demonstrated that patterns of socioemotional development, neuroendocrine responsiveness, and neurotransmitter metabolism alike can be modified substantially by certain early social experiences, especially those involving early attachment relationships.

Some of the most compelling evidence comes from studies of rhesus monkey infants raised with peers instead of their biological mothers. During their initial weeks of life peer-reared infants readily establish strong social bonds with each other, much as mother-reared infants develop attachments to their own mothers (Harlow, 1969). However, because peers are not nearly as effective as typical monkey mothers in reducing fear in the face of novelty or in providing secure bases for environmental exploration, the attachment relationships that these peer-reared infants develop are almost always "anxious" in nature (Suomi, 1995). As a result, while peer-reared monkeys show completely normal physical and motor development, most appear to be excessively fearful – their early exploratory behaviour tends to be somewhat limited, they seem reluctant to approach novel objects, and they tend to be shy in initial encounters with unfamiliar peers (Suomi, 1991b).

Social play among peer-reared monkeys occurs less frequently and tends to be less complex with respect to the duration, the diversity of specific behaviours incorporated, and the number of partners involved in most play episodes than is typically shown by their mother-reared counterparts. One explanation for their relatively poor play performance is that their partners have to serve both as attachment figures and playmates, dual roles that neither mothers nor mother-reared peers have to fulfil. Another obstacle to developing sophisticated play repertoires faced by peer-reared monkeys is that all of their early play bouts involve partners who are basically as incompetent socially as they are. Perhaps as a result of these factors, peer-reared youngsters typically drop to the bottom of their respective dominance hierarchies when they are subsequently housed with mother-reared monkeys their own age (Higley, Suomi, & Linnoila, 1996).

Several prospective longitudinal studies have found that peer-reared monkeys consistently exhibit more extreme behavioural, adrenocortical, and noradrenergic reactions to social separations than do their mother-reared cohorts, even after they have been living in the same social groups for extended periods (e.g., Higley & Suomi, 1989; Higley, Suomi, & Linnoila, 1992). Such differences in prototypical biobehavioural reactions to separation persist from infancy to adolescence, if not beyond. Interestingly, the general nature of the separation reactions exhibited by peer-reared monkeys seems to mirror that shown by "naturally occurring" highly fearful mother-reared subjects. In this sense, early rearing with peers appears to have the effect of making rhesus monkey infants generally more fearful than they might have been if reared by their biological mothers (Suomi, 1991b).

Early peer-rearing has another long-term developmental consequence for rhesus monkeys: it tends to make them more impulsive, especially if they are males. Like the previously described impulsive monkeys growing up in the wild, peer-reared males initially exhibit overly aggressive tendencies in the context of juvenile play; as they approach puberty, the frequency and severity of their aggressive episodes typically exceed those of mother-reared group members of similar age. Peer-reared females tend to groom (and be groomed by) others in their social group less frequently and for shorter durations than their mother-reared counterparts, and they usually stay at the bottom of their respective dominance hierarchies. These differences between peer-reared and mother-reared age mates in aggression, grooming, and dominance remain relatively robust throughout the preadolescent and adolescent years (Higley, Suomi, & Linnoila, 1996). Peer-reared monkeys also consistently show lower CSF concentrations of 5-HIAA than their mother-reared counterparts. These group differences in 5-HIAA concentrations appear well before 6 months of age, and they remain stable at least throughout adolescence and into early adulthood (Higley & Suomi, 1996). Thus peer-reared monkeys exhibit the same general tendencies that characterize excessively impulsive wild-living (and mother-reared) rhesus monkeys, not only behaviourally but also in terms of decreased serotonergic functioning.

Gene–environment interactions

Studies examining the effects of peer-rearing and other variations in early rearing history (e.g., Harlow & Harlow, 1969), along with the previously cited heritability findings, clearly provide compelling evidence that *both* genetic and early experiential factors can affect a monkey's capacity to regulate expression of fear and aggression. Do these factors operate independently, or do they interact in some fashion in shaping individual developmental trajectories? Ongoing research capitalizing on the discovery of polymorphisms in one specific gene – the serotonin transporter gene – suggests that gene–environment interactions not only occur but also can be expressed in multiple forms.

The serotonin transporter gene (5-HTT), considered by biological psychiatrists to be a "candidate" gene for impaired serotonergic function (Lesch et al., 1996), has length variation in its promoter region that results in allelic variation in serotonin expression. A heterozygous "short" allele (LS) confers low transcriptional efficiency to the 5-HTT promoter relative to the homozygous "long" allele (LL), raising the possibility that low 5-HTT expression may result in decreased serotonergic functioning (Heils et al., 1996), although evidence in support of this hypothesis in humans has been decidedly mixed to date (e.g., Furlong et al., 1998). The 5-HTT polymorphism was first characterized in humans but, as was previously mentioned, it also appears in a largely homologous form in rhesus monkeys – but interestingly *not* in many other species of primates and not in any other mammals studied to date (Lesch et al., 1997).

We recently utilized polymerase chain reaction (PCR) techniques to characterize the 5-HTT allelic status of monkeys used in our studies comparing peer-reared monkeys with mother-reared controls described above. Because extensive observational data and biological samples had been previously collected from these monkeys throughout development, it was possible to examine a wide range of behavioural and physiological measures for potential

5-HTT polymorphism interactions with early rearing history. Analyses completed to date suggest that such interactions are widespread and diverse.

For example, Bennett et al. (2002) found that CSF 5-HIAA concentrations did not differ as a function of 5-HTT status for mother-reared subjects, whereas among peer-reared monkeys individuals with the LS allele had significantly lower CSF 5-HIAA concentrations than those with the LL allele. One interpretation of this interaction is that mother-rearing appeared to "buffer" any potentially deleterious effects of the LS allele on serotonin metabolism. Barr et al. (2003) reported a similar buffering effect with respect to aggression: High levels of aggression were found in peer-reared monkeys with the LS allele, whereas mother-reared LS monkeys exhibited low levels that were comparable to those of both mother- and peer-reared LL monkeys. Additionally Barr et al. (2004) found a parallel pattern of maternal buffering with respect to HPA activity in response to social separation: LS peer-reared juveniles had significantly higher ACTH concentrations than LS mother-reared, LL mother-reared, and LL peer-reared juveniles. Finally, Champoux et al. (2002) examined the relationship between early rearing history and serotonin transporter gene polymorphic status on measures of neonatal neurobehavioural development during the first month of life and found further evidence of maternal buffering. Specifically, infants possessing the LS allele who were being reared in the laboratory neonatal nursery showed significant deficits in measures of attention, activity, and motor maturity relative to nursery-reared infants possessing the LL allele, whereas both LS and LL infants who were being reared by competent mothers exhibited normal values for each of these measures.

In sum, the consequences of having the LS allele differed dramatically for peer-reared and mother-reared monkeys. Peer-reared individuals with the LS allele exhibited deficits in measures of neurobehavioural functioning during their initial weeks of life, increased HPA activity and high levels of aggression as juveniles, and reduced serotonin metabolism as adolescents. Mother-reared subjects with the very same allele developed normal early neurobehavioural functioning, HPA activity, regulation of aggression, and serotonin metabolism. Indeed, it could be argued on the basis of these findings that having the LS allele may well lead to psychopathology among monkeys with poor early rearing histories but might actually be adaptive for monkeys who develop secure early attachment relationship with their mothers.

The implications of these recent findings are considerable with respect to the potential for cross-generational transmission of these biobehavioural characteristics. Among the most intriguing aspects of the long-term consequences of different early attachment experiences is the apparent transfer of specific features of maternal behaviour across successive generations. Several studies of rhesus monkeys and other non-human primate species have demonstrated strong continuities between the type of attachment relationship a female infant develops with her mother and the type of attachment relationship she develops with her own infant(s) when she becomes a mother herself (Suomi, 1999). In particular, the pattern of ventral contact a female infant has with her mother (or mother substitute) during her initial months of life is a powerful predictor of the pattern of ventral contact she will have with her own infants during their first 6 months of life (Champoux, Byrne, Delizio, & Suomi, 1992; Fairbanks, 1989). This predictive cross-generational relationship is as strong in females who were foster-reared from birth by unrelated multiparous females as it is for females reared by their biological mothers, strongly suggesting that such cross-generational transmission necessarily involves non-genetic mechanisms (Suomi & Levine, 1998).

If similar maternal buffering is indeed experienced by the next generation of infants carrying the LS 5-HTT polymorphism, then having had their mothers develop a secure attachment relationship with their own mothers when they were infants themselves might well provide the basis for a non-genetic means of transmitting its apparently adaptive consequences to that new generation of monkeys. On the other hand, if contextual factors such as changes in maternal dominance rank, instability within the troop, or changes in the availability of food were to alter a young mother's care of her infants in a way that compromised any such buffering, then one might well expect any offspring carrying the LS 5-HTT polymorphism to develop some of the problems described above. What the relevant non-genetic mechanisms might be, and through what developmental processes they might act, are questions at the heart of ongoing investigations.

We are currently carrying out parallel studies focusing on other potential gene–environment interactions involving not only 5-HTT polymorphisms but also polymorphisms in other "candidate" genes such as monoamine oxidase A (MAOA), and our findings to date suggest that such interactions are ubiquitous and can occur at a variety of points throughout development. We are also currently involved in collaborative studies investigating patterns of gene expression in different brain regions and how such patterns might be influenced by early experience. At the very least, our findings suggest that the social context in which a rhesus monkey infant is reared can have far-ranging consequences throughout the whole of development – not only at the levels of behavioural functioning and socio-emotional regulation, but also at the levels of neurohormonal responsiveness, neurotransmitter metabolism, and perhaps even gene expression. Clearly, the context in which development takes place matters a great deal for rhesus monkeys. It is hard to imagine how it could be less so for human development.

Note

1 This chapter has been previously published as: Suomi, S. J. (2004). How gene environment interactions shape biobehavioral development: Lessons from studies with rhesus monkeys. *Research in Human Development*, *1*, 205–222.

References

Altmann, J. (1980). *Baboon mothers and infants*. Cambridge, MA: Harvard University Press.

Andrews, M. W., & Rosenblum, L. A. (1991). Security of attachment in infants raised in variable or low-demand environments. *Child Development, 62,* 686–693.

Barr, C. S., Newman, T. K., Becker, M. L., Parker, C. C., Champoux, M., Lesch, K. P., et al. (2003). The utility of the non-human primate model for studying gene by environment interactions in behavioral research. *Genes, Brain, and Behavior, 2,* 336–340.

Barr, C. S., Newman, T. K., Shannon, C, Parker, C., Dvoskin, R. L., Becker, M. L., et al. (2004). Rearing condition and rh5-HTTLPR interact to influence LHPA-axis response to stress in infant macaques. *Biological Psychiatry, 55,* 733–739.

Bennett, A. J., Lesch, K. P., Heils, A., Long, J., Lorenz, J., Shoaf, S. E., et al. (2002). Early experience and serotonin transporter gene variation interact to influence primate CNS function. *Molecular Psychiatry, 17,* 118–122.

Bennett, A. J, Tsai, T., Hopkins, W. D., Lindell, S. G., Pierre, P. J., Champoux, M., & Shoaf, S. E. (1999). Early social environment influences acquisition of a computerized joystick task in rhesus monkeys (*Macaca mulatta*). *American Journal of Primatology, 49,* 33–34.

Berard, J. (1989). Male life histories. *Puerto Rican Health Sciences Journal, 8,* 47–58.

Berman, C. M., Rasmussen, K. L. R., & Suomi, S. J. (1993). Reproductive consequences of maternal care patterns during estrus among free-ranging rhesus monkeys. *Behavioral Ecology and Sociobiology, 32,* 391–399.

Berman, C. M., Rasmussen, K. L. R., & Suomi, S. J. (1994). Responses of free-ranging rhesus monkeys to a natural form of maternal separation: I. Parallels with mother–infant separation in captivity. *Child Development, 65,* 1028–1041.

Berman, C. M., Rasmussen, K. L. R., & Suomi, S. J. (1997). Group size, infant development, and social networks: A natural experiment with free-ranging rhesus monkeys. *Animal Behavior, 53,* 405–421.

Bowlby, J. (1969). *Attachment*. New York: Basic Books.

Bowlby, J. (1973). *Separation*. New York: Basic Books.

Caspi, A., Sugen, K., Moffitt, T. E., Taylor, A., Craig, I. W., Harrington, H., et al. (2003). Influence of life stress on depression: moderation by a polymorphism in the 5-HTT gene. *Science, 301,* 386–389.

Champoux, M., Bennett, A. J., Lesch, K. P., Heils, A., Nielsen, D. A., Higley, J. D., & Suomi, S. J. (2002). Serotonin transporter gene polymorphism and neurobehavioral development in rhesus monkey neonates. *Molecular Psychiatry, 7,* 1058–1063.

Champoux, M., Byrne, E., Delizio, R. D., & Suomi, S. J. (1992). Motherless mothers revisited: Rhesus maternal behavior and rearing history. *Primates, 33,* 251–255.

Champoux, M., Suomi, S. J., & Schneider, M. L. (1994). Temperamental differences between captive Indian and Chinese-Indian hybrid rhesus macaque infants. *Laboratory Animal Science, 44,* 351–357.

Collins, W. A., Maccoby, E. E., Steinburg, L., Hetherington, E. M., & Bornstein, M. H. (2000). Contemporary research on parenting: The case for nature *and* nurture. *American Psychologist, 55,* 218–232.

Dittus, W. P. J. (1979). The evolution of behaviours regulating density and age-specific sex ratios in a primate population. *Behaviour, 69,* 265–302.

Fahlke, C., Lorenz, J. G., Long, J., Champoux, M., Suomi, S. J., & Higley, J. D. (2000). Rearing experiences and stress-induced plasma cortisol as early risk factors for excessive alcohol consumption in nonhuman primates. *Alcoholism: Clinical and Experimental Research, 24*, 644–650.

Fairbanks, L. A. (1989). Early experience and cross-generational continuity of mother–infant contact in vervet monkeys. *Developmental Psychobiology, 22*, 669–681.

Furlong, R. A., Ho, L., Walsh, C., Rubinsztein, J. S., Jain, S., Pazkil, E. S., et al. (1998). Analysis and meta-analysis of two serotonin transporter gene polymorphisms in bipolar and unipolar affective disorders. *American Journal of Medical Genetics, 81*, 58–63.

Harlow, H. F. (1969). Age-mate or peer affectional system. In D. S. Lehrman, R. A. Hinde, & E. Shaw (Eds.), *Advances in the study of behavior* (Vol. 2, pp. 333–383). New York: Academic Press.

Harlow, H. F., & Harlow, M. K. (1969). Effects of various mother–infant relationships on rhesus monkey behaviors. In B. M. Foss (Ed.), *Determinants of infant behaviour* (Vol. 4, pp. 15–36). London: Methuen.

Harlow, H. F., Harlow, M. K., & Hansen, E. W. (1963). The maternal affectional system of rhesus monkeys. In H. L. Rheingold (Ed.), *Maternal behavior in mammals* (pp. 254–281). New York: Wiley.

Harlow, H. F., Suomi, S. J., & Gluck, J. P. (1972). Generalization of behavioral data between nonhuman and human animals. *American Psychologist, 27*, 709–716.

Heils, A. Teufel, A., Petri, S., Stober, G., Riederer, P. Bengel, B., & Lesch, K. P. (1996). Allelic variation of human serotonin transporter gene expression. *Journal of Neurochemistry, 6*, 2621–2624.

Higley, J. D., King, S. T., Hasert, M. F., Champoux, M., Suomi, S. J., & Linnoila, M. (1996a). Stability of individual differences in serotonin function and its relationship to severe aggression and competent social behavior in rhesus macaque females. *Neuropsychopharmacology, 14*, 67–76.

Higley, J. D., Mehlman, P. T., Taub, D. M., Higley, S., Fernald, B., Vickers, J. H., et al. (1996b). Excessive mortality in young free-ranging male nonhuman primates with low CSF 5-HIAA concentrations. *Archives of General Psychiatry, 53*, 537–543.

Higley, J. D., Mehlman, P. T., Taub, D. M., Higley, S. B., Vickers, J. H., Suomi, S. J., & Linnoila, M. (1992). Cerebrospinal fluid monoamine and adrenal correlates of aggression in free-ranging rhesus monkeys. *Archives of General Psychiatry, 49*, 436–444.

Higley, J. D., & Suomi, S. J. (1989). Temperamental reactivity in nonhuman primates. In G. A. Kohnstamm, J. E. Bastes, & M. K. Rothbard (Eds.), *Handbook of temperament in children* (pp. 153–167). New York: Wiley.

Higley, J. D., & Suomi, S. J. (1996). Reactivity and social competence affect individual differences in reaction to severe stress in children: Investigations using nonhuman primates. In C. R. Pfeffer (Ed.), *Intense stress and mental disturbance in children* (pp. 3–58). Washington, DC: American Psychiatric Press.

Higley, J. D., Suomi, S. J., & Linnoila, M. (1992). A longitudinal assessment of CSF monoamine metabolite and plasma cortisol concentrations in young rhesus monkeys. *Biological Psychiatry, 32*, 127–145.

Higley, J. D., Suomi, S. J., & Linnoila, M. (1996). A nonhuman primate model of Type II alcoholism? Part 2: Diminished social competence and excessive aggression correlates with low CSF 5-HIAA concentrations. *Alcoholism: Clinical and Experimental Research, 20*, 643–650.

Higley, J. D., Thompson, W. T., Champoux, M., Goldman, D., Hasert, M. F., Kraemer, G. W., et al. (1993). Paternal and maternal genetic and environmental contributions to CSF monoamine metabolites in rhesus monkeys (*Macaca mulatta*). *Archives of General Psychiatry, 50*, 615–623.

Hinde, R. A., & Spencer-Booth, Y. (1967). The behaviour of socially living rhesus monkeys in their first two and a half years. *Animal Behaviour, 15*, 169–176.

Lesch, K. P., Bengel, D., Heils, A., Sabol, S. Z., Greenberg, B. D., Petri, S., et al. (1996). Association of anxiety-related traits with a polymorphism in the serotonin transporter gene regulatory region. *Science, 274*, 1527–1531.

Lesch, K. P., Meyer, J., Glatz, K., Flugge, G., Hinney, A., Hebebrand, J., et al. (1997). The 5-HT transporter gene-linked polymorphic region (5-HTTLPR) in evolutionary perspective: Alternative biallelic variation in rhesus monkeys. *Journal of Neural Transmission, 104*, 1259–1266.

Lindburg, D. G. (1971). The rhesus monkey in north India: An ecological and behavioral study. In L. A. Rosenblum (Ed.), *Primate behavior: Developments in field and laboratory research* (Vol. 2, pp. 1–106). New York: Academic Press.

Mehlman, P. T., Higley, J. D., Faucher, I., Lilly, A. A., Taub, D. M., Vickers, J. H., et al. (1994). Low cerebrospinal fluid 5 hydroxyindoleacetic acid concentrations are correlated with severe aggression and reduced impulse control in free-ranging primates. *American Journal of Psychiatry, 151*, 1485–1491.

Mehlman, P. T., Higley, J. D., Faucher, I., Lilly, A. A., Taub, D. M., Vickers, J. H., et al. (1995). CSF 5-HIAA concentrations are correlated with sociality and the timing of emigration in free-ranging primates. *American Journal of Psychiatry, 152*, 901–913.

Novak, M. A., & Suomi, S. J. (1991). Social interaction in nonhuman primates: An underlying theme for primate research? *Laboratory Animal Science, 41*, 308–314.

Plomin, R. (1990). *Nature and nurture: An introduction to human behavioral genetics.* Pacific Grove, CA: Brooks/Cole.

Rasmussen, K. L. R., Fellows, J. R., & Suomi, S. J. (1990). Physiological correlates of emigration behavior and mortality in adolescent male rhesus monkeys on Cayo Santiago. *American Journal of Primatology, 20*, 224–225.

Rasmussen, K. L. R., Timme, A., & Suomi, S. J. (1997). Comparison of physiological measures of Cayo Santiago rhesus monkey females within and between social groups. *Primate Reports, 47*, 49–55.

Reiss, D., Neiderhiser, J. M., Hetherington, E. M., & Plomin, R. (2000). *The relationship code: Deciphering genetic and social influences on adolescent development.* Cambridge, MA: Harvard University Press.

Ruppenthal, G. C., Harlow, M. K., Eisele, C. D., Harlow, H. F., & Suomi, S. J. (1974). Development of peer interactions of monkeys reared in a nuclear family environment. *Child Development, 45*, 670–682.

Rutter, M. (2001). How can we know environment really matters? In F. Lamb-Parker, J. Hagen, & R. Robinson (Eds.), *Developmental and contextual transition of children and families: Implications for research, policy, and practice* (pp. 3–18). New York: Columbia University Press.

Sameroff, A. J., & Suomi, S. J. (1996). Primates and persons: a comparative developmental understanding of social organization. In R. B. Cairns, G. H. Elder, & E. J. Costello (Eds.), *Developmental science* (pp. 97–120). Cambridge: Cambridge University Press.

Suomi, S. J. (1986). Anxiety-like disorders in young primates. In R. Gittelman (Ed.), *Anxiety disorders of childhood* (pp. 1–23). New York: Guilford Press.

Suomi, S. J. (1991a). Primate separation models of affective disorders. In J. Madden (Ed.), *Neurobiology of learning, emotion, and affect* (pp. 195–214). New York: Raven Press.

Suomi, S. J. (1991b). Up-tight and laid-back monkeys: Individual differences in the response to social challenges. In S. Brauth, W. Hall, & R. Dooling (Eds.), *Plasticity of development* (pp. 27–56). Cambridge, MA: MIT Press.

Suomi, S. J. (1995). Influence of Bowlby's attachment theory on research on nonhuman primate biobehavioral development. In S. Goldberg, R. Muir, & J. Kerr (Eds.), *Attachment theory: Social, developmental, and clinical perspectives* (pp. 185–201). Hillsdale, NJ: Analytic Press.

Suomi, S. J. (1997). Early determinants of behaviour: Evidence from primate studies. *British Medical Bulletin, 53*, 170–184.

Suomi, S. J. (1998). Conflict and cohesion in rhesus monkey family life. In M. Cox & J. Brooks-Gunn (Eds.), *Conflict and cohesion in families* (pp. 283–296). Mahwah, NJ: Lawrence Erlbaum Associates, Inc.

Suomi, S. J. (1999). Attachment in rhesus monkeys. In J. Cassidy & P. R. Shaver (Eds.), *Handbook of attachment: Theory, research, and clinical applications* (pp. 181–197). New York: Guilford Press.

Suomi, S. J. (2000a). A biobehavioral perspective on developmental psychopathology: Excessive aggression and serotonergic dysfunction in monkeys. In A. J. Sameroff, M. Lewis, & S. Miller (Eds.), *Handbook of developmental psychopathology* (pp. 237–256). New York: Plenum Press.

Suomi, S. J. (2000b). Behavioral inhibition and impulsive aggressiveness: Insights from studies with rhesus monkeys. In L. Balter & C. Tamis-Lamode (Eds.), *Child psychology: A handbook of contemporary issues* (pp. 510–525). New York: Taylor & Francis.

Suomi, S. J., & Levine, S. (1998). Psychobiology of intergenerational effects of trauma: Evidence from animal studies. In Y. Daniele (Ed.), *International handbook of multigenerational legacies of trauma* (pp. 623–637). New York: Plenum Press.

Suomi, S. J., & Ripp, C. (1983). A history of motherless mother monkey mothering at the University of Wisconsin Primate Laboratory. In M. Reite & N. Caine (Eds.), *Child abuse: The nonhuman primate data* (pp. 49–77). New York: Alan R. Liss.

Williamson, D. E., Coleman, K., Bacanu, S. A., Devlin, B. J., Rogers, J., Ryan, N. D., & Cameron, J. L. (2003). Heritability of fearful-anxious endophenotypes in infant rhesus macaques: A preliminary report. *Biological Psychiatry, 53*, 284–291.

Zajicek, K., Higley, J. D., Suomi, S. J., & Linnoila, M. (1997). Rhesus macaques with high CSF 5-HIAA concentrations exhibit early sleep onset. *Psychiatric Research, 77*, 15–25.

3   Epigenetics and behaviour[1]

Moshe Szyf, Ian Weaver, Nadine Provencal,
Patrick O. McGowan, Richard E. Tremblay and
Michael J. Meaney

Epigenetics and inter-individual differences in behaviour

Genes, gene expression programmes and phenotype

The comprehensive sequencing of the human genome has generated great
anticipation that by comparing the DNA sequence between individuals we
will be able to understand the basis of phenotypic diversity between individuals, including the reasons for differences in behaviour such as diversity of
levels of aggression amongst individuals. However, our current understanding of how the genome functions suggests that this might not be the complete
story. The genome has to be programmed to express its unique patterns of
gene expression. Different cell types execute distinctive plans of gene expression, which are highly responsive to developmental, physiological, pathological and environmental cues. The combinations of mechanisms, which
confer long-term programming to genes and could bring about a change in
gene function without changing gene sequence, are termed here epigenetic
changes. Thus, many of the phenotypic variations seen in human populations
might be caused by differences in long-term programming of gene function
rather than the sequence *per se*. Therefore, looking at sequence variations
and polymorphisms *per se* might miss the mark. Thus, any future study
of the basis for inter-individual phenotypic diversity should consider epigenetic variations in addition to genetic sequence polymorphisms (Meaney
& Szyf, 2005).

    The dynamic nature of epigenetic regulation in difference from the static
nature of the gene sequence provides a mechanism for reprogramming gene
function in response to changes in life style trajectories. Thus, epigenetics
could provide an explanation for well-documented gene × environment interactions. An important implication of the possible involvement of epigenetics
in defining behavioural patterns is the potential for therapeutic intervention.
Epigenetic mechanisms are dynamic and potentially reversible and are therefore amenable to therapeutic intervention (Szyf, 2001). Drugs that target the
epigenetic machinery are currently tested in clinical trials in cancer (Kramer,
Gottlicher, & Heinzel, 2001; Weidle & Grossmann, 2000) and psychiatry

disorders (Simonini et al., 2006). Moreover, once we understand the rules through which different environmental exposures modify the epigenetic processes we might be able to design behavioural strategies to prevent and revert deleterious environmentally driven epigenetic alterations.

Definition of epigenetics

The classic definition of epigenetics emphasizes heritability. Epigenetic change is defined as a heritable change in gene function that does not involve a change in the DNA sequence. This emphasis on heritability in its classical interpretation, which implies trans-generational inheritance, limits the scope of epigenetics to trans-generational effects. A broader definition of heritability includes any event of DNA replication and cell division at the cellular level. This definition extends epigenetics to cancer and cancer cells, as well as some normal cell types that divide and grow. This definition covers therefore changes in gene function, which are passed from a cell to a daughter cell. However, it leaves postmitotic tissues such as brain, heart and others, which do not replicate their DNA, outside the epigenetic sphere. Nevertheless, it is now becoming clear that long-term changes in gene function and the resulting phenotypic variations might take place in postmitotic tissues such as the brain. Epigenetic changes are responsive to environmental cues after birth and these changes are not passed through the germ line (Meaney & Szyf, 2005). We therefore propose here a broader definition of epigenetics, which includes any long-term change in gene function that does not involve a change in gene sequence or structure in both dividing and non-dividing cells. In summary, epigenetic changes occur either in the germ line and result in heritable and trans-generational transmission of alterations in gene function, or in dividing cells and are heritable from cell to daughter cells but are not inherited through the germ line or in postmitotic cells such as neurons and are therefore not heritable.

Genetic polymorphisms and epigenetic alterations could have similar consequences

During the normal processes of development and cellular differentiation a cell type-specific pattern of epigenetic marks is generated (Razin & Riggs, 1980). This normal "pattern" of epigenetic marks defines the normal pattern of gene function in each tissue and cell type (Razin & Szyf, 1984). The normal pattern of gene function is critical for the execution of the normal life necessities: physiological and behavioural functions. A change in the normal pattern of gene function would result in phenotypic differences. Gene function could change by sequence alterations that either completely eliminate the function of the gene or alter the function of the protein encoded by the gene, resulting in either increase or decrease in its activity. Many polymorphisms in gene sequences between individuals were discovered to date and some of these known sequence differences were associated with behavioural pathologies (Caspi et al., 2003; Gillespie, Whitfield, Williams, Heath, & Martin, 2005). However, gene function may well be changed also by an epigenetic process that could lead to phenotypic differences that are indistinguishable from those caused by gene mutation. Epigenetic changes could be environmentally driven, may occur in response to triggers at different points in life and are potentially reversible, whereas genetic differences are germ line transmitted, are fixed and irreversible.

A paradigm of epigenetic silencing is the case of "tumour suppressor" genes in cancer. Tumour suppressor genes are normally active and protect our cells from abnormal growth. The first tumour suppressor gene that was characterized was the *RETINOBLASTOMA* gene, a recessive mutation leading to childhood tumours in either one or two eyes (Neel & Falls, 1951; Sparkes et al., 1983). All tumour suppressor genes were originally discovered as a result of a recessive mutation, which led to a specific type of cancer. It was later found that many of these tumour suppressor genes were silenced by epigenetic inactivation in many cancers rather than by genetic lesions (Gonzalez-Zulueta et al., 1995). Thus, epigenetic silencing and genetic silencing could have similar phenotypic consequences. Therefore, epigenetic mapping is potentially as important as genetic mapping in our quest to understand phenotypic differences in human behaviour. Moreover, while nothing could be done to activate a tumour suppressor gene silenced by genetic lesions, epigenetic drugs were shown to activate silenced tumour suppressor genes and are now being tested in clinical trials in cancer therapy (Momparler, 2005; Szyf, 1994, 2001). Thus, identifying epigenetic changes that are associated with behavioural pathologies might lead to new therapeutic interventions.

In summary, understanding epigenetic alterations, which are associated with behavioural disorders, is important for a number of reasons. First, identifying epigenetic alterations in specific genes enables the generation of hypotheses as to the immediate mechanisms involved in a behavioural pathology. Second, by defining the relationship between epigenetic changes and specific environmental exposures we will be able to decipher the mechanisms involved in gene × environment interactions. Third, by understanding the mechanisms responsible for the epigenetic aberrations we might be able to either prevent or reverse these changes. In this chapter we will describe the path that we have taken to delineate the mechanisms involved in epigenetic programming by maternal care in rats as a paradigm for unravelling the epigenetic basis of phenotypic differences in behaviour. We also discuss some of our preliminary foray into understanding epigenetic differences associated with differences in human aggression.

The epigenome

Chromatin

The epigenome consists of the chromatin and its modifications as well as a covalent modification by methylation of cytosine rings found at the dinucleotide sequence CG (Figure 3.1) (Razin, 1998). The epigenome determines the accessibility of the transcription machinery, which transcribes the genes into messenger RNA, to the DNA. Inaccessible genes are therefore silent whereas accessible genes are transcribed. We therefore distinguish between open and closed configurations of chromatin (Groudine, Eisenman, Gelinas, & Weintraub, 1983; Grunstein, 1997; Marks, Sheffery, & Rifkind, 1985; Ramain, Bourouis, Dretzen, Richards, Sobkowiak, & Bellard, 1986; Varga-Weisz & Becker, 2006). Densely packaged chromatin could be visualized microscopically and is termed heterochromatin while open accessible chromatin is termed euchromatin. Recently another new level of epigenetic regulation by small non-coding RNAs termed microRNA has been discovered (Bergmann & Lane, 2003). MicroRNAs regulate gene expression at different levels: silencing of chromatin, degradation of mRNA and blocking translation. MicroRNAs were found to play an important role in cancer (Zhang,

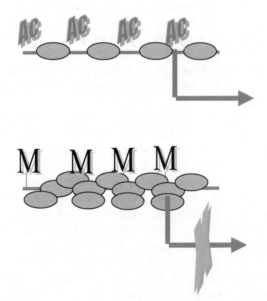

Figure 3.1 Chromatin structure, gene expression and DNA methylation are correlated; DNA methylation and chromatin programme to control gene expression. The scheme shows that a gene could be found in either an open chromatin structure and active state (top) or a closed chromatin structure and an inactive state (bottom). Other intermediate states are possible as well. Ac = acetylation, the ovals represent nucleosomes, M = DNA methylation and horizontal arrows represent transcription into mRNA.

Pan, Cobb, & Anderson, 2007) and could potentially play an important role in behavioural pathologies as well (Vo et al., 2005).

The histone code

The DNA is wrapped around a protein-based structure termed chromatin. The basic building block of chromatin is the nucleosome, which is formed of an octamer of histone proteins. There are five basic forms of histone proteins termed H1, H2A, H2B, H3 and H4 (Finch et al., 1977), as well as other minor variants that are involved in specific functions such as DNA repair or gene activation (Sarma & Reinberg, 2005). The octamer structure of the nucleosome is composed of an H3-H4 tetramer flanked on either side with an H2A-H2B dimer (Finch et al., 1977). The N-terminal tails of these histones are extensively modified by methylation (Jenuwein, 2001), phosphorylation, acetylation (Wade, Pruss, & Wolffe, 1997) and ubiquitination (Shilatifard, 2006). The state of modification of these tails plays an important role in defining the accessibility of the DNA wrapped around the nucleosome core. It was proposed that the amino terminal tails of H3 and H4 histones that are positively charged form tight interactions with the negatively charged DNA backbone, thus blocking the interaction of transcription factors with the DNA. Modifications of the tails neutralize the charge on the tails, thus relaxing the tight grip of the histone tails. Different histone variants, which replace the standard isoforms, also play a regulatory role and serve to mark active genes in some instances (Henikoff, McKittrick, & Ahmad, 2004). The specific pattern of histone modifications was proposed to form a "histone code" that delineates the parts of the genome to be expressed at a given point in time in a given cell type (Jenuwein & Allis, 2001). A change in histone modifications around a gene will change its level of expression and could convert an active gene to become silent, resulting in "loss of function", or switch a silent gene to be active, leading to "gain of function".

Histone modifying enzymes

The most-investigated histone modifying enzymes are histone acetyltransferases (HAT), which acetylate histone H3 at the K9 residue as well as other residues and H4 tails at a number of residues, and histone deacetylases (HDAC), which deacetylate histone tails (Kuo & Allis, 1998). Histone acetylation is believed to be a predominant signal for an active chromatin configuration (Lee, Hayes, Pruss, & Wolffe, 1993; Perry & Chalkley, 1982). Deacetylated histones signal inactive chromatin, chromatin associated with inactive genes. Many repressors and repressor complexes recruit HDACs to genes, thus causing their inactivation (Wolffe, 1996). Histone tail acetylation is believed to enhance the accessibility of a gene to the transcription machinery whereas deacetylated tails are highly charged and believed to be tightly associated with the DNA backbone, thus limiting accessibility of genes to transcription factors (Kuo & Allis, 1998).

Histone modification by methylation is catalysed by different histone methyltransferases. Some specific methylation events are associated with gene silencing and some with gene activation. For example methylation of the K9 residue of H3-histone tails is catalysed by the histone methyltransferase SUV3-9 and is associated with silencing of the associated gene (Lachner, O'Carroll, Rea, Mechtler, & Jenuwein, 2001). Particular factors recognize histone modifications and further stabilize an inactive state. For example, the heterochromatin-associated protein HP-1 binds H3-histone tails methylated at the K9 residue and precipitates an inactive chromatin structure (Lachner et al., 2001). Recently described histone demethylases remove the methylation mark, causing either activation or repression of gene expression (Shi et al., 2004; Tsukada et al., 2006).

Chromatin remodelling

Chromatin remodelling complexes, which are ATP dependent, alter the position of nucleosomes around the transcription initiation site and define its accessibility to the transcription machinery (Varga-Weisz & Becker, 2006). It is becoming clear now that there is an interrelationship between chromatin modification and chromatin remodelling. For example, the presence of BRG1 (the catalytic subunit of SWI/SNF-related chromatin remodelling complexes) is required for histone acetylation and regulation of β-globin expression during development (Bultman, Gebuhr, & Magnuson, 2005).

Targeting of chromatin modifying enzymes to specific genes

A basic principle in epigenetic regulation is targeting. Histone modifying enzymes are generally not gene specific. Specific transcription factors and transcription repressors recruit histone modifying enzymes to specific genes and thus define the gene-specific profile of histone modification (Jenuwein & Allis, 2001). Transcription factors and repressors recognize specific *cis*-acing sequences in genes, bind to these sequences and attract the specific chromatin modifying enzymes to these genes through protein–protein interactions. The *cis*-acting sequences act as area codes while the transcription factors that read these codes deliver a load of chromatin modifying and remodelling enzymes. Specific transacting factors are responsive to cellular signalling pathways. Signal transduction pathways, which are activated by cell-surface receptors, could thus serve as conduits for epigenetic change linking the environmental trigger at cell surface receptors with gene-specific chromatin alterations and reprogramming of gene activity. For example, numerous signalling pathways, including those triggered by G protein-coupled cell surface receptors in the brain, alter the concentration of cAMP in the cell. One of the transcription factors that responds to increased cAMP is CREB (cAMP response element binding protein). CREB binds cAMP response elements in certain genes and also recruits CREB binding protein CBP. CBP is a HAT that acetylates histones (Ogryzko, Schiltz, Russanova, Howard, & Nakatani, 1996). Thus, elevation of cAMP levels in response to an extracellular signal would result in a change in the state of histone acetylation in specific genes. Obviously environmental or physiological events that interfere at any point along the signalling pathway might result in chromatin alterations. An example of such a pathway that leads from maternal behaviour to long-term programming of gene expression in the hippocampus will be discussed in detail in this chapter (Meaney & Szyf, 2005).

DNA methylation

In addition to chromatin, which is associated with DNA, the DNA molecule itself is chemically modified by methyl residues at the 5′ position of the cytosine rings in the dinucleotide sequence CG in vertebrates (Figure 3.2) (Razin, 1998). What distinguishes DNA methylation in vertebrate genomes is the fact that not all CGs are methylated in any given cell type (Razin, 1998). Distinct CGs are methylated in different cell types, generating cell type-specific patterns of methylation. Thus, the DNA methylation pattern confers upon the genome its cell type identity (Razin, 1998). Since DNA methylation is part of the chemical structure of the DNA itself, it is more stable than other epigenetic marks and thus it has extremely important diagnostic potential (Beck, Olek, & Walter, 1999) that is yet to be taken advantage of in behavioural disorders.

The DNA methylation pattern is established during development and is then maintained faithfully through life by the maintenance DNA methyltransferase (Figure 3.3) (Razin & Riggs, 1980). The DNA methylation reaction was believed to be irreversible, thus the common consensus was that the only manner by which methyl residues could be lost was through replication in the absence of DNA methyltransferase by passive demethylation (Razin &

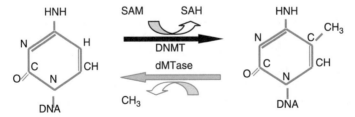

Figure 3.2 The reversible DNA methylation reaction. DNA methyltransferases (DNMT) catalyse the transfer of methyl groups from the methyl donor *S*-adenosylmethionine (SAM) to DNA, releasing *S*-adenosylhomocysteine (SAH). Demethylases release the methyl group from methylated DNA. It was originally proposed that the methyl group is released as methanol but recent data suggests that the methyl group is released as formaldehyde.

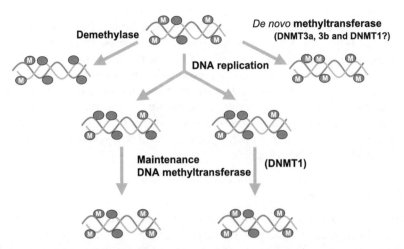

Figure 3.3 DNA methylation reactions. Early after fertilization many of the methylation marks are removed by demethylases (methyl groups are indicated by M, potential methylatable sites are indicated by an open circle). *De novo* DNA methyltransferases (DNMT) add methyl groups. Once a pattern is generated it is inherited by maintenance DNMTs that copy the methylation pattern.

Riggs, 1980). Recent data supports the idea that, similar to chromatin modification, DNA methylation is also potentially reversible (Ramchandani, Bhattacharya, Cervoni, & Szyf, 1999) even in postmitotic tissues (Weaver et al., 2004a). The DNA methylation pattern is not copied by the DNA replication machinery but by independent enzymatic machinery, DNA methyltransferase(s) (DNMT; Figures 3.2 and 3.3) (Razin & Cedar, 1977). DNA methylation patterns in vertebrates are distinguished by their correlation with chromatin structure. Active regions of the chromatin, which enable gene expression, are associated with hypomethylated DNA whereas hypermethylated DNA is packaged in inactive chromatin (Razin, 1998; Razin & Cedar, 1977).

It is generally accepted that DNA methylation plays an important role in regulating gene expression (Figure 3.4). DNA methylation in distinct regulatory regions is believed to mark silent genes. Thus, aberrant methylation will silence a gene resulting in loss of function, which will have a similar consequence to loss of function by a genetic mechanism such as mutation, deletion or rearrangement (Figure 3.4). A recent whole epigenomic screening of three human chromosomes suggests that a third of the genes analysed show inverse correlation between the state of DNA methylation at the 5′ regulatory regions and gene expression (Eckhardt et al., 2006). There is now overwhelming data indicating that aberrant silencing of tumour suppressor genes by DNA methylation is a common mechanism in cancer (Baylin, Esteller, Rountree, Bachman, Schuebel, & Herman, 2001).

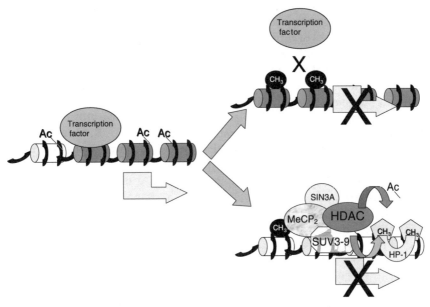

Figure 3.4 Two mechanisms of silencing gene expression by DNA methylation. An expressed gene (transcription indicated by horizontal arrow) is usually associated with acetylated histones and is unmethylated. An event of methylation would lead to methylation by two different mechanisms. The methyl group (CH₃) interferes with the binding of a transcription factor that is required for gene expression, resulting in blocking of transcription. The second mechanism shown in the bottom right is indirect. Methylated DNA attracts methylated DNA binding proteins such as MeCP2, which in turn recruits co-repressors such as SIN3A, histone methyltransferases such as SUV3-9 that methylates histones and histone deacetylases (HDAC) that remove the acetyl groups from histone tails. Methylated histones (K9 residue of histone tails) recruit heterochromatin proteins such as HP-1, which contributes to a closed chromatin configuration and silencing of the gene.

Current data suggests a bilateral relation between chromatin structure and DNA methylation. This interrelationship of chromatin modification state and DNA methylation has important implications for our understanding of how the epigenome is generated, and its utility as a diagnostic and as a therapeutic target.

DNA methylation enzymes

The DNA methylation pattern is not copied by the DNA replication machinery, but by independent enzymatic machinery: DNA methyltransferase(s) (DNMT; Figures 3.2 and 3.3). The DNA methylation machinery in vertebrates has two main roles. First, it has to establish new cell type-specific DNA methylation patterns during development and possibly during adulthood in response to new signals. Second, it has to maintain these patterns during downstream cell divisions and after DNA repair. The different enzymes and proteins of the DNA methylation machinery must address these different tasks. The methylation of DNA occurs immediately after replication by transfer of a methyl moiety from the donor S-adenosyl-L-methionine (AdoMet) in a reaction catalysed by DNMT (Figure 3.2). Most of our structural and mechanistic understanding of DNMTs is derived from structural work done on bacterial DNMTs, particularly the 5-methylcytosine DNMT HhaI (Cheng, Kumar, Posfai, Pflugrath, & Roberts, 1993). Razin and Riggs proposed more than two decades ago that the maintenance DNMT1 prefers a hemimethylated substrate (Razin & Riggs, 1980). Since hemimethylated sites are generated during DNA replication when a nascent unmethylated C is synthesized across a methylated C in the template parental strand, the DNMT accurately copies the methylation pattern of the template strand (Figure 3.3). Three distinct phylogenic DNMTs were identified in mammals: DNMT1 shows preference for hemimethylated DNA *in vitro*, which is consistent with its role as a maintenance DNMT, whereas DNMT3a and DNMT3b methylate unmethylated and methylated DNA at an equal rate that is consistent with a *de novo* DNMT role (Okano, Xie, & Li, 1998). Two additional DNMT homologues were found: DNMT2, whose substrate and methylation activity is unclear (Vilain, Apiou, Dutrillaux, & Malfoy, 1998); and DNMT3L, which belongs to the DNMT3 family of DNMTs by virtue of its sequence and is essential for the establishment of maternal genomic imprints but lacks key methyltransferase motifs, and is possibly a regulator of methylation rather than an enzyme that methylates DNA (Bourc'his, Xu, Lin, Bollman, & Bestor, 2001). Knock-out mouse data indicates that DNMT1 is responsible for a majority of DNA methylation marks in the mouse genome (Li, Bestor, & Jaenisch, 1992) whereas DNMT3a and DNMT3b are responsible for some but not all *de novo* methylation during development (Okano, Bell, Haber, & Li, 1999).

The DNA methylation pattern is reversible; DNA demethylation enzymes

It was a long held belief that the DNA methylation pattern is solely dependent on DNMTs and that the reverse reaction cannot occur. Thus, according to the classic model DNA methylation patterns were generated during development but were then copied faithfully by the maintenance DNMT. The only reaction that takes place according to this model in differentiated cells is maintenance DNA methylation during cell division. The answer to the question of whether the DNA methylation is reversible or not has important implications on the possibility that DNA methylation is dynamic and responsive to physiological and environmental signals throughout life. This issue of the reversibility of the DNA methylation reaction has important implications for our understanding of the role of DNA methylation in non-dividing tissues such as neurons. If DNA methylation only happens when DNMT is copying DNA methylation patterns during cell division, as suggested by the classic model, there is no need for DNMTs in neurons. Nevertheless, DNMTs are present in neurons (Goto, Numata, Komura, Ono, Bestor, & Kondo, 1994) and there is data suggesting that DNMT levels in neurons change in certain pathological conditions such as schizophrenia (Veldic, Guidotti, Maloku, Davis, & Costa, 2005). The presence of DNMT in neurons would make sense only if the DNA methylation is dynamic in postmitotic tissues and is a balance of methylation and demethylation reactions (Szyf, 2001). Without active demethylation there is no need for DNA methylation in neurons.

We have proposed a while ago that the DNA methylation pattern is a balance of methylation and demethylation reactions that are responsive to physiological and environmental signals and thus forms a platform for gene–environment interactions (Figure 3.2) (Ramchandani et al., 1999). There is a long list of data from both cell culture and early mouse development supporting the hypothesis that active methylation occurs in embryonal and somatic cells. There are now convincing examples of active, replication-independent DNA demethylation during development as well as in somatic tissues. Active demethylation was reported for the *myosin* gene in differentiating myoblast cells (Lucarelli, Fuso, Strom, & Scarpa, 2001), the interleukin-2 (IL-2) gene upon T cell activation (Bruniquel & Schwartz, 2003), the interferon β-gene upon antigen exposure of memory CD8 T cells (Kersh et al., 2006) and in the glucocorticoid receptor gene promoter in adult rat brains upon treatment with the HDAC inhibitor TSA (Weaver et al., 2004a).

The main challenge of the field is identifying the enzymes responsible for demethylation. The characteristics of the enzymes responsible for active demethylation are controversial. One proposal has been that a G/T mismatch repair glycosylase also functions as a 5-methylcytosine DNA glycosylase, recognizes methylcytosines and cleaves the bond between the sugar and the base. The abasic site is then repaired and replaced with a non-methylated cytosine, resulting in demethylation (Jost, 1993). An additional protein with a similar activity was recently identified, the methylated DNA binding protein 4 (MBD4) (Zhu et al., 2000). While such a mechanism can explain site-specific demethylation, global demethylation by a glycosylase would involve extensive damage to DNA that would compromise genomic integrity. Another report has proposed that methylated binding protein 2 (MBD2) has demethylase activity. MBD2b (a shorter isoform of MBD2) was shown to directly remove the methyl group from methylated cytosine in methylated CpGs (Bhattacharya, Ramchandani, Cervoni, & Szyf, 1999). This enzyme was therefore proposed to reverse the DNA methylation reaction. However, other groups disputed this finding (Ng et al., 1999). Very recent data suggests that active demethylation early in embryogenesis, as well as in somatic cells, is catalysed by a nucleotide excision repair mechanism whereby methylated cytosines are replaced by unmethylated cytosines, which involves the growth arrest and damage response protein Gadd45a and the DNA repair endonuclease XPG (Barreto et al., 2007). The main problem with this mechanism is that it involves the risk of extensive damage to the DNA. Although a number of biochemical processes were implicated in demethylation, it is unclear how and when these different enzymes participate in shaping and maintaining the overall pattern of methylation and how these activities respond to different environmental exposures.

Targeting DNA methylation and demethylation; chromatin and DNA methylation

The classic model of maintenance DNA methylation did not require targeting. According to this model the DNA methylation pattern is copied automatically on the basis of the methylation pattern of the paternal DNA (Razin & Riggs, 1980). However, if DNA methylation patterns are dynamic and responsive throughout life they cannot be just automatically copied and preserved. The methylation and demethylation enzymes do not have exquisite sequence specificity, so how could these enzymes maintain highly specific DNA methylation patterns? Methylation and demethylation enzymes have to be targeted to specific genes to either preserve or change in a regulated manner their pattern of methylation. The picture that is currently emerging is that the DNA methylation pattern is tightly coordinated with the chromatin structure. That is, "opening" of chromatin leads to demethylation and a "closed configuration" of chromatin leads to methylation. Thus, we propose that the direction of the DNA methylation reaction is defined by the state of chromatin, as discussed above. The gene specificity of the state of chromatin is defined by sequence-specific *trans*-acting factors that recruit chromatin modifying enzymes to specific genes. Chromatin configuration then gates the accessibility of genes to DNA methylation or demethylation machineries (Cervoni & Szyf, 2001; D'Alessio & Szyf, 2006). In support of this hypothesis we have previously shown that the histone deacetylase inhibitor (HDACi) trichostatin A, which causes histone hyperacetylation, also causes active DNA demethylation (Figure 3.5) (Cervoni & Szyf, 2001). A change in histone acetylation is normally caused by transcription factors, which recruit histone acetyltransferases (HATs). Thus, binding of transcription factors to a specific sequence in a gene could recruit HATs, which would cause histone acetylation, facilitating in turn demethylation. In summary, we propose the following model. Factors that target specific chromatin modification events to genes define the direction of the DNA methylation equilibrium either by recruiting DNA methylation enzymes or by facilitating demethylation. We will illustrate how this might be working using gene expression programming by maternal care as a paradigm for behavioural programming of DNA methylation below.

There is evidence to support different elements of this model. Histone modifying enzymes interact with DNA methylating enzymes and participate in recruiting them to specific targets. A growing list of histone modifying

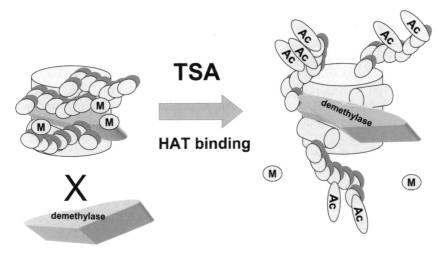

Figure 3.5 Demethylation is directed by the state of chromatin structure. Histone acetylation (Ac) triggered by a pharmacological inhibitor of histone deacetylase (TSA) facilitates the interaction of demethylases with methylated DNA, allowing for demethylation.

enzymes has been shown to interact with DNMT1, such as HDAC1 and HDAC2, the histone methyltransferases SUV3-9 and EZH2, a member of the multi-protein Polycomb complex PRC2 that methylates H3 histone at the K27 residue (Fuks, Burgers, Brehm, Hughes-Davies, & Kouzarides, 2000; Fuks, Hurd, Wolf, Nan, Bird, & Kouzarides, 2003; Rountree, Bachman, & Baylin, 2000; Vire et al., 2005). DNMT3a was recently also shown to interact with EZH2 which targets the DNA methylation-histone modification multi-protein complexes to specific sequences in DNA (Vire et al., 2005).

Trans-acting repressors target both histone modifying enzymes and DNMTs to specific *cis*-acting signals in regulatory regions of particular genes causing gene-specific DNA methylation and chromatin modification. For example, the promyelocytic leukaemia PML-RAR fusion protein engages histone deacetylases and DNMTs to its target binding sequences and produces *de novo* DNA methylation of adjacent genes (Di Croce et al., 2002). There are also documented interactions between proteins that read the DNA methylation and histone methylation marks and either histone or DNA modifying enzymes. The methylated DNA binding protein MeCP2 interacts with the HMT SUV3-9 (Fuks et al., 2003) and in plants it was shown that chromomethylase-3 (CMT3), a plant CNG-specific DNMT, interacts with an arabidopsis homologue of HP-1, a protein that binds histone H3 methylated at lysine 9 (Jackson, Lindroth, Cao, & Jacobsen, 2002).

Evidence is emerging that supports the hypothesis that sequence-specific transcription factors target demethylation to specific genes. Transcription factors recruit HATs to specific genes causing gene specific acetylation and thus facilitate their demethylation. For example, the intronic kappa chain enhancer and the transcription factor NF-kappaB are required for B cell-specific demethylation of the kappa immunoglobulin gene (Lichtenstein, Keini, Cedar, & Bergman, 1994). The demethylation of the maize suppressor-mutator (Spm) transposon is mediated by the transposon-encoded transcriptional activator TnpA protein (Bruniquel & Schwartz, 2003). We will discuss below how maternal care is employing this mechanism to programme gene expression through recruitment of the transcription factor NGFI-A to one of the *GLUCOCORTICOID RECEPTOR* (GR) gene promoters in the hippocampus (Weaver et al., 2007).

In summary, in difference from the original dogma that has dominated the field for some time we propose that the DNA methylation and chromatin structures are found in a dynamic balance through life. The direction of the balance is maintained and defined by sequence-specific factors that deliver histone modification and DNA modification enzymes to genes. These factors are responsive to signalling pathways in the cell. Methylation patterns are maintained as long as this equilibrium of sequence-specific factor engagement of the genes is maintained. The state of this equilibrium is defined during development and in the process of cellular differentiation. Physiological or environmental signals, which alter the signalling pathways in the cell, would result in tilting of this balance by activating or suppressing specific *trans*-acting factors. This mechanism could provide an explanation for how the environment sculpts our genome (see model in Figures 3.5 and 3.6).

How does DNA methylation silence gene expression?

DNA methylation in critical regulatory regions serves as a signal to silence gene expression. There are two main mechanisms by which cytosine methylation suppresses gene expression (Figure 3.4). The first mechanism involves direct interference of the methyl residue with the binding of a transcription factor to its recognition element in the gene. The interaction of transcription factors with genes is required for activation of the gene; lack of binding of a transcription factor would result in silencing of gene expression (Comb & Goodman, 1990; Inamdar, Ehrlich, & Ehrlich, 1991). This form of inhibition of transcription by methylation requires that the methylation events occur within the recognition sequence for a transcription factor. A second mechanism is indirect. A certain density of DNA methylation moieties in the region of the gene attracts the binding of methylated-DNA binding proteins such as MeCP2 (Nan, Campoy, & Bird, 1997). MeCP2 recruits other proteins such as SIN3A and histone modifying enzymes, which lead to the formation of a "closed" chromatin configuration and silencing of gene expression (Nan et al., 1997). Several methylated-DNA binding proteins such as MBD1, MBD2 and MBD3 suppress gene expression by a similar mechanism (Fujita et al., 1999; Hendrich & Bird, 1998; Ng et al., 1999).

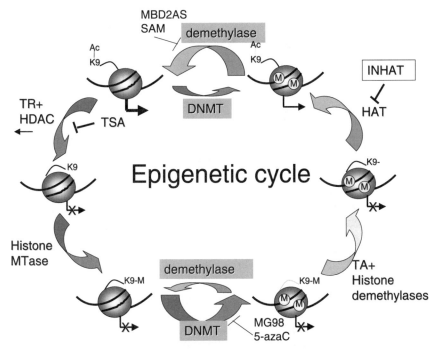

Figure 3.6 The epigenetic cycle. A gene could be found in either of the epigenetic states from highly active to stably inactive. The transition from one state to the other involves recruitment of chromatin modifying enzymes to *cis*-acting signals in the gene regulatory region by *trans*-acting repressors (TR) or *trans*-acting activators (TA). The state of chromatin facilitates interaction of either DNA methyltransferases (DNMT) or demethylases, which alter the state of DNA methylation. Ac = acetylation, K9 = the lysine residue at the 9th position of the H3-histone tails, M = methylation, horizontal arrow-transcription to mRNA, HDAC = histone deacetylases, Histone MTase = histone methyltransferases, HAT = histone acetyltransferases, INHAT = inhibitors of HAT, MBD2 AS = antisense inhibitors of MBD2, MG98 = an antisense oligonucleotide inhibitor of DNMT1, 5-azaC = DNA methyltransferase inhibitor 5-azacytidine, SAM = *S*-adenosylmethionine.

Bilateral relationship between chromatin structure and DNA methylation

The second mechanism described in the previous section illustrates how DNA methylation could define chromatin structure by recruiting chromatin modifying enzymes. Similarly, loss of DNA methylation will result in a change in chromatin structure in the opposite direction, resulting in an increased level of histone acetylation and "opening" of chromatin configuration. Thus, chromatin structure and DNA methylation exhibit a bilateral relationship creating a positive-feedback loop whereby increased DNA methylation further

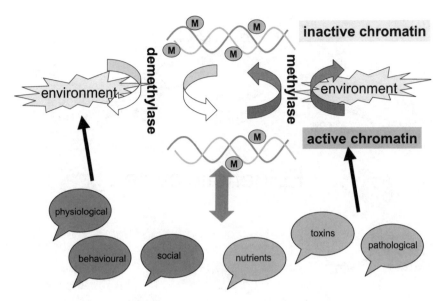

Figure 3.7 Hypothesis: The steady state methylation pattern is a dynamic equilibrium between methylase and demethylase activities, defined by the state of chromatin. Different environmental exposures could tilt the balance of chromatin state and DNA methylation state.

enhances chromatin inactivation, which further facilitates DNA methylation. Similarly, demethylation increases chromatin activation, which further enhances DNA demethylation (Figures 3.5–3.7).

Mechanisms of epigenetic programming by maternal care

The maternal care model and its implication on epigenetics as a mediator and effector of behaviour

The best-documented case to date of epigenetic programming triggered by the social environment is the long-term impact that maternal care has on expression of the glucocorticoid receptor gene in the hippocampus of the offspring in the rat. In the rat, the adult offspring of mothers that exhibit increased levels of pup licking/grooming (i.e., High LG mothers) over the first week of life show increased hippocampal GR expression, enhanced glucocorticoid feedback sensitivity, decreased hypothalamic corticotrophin releasing factor (CRF) expression and more modest HPA stress responses compared to animals reared by Low LG mothers (Francis, Diorio, Liu, & Meaney, 1999; Liu et al., 1997). Cross-fostering studies suggest direct effects of maternal care on both gene expression and stress responses (Francis et al., 1999; Liu et al., 1997). These studies supported an epigenetic mechanism rather than a genetic mechanism since the fostering mother and not the biological mother defined the stress response of its adult offspring. The critical question was obviously mechanism. How could the behaviour of the caregiver cause a stable change in gene expression in the offspring long after the caregiver is gone? We postulated an epigenetic mechanism. That is, we hypothesized that the maternal behaviour of the caregiver triggered an epigenetic change in the brain of the offspring (Meaney & Szyf, 2005).

This model has two nodal implications on our understanding of the relationship between behaviour and epigenetics. First, the social behaviour of one subject can affect epigenetic programming in another subject. Thus our model provides a molecular mechanism mediating the effects of nurture on nature. Second, epigenetic programming can have long-term impact on behaviour. This highlights the significance of epigenetic mechanisms in the establishment of inter-individual differences in behaviour.

Maternal care epigenetically programmes stress responses in the offspring

We have previously published evidence to support the hypothesis that epigenetic mechanisms mediate the maternal effect on stress response. Increased maternal LG is associated with demethylation of the nerve growth factor-inducible protein A (NGFI-A) transcription factor response element located within the exon 1_7 GR promoter (Figure 3.8) (Weaver et al., 2004a). The difference in the methylation status of this CpG site between the offspring of High and Low LG mothers emerges over the first week of life, is reversed with cross-fostering, persists into adulthood and is associated with altered histone acetylation and NGFI-A binding to the GR promoter (Weaver et al., 2004a). Thus maternal care affects the chromatin, DNA methylation and transcription factor binding to the GR exon 1_7 promoter, illustrating the basic principles of epigenetic regulation discussed above. We have also shown that maternal care early in life affected the expression of hundreds of genes in the adult hippocampus (Weaver, Meaney, & Szyf, 2006), thus illustrating the profound effect of the social environment early in life on gene expression programming throughout life. These results have quite tantalizing implications. They imply that differences in maternal care early in life can result in

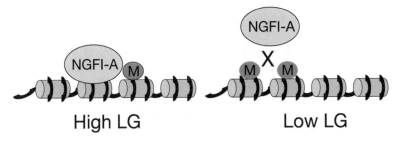

Figure 3.8 Methylation of the hippocampal glucocorticoid receptor GR exon 1_7 promoter blocks the binding of the transcription factor NGFI-A.

gene expression changes that remain persistent into adulthood in numerous genes. This range of change in gene expression would have required simultaneously mutating hundreds of genes if it had been accomplished by genetic means. This illustrates the potential power of epigenetic processes in modulating our genomic inheritance

Epigenetic programming by maternal care is reversible in the adult animal

Although epigenetic programming by maternal care is highly stable and results in long-term changes in gene expression, it is nevertheless reversible. The combination of reversibility and stability is one of the appealing aspects of epigenetics. The possibility that certain adverse gene expression programming of behaviourally relevant genes could be reversed by either epigenetic drugs or perhaps even by behavioural intervention has obvious implications. To test this hypothesis we used the well-documented histone deacetylase (HDAC) inhibitor TSA (Yoshida, Kijima, Akita, & Beppu, 1990). Since the state of histone acetylation is a balance of histone deacetylation and histone acetylation reactions, inhibition of HDAC activity would tilt the equilibrium toward acetylation and as a consequence bring about increased acetylation of histones, leading to open chromatin configuration. We have previously proposed, as discussed above, that chromatin states and DNA methylation states are linked so that opening up of chromatin by increasing histone acetylation would tilt the balance of the DNA methylation equilibrium toward demethylation (Figures 3.5 and 3.7) (Cervoni & Szyf, 2001; Cervoni, Detich, Seo, Chakravarti, & Szyf, 2002). Treating adult offspring of low LG-ABN (arched back nursing) maternal care with TSA reversed the epigenetic marks on the GR exon 1_7 promoter: histone acetylation increased, the gene was demethylated and there was increased occupancy of the promoter with the transcription factor NGFI-A, resulting in increased GR exon 1_7 promoter expression. The epigenetic reversal was accompanied by a behavioural change so that the stress response of the TSA-treated adult offspring of low LG-ABN was indistinguishable from the offspring of high LG-ABN (Weaver, Diorio, Seckl, Szyf, & Meaney, 2004b). This was the first illustration of reversal of early life behavioural programming by pharmacological modulation of the epigenome during adulthood. TSA is not a DNA methylation inhibitor but nevertheless TSA treatment resulted in demethylation as we predicted. We propose that increased histone acetylation triggered by the HDAC inhibitor facilitated the interaction of a resident demethylase with the GR exon 1_7 promoter (Figures 3.5 and 3.9). This data illustrates the tight association between the DNA methylation and histone acetylation equilibrium in the adult brain and the potential reversibility of the DNA methylation pattern in the non-dividing adult neuron.

Histone acetylation could be altered not only by pharmacological modulation but also by neurotransmitter activation of signalling pathways whose downstream targets include histone acetyltransferases. Thus, behavioural interventions that lead to firing of neurons and consistent and repetitive activation of signalling pathways might also lead to a change in DNA methylation of specific genes in the adult brain. In addition, drugs that are used for entertainment or therapeutic process and reach the central nervous system (CNS) might potentially alter DNA methylation patterns of genes in the brain by similar mechanisms. An interesting example of such a drug is the antiepileptic and mood stabilizing agent valproic acid. This drug was found to be an HDAC inhibitor. We have shown that valproate triggered replication-independent DNA demethylation in tissue culture (Detich, Bovenzi, & Szyf, 2003b; Milutinovic, D'Alessio, Detich, & Szyf, 2006) and valproate was shown to inhibit DNA methylation in the brain in an animal model (Tremolizzo et al., 2002).

If the DNA methylation state remains in methylation–demethylation equilibrium in adult neurons throughout life it should be possible also to reverse the DNA methylation in the opposite direction by increasing DNA methylation. We have previously demonstrated that the methyl donor *S*-adenosylmethionine (SAM) inhibits the demethylation reaction (Detich, Hamm, Just, Knox, & Szyf, 2003a). Thus, changing SAM levels would alter the DNA methylation equilibrium by either increasing the rate of the DNA methylation reaction or by inhibiting the demethylation reaction, or both (Figure 3.9). Since SAM is an unstable compound we injected the precursor of SAM, the amino acid L-methionine, into the brain of adult offspring of either high or low maternal LG-ABN. Systemic injection of methionine was previously shown to increase SAM concentrations in the brain (Tremolizzo et al., 2002). Injection of methionine to the brain led to hypermethylation and reduced expression of the GR exon 1_7 expression in the adult hippocampus of offspring of high LG-ABN and reversal of its stress response to a pattern that

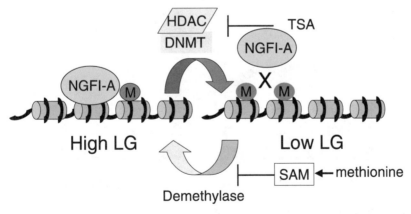

Figure 3.9 The epigenetic programming of the GR exon 1_7 promoter expression by maternal care is reversible later in life by either the HDAC inhibitor TSA or the methyl donor SAM.

was indistinguishable from offspring of low LG-ABN (Weaver et al., 2005). Thus, maternal epigenetic programming could be reversed later in life in both directions. Methionine is especially interesting since the levels of methionine in cells are influenced by diet. Thus, this might provide an example of a potential link between dietary intake and alteration in epigenetic programming in the brain (Figure 3.9).

Mechanisms leading from maternal care to epigenetic programming

In order to fully appreciate the potential role and significance of epigenetic programming in determining and altering behaviour, it is critical to start deciphering the mechanisms leading from social behaviour to epigenetic change. How would LG-ABN result in distinct epigenetic changes in certain genes? We proposed above that transcription factors that respond to signalling pathways play a role in directing the chromatin and DNA methylation modifying enzymes to specific targets. Our working hypothesis was that maternal LG-ABN activated a signalling pathway, which led to delivery of a *cis*-acting transcription factor to the GR exon 1_7 promoter (Figure 3.10).

In vivo and *in vitro* studies suggest that maternal LG or postnatal handling, which increases maternal LG, increase GR gene expression in the offspring

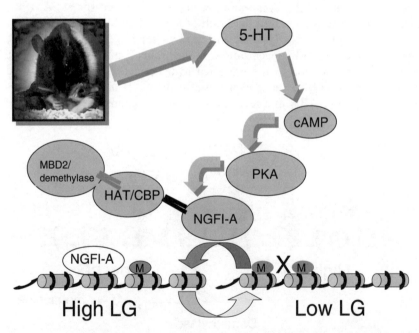

Figure 3.10 Behavioural gene programming by maternal care. The sequence of events leading from maternal licking and grooming behaviour to epigenetic programming of the GR exon 1_7 promoter. CBP = cAMP recognition element binding protein.

through a thyroid hormone-dependent increase in serotonin (5-HT) activity at 5-HT_7 receptors, and the subsequent activation of cyclic adenosine 3′, 5′-monophosphate (cAMP) and cAMP-dependent protein kinase A (PKA) (Laplante, Diorio, & Meaney, 2002; Meaney, Aitken, & Sapolsky, 1987; Meaney et al., 2000). Both the *in vitro* effects of 5-HT and the *in vivo* effects of maternal behaviour on GR mRNA expression are accompanied by increased hippocampal expression of NGFI-A transcription factor. The GR exon 1_7 promoter region contains a binding site for NGFI-A (McCormick et al., 2000). Interestingly, NGFI-A was previously shown to interact with the transcriptional co-activator and histone acetyltransferase CREB binding protein (CBP). Signalling pathways that result in increased cAMP also activate CBP. Recruitment of CBP to the GR exon 1_7 promoter in response to maternal care could explain the increased acetylation and demethylation observed in offspring of high LG-ABN. We therefore examined whether high maternal LG-ABN resulted in increased occupancy of the GR exon 1_7 promoter by NGFI-A in day 6 pups. Second, we tested the hypothesis that increased NGFI-A occupancy at the GR exon 1_7 promoter would result in recruitment of CBP and epigenetic reprogramming.

Maternal care results in increased recruitment of NGFI-A and CBP to the GR exon 17 promoter in the hippocampi of day 6 pups

To test whether NGFI-A engaged the GR exon 1_7 promoter in the hippocampus of day 6 embryos we performed a chromatin immunoprecipitation (ChIP) assay. In this assay the chromatin is fixed to the DNA by formaldehyde perfusion. This method conserves all the protein–chromatin–DNA interactions *in vivo* as they are at the moment of sacrifice. In order to look at interactions between a specific protein and a specific gene sequence, the fixed DNA–chromatin complex is immunoprecipitated with an antibody that recognizes the specific protein, and the specific gene sequence is amplified by polymerase chain reaction (PCR). We performed a ChIP analysis of CBP association, histone H3-K9 acetylation and NGFI-A protein binding to the exon 1_7 GR promoter in the native chromatin environment *in vivo* in intact hippocampi from day 6 offspring of High and Low LG mothers. The results indicated significantly greater binding of NGFI-A, increased CBP association and greater histone H3-K9 acetylation of the hippocampal exon 1_7 GR promoter in the neonatal offspring of High compared with Low LG mothers. Thus, maternal programming of the exon 1_7 GR promoter is associated with differences in NGFI-A binding, CBP association and histone H3-K9 acetylation in the neonatal offspring of High and Low LG mothers (Figure 3.10).

If indeed NGFI-A interaction with the GR exon 1_7 promoter in the hippocampi of the pups targets these genes for demethylation, then the copies of GR exon 1_7 promoter sequences, which are bound to NGFI-A in the hippocampi of day 6 pups, should be demethylated. We used a combination of ChIP and DNA methylation mapping to confirm that. The chromatin was first immunoprecipitated with an antibody directed against NGFI-A, the DNA bound to NGFI-A was purified and the state of methylation of the GR exon 1_7 promoter was deciphered by sodium bisulfite mapping. The 5′ and 3′ CpG dinucleotides within the NGFI-A response element on the exon 1_7 GR promoter bound to NGFI-A were found to be significantly unmethylated in comparison to the non-immunoprecipitated (i.e., sequences not bound to NGFI-A) "Input" DNA. These findings are consistent with the hypothesis that maternal LG-ABN results in increased targeting of NGFI-A to the GR exon 1_7 promoter and that this targeting leads to increased binding of CBP, increased acetylation and DNA demethylation (Weaver et al., 2007).

Increased binding of NGFI-A to the methylated GR exon 1_7 promoter in cell cultures leads to enhanced CBP binding, histone acetylation and demethylation

To test a causal link between NGFI-A binding and epigenetic reprogramming of the GR exon 1_7 promoter we resorted to cell culture experiments. We used the human cell line HEK 293 because these cells are readily transfected with foreign DNA and because it is not anticipated that they express neuron-specific factors. This model therefore enables studying the specific contribution of NGFI-A and other defined candidate proteins to demethylation. We also used a transient transfection assay in order to measure the immediate effects of NGFI-A on the state of methylation of the promoter and to avoid the possibility that DNA methylation will be lost passively through DNA replication in the absence of DNA methylation. The GR exon 1_7 promoter was introduced into a reporter vector that contained the cDNA encoding the firefly luciferase enzyme under its direction to report for the transcriptional activity of this promoter. The promoter was methylated with a CG-specific bacterial DNA methyltransferase *in vitro* to completion and thus all the CG dinucleotides in the plasmids were methylated. Note that the main dinucleotide sequence methylated in mammalian DNA is CG. The methylated reporter plasmid was then introduced into HEK 293 cells using the calcium-phosphate precipitation method in either the presence or absence of a vector expressing NGFI-A. The cells were harvested 72 hours after transfection. The transcriptional activity of the GR exon 1_7 promoter was determined by measuring luciferase activity. The interactions of NGFI-A and CBP and the state of histone acetylation of the transfected promoter were determined using ChIP assays. The state of methylation of GR exon 1_7 promoter was delineated by sodium bisulfite mapping.

Our results show that in cell culture DNA methylation causes a significant inhibition of GR exon 1_7 promoter–luciferase transcription activity, reduced NGFI-A binding, reduced CBP binding and reduced histone acetylation when transfected into HEK 293 cells, thus confirming that DNA methylation plays a causal role in the silencing of GR exon 1_7 promoter. Nevertheless, if an expression vector expressing high levels of NGFI-A is co-transfected with the methylated GR exon 1_7 promoter–luciferase, the transcription activity of the promoter is induced, there is an increased recruitment of NGFI-A to the promoter as expected, increased recruitment of CBP and increased histone acetylation and methylation mapping, indicating that the GR exon 1_7 promoter was demethylated. We suggest that the role that NGFI-A plays in regulation of the GR exon 1_7 promoter is bimodal. Under low concentrations of NGFI-A, binding to the target sequence is inhibited by DNA methylation. However, under conditions of high NGFI-A activity some NGFI-A interacts with the methylated GR exon 1_7 promoter, launching a cascade of events leading to demethylation of the promoter. Thus, increased activation of NGFI-A triggered by a repetitive and frequent behaviour such as maternal LG leads to binding of NGFI-A to the methylated promoter and recruitment of CBP. We proposed that the recruitment of CBP led to increased histone acetylation, which resulted in demethylation (Weaver et al., 2007). This sequence of events is consistent with our working hypothesis on the relationship between histone acetylation and DNA demethylation (Cervoni & Szyf, 2001; Cervoni et al., 2002). Thus we show that, similar to acetylation in response to pharmacological administration of TSA, targeted acetylation by recruitment of a transcription factor leads to demethylation of DNA (Weaver et al., 2007).

To demonstrate that NGFI-A physical interaction with the GR exon 1_7 promoter rather than an indirect effect of NGFI-A expression through other targets is required for reprogramming of GR exon 1_7 promoter, we resorted to site-directed mutagenesis. We showed that mutation of the 3′-CG of the NGFI-A recognition element to AG abolished NGFI-A binding to its recognition element *in vitro* and in living cells. When a 3′-mutated GR exon 1_7 promoter was methylated and transfected into HEK 293 cells with NGFI-A, no transcriptional activation, CBP binding, histone acetylation or demethylation of the GR exon 1_7 promoter was observed, demonstrating that physical interaction between NGFI-A and the methylated GR exon 17 promoter is required for epigenetic reprogramming (Weaver et al., 2007).

In summary, our studies establish a first working hypothesis on how maternal behaviour can result in an epigenetic reprogramming in the offspring. Neurotransmitter release results in activation of a signalling pathway that leads to recruitment of particular transcription factors such as NGFI-A to their recognition elements in front of specific genes. The transcription factors recruit histone acetyltransferases, which in turn reprogramme the chromatin and facilitate demethylation.

MBD2 targets demethylation to the GR exon 1_7 promoter in concert with NGFI-A

The data discussed in the previous section provides a molecular link between maternal LG-ABN and histone acetylation of the GR exon 1_7 promoter. Histone acetylation was shown before to target demethylation (Cervoni &

Szyf, 2001) and we proposed that histone acetylation facilitated the accessibility of a demethylase to the target sequence. The remaining question was to identify the protein(s) involved in demethylation of DNA. Some of us have previously proposed that the methylated DNA binding protein 2 (MBD2) was a DNA demethylase that could bring about DNA demethylation *in vitro* (Bhattacharya et al., 1999). Other groups (Ng et al., 1999) hotly contested the *in vitro* demethylation activity of MBD2 but more recent data from our laboratory supported a demethylation role for MBD2 (Detich, Theberge, & Szyf, 2002; Detich et al., 2003a). We therefore tested the hypothesis that MBD2 mediated the demethylation of GR exon 1_7 promoter. We first tested whether MBD2 interacted with the GR exon 1_7 promoter in the hippocampi of day 6 pups. Our results indicate that MBD2 binds the GR exon 1_7 promoter in the hippocampi of day 6 pups and that this binding is increased with high maternal LG-ABN. We also showed, using a combination of ChIP with an anti-MBD2 antibody and bisulfite mapping of DNA methylation, that the GR exon 1_7 promoter molecules bound to MBD2 were unmethylated in comparison with the total DNA. This supports the hypothesis that MBD2 mediates demethylation in response to maternal LG-ABN (Figure 3.10). Using a transient transfection assay similar to the one described in the previous section we show that ectopically expressed MBD2 transcriptionally activates *in vitro* methylated GR exon 1_7 promoter–luciferase promoter, increases the interaction of CBP and increases histone acetylation. A combination of ChIP and bisulfite mapping of DNA methylation indicated that MBD2-bound GR exon 1_7 promoter molecules were demethylated at a CG site found in the NGFI-A recognition element. We then determined whether binding of NGFI-A was required for demethylation, as predicted by our hypothesis discussed in the above section. We first showed that co-expressing NGFI-A and MBD2 enhances the binding of MBD2 to GR exon 1_7 promoter. We then showed that binding of NGFI-A to its response element was required for MBD2 action since a mutation that abolished NGFI-A binding also prevented MBD2 binding, activation of gene expression and demethylation. Finally if NGFI-A targeted the GR exon 1_7 promoter for MBD2 binding, as predicted by our hypothesis, then both proteins should be bound to the same promoter molecules. Using a double ChIP approach, which involves immunoprecipitation sequentially with both NGFI-A and MBD2 antibodies, we show that both proteins simultaneously bind the same GR exon 1_7 promoter molecule (Weaver et al., unpublished data).

In summary, our data shows a causal relationship between MBD2 binding, demethylation and activation of GR exon 1_7 promoter and is consistent with the hypothesis that binding of NGFI-A facilitates the interaction of MBD2 with its target. Our hypothesis is that NGFI-A facilitates MBD2 interaction through recruitment of CBP and that the ensuing increased acetylation of the GR exon 1_7 promoter opens up the chromatin configuration, thus increasing the accessibility of the sequence to MBD2 (Figure 3.10). As discussed in the introduction of this chapter, we propose that the gene specificity of epigenetic programming by DNA methylation–demethylation as well as histone acetylation–deacetylation is defined by sequence-specific factors that reside downstream of the signal transduction pathways (Figures 3.6 and 3.10).

Epigenetic programming and human aggression

Specific challenges for studying epigenetic programming of human behaviour

A fundamental question that remains to be answered is whether a mechanism similar to the mechanism described in the rat operates in generating inter-individual differences in human behaviour (Figure 3.11). The hypothesis is obviously attractive; social adversity in early childhood similar to low LG-ABN might result in aberrant epigenetic programming causing changes in gene expression, which will stably impact on behaviour later in life. Similarly, strong environmental exposures later in life might reverse or alter epigenetic programming of genes regulating human behaviour. The main impediment in studying epigenetic programming in living humans is obviously the inaccessibility of the brain to epigenetic analysis. The critical question is whether epigenetic alterations that are relevant to human behaviour occur in peripheral tissue. The best candidates are probably white blood cells. Cytokines secreted by different types of blood cells were shown to interact with receptors in the CNS, and crosstalk between the immune system and the brain has been proposed for some time to play a role in human behaviours such as the stress response. For example, the cytokine IL-1β is expressed in peripheral blood cells, but receptors for IL-1β are present in the brain (Takao, Tracey, Mitchell, & De Souza, 1990; Takao, Culp, Newton, & De Souza, 1992; Takao, Culp, & De Souza, 1993). IL-1β was proposed to interact with the HPA axis activities and thus it stands to reason that differences in IL-1β might have an impact on stress responsivity as well as other behaviours. Notably, several cytokines were previously shown to be regulated by DNA methylation (Bruniquel & Schwartz, 2003; Falek, Ben-Sasson, & Ariel, 2000;

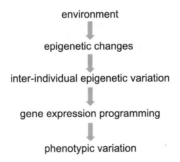

Figure 3.11 A scheme for environmentally driven epigenetic states, inter-individual phenotypic variance in behaviour and susceptibility to disease in humans.

Fitzpatrick, Shirley, & Kelso, 1999; Northrop, Thomas, Wells, & Shen, 2006; Reid, Merigan, & Basham, 1992) and expression of IL-1β was induced by treatment of human monocyte cell lines with the DNA methylation inhibitor 5-azacytidine (Kovacs, Oppenheim, Carter, & Young, 1987). However, although these candidate genes are interesting, a non-biased approach might identify other unanticipated candidates. Thus, whole epigenome analyses should enable the identification of hitherto unknown epigenetic markers of human behaviour patterns. The question of whether there are markers of epigenetic alteration in peripheral tissues is obviously of utmost importance for the progress of the study of epigenetics in human behaviour.

Trajectories of human aggression

Four trajectories of development of human aggression were previously char-acterized: a chronic problem trajectory, a high-level near-desister trajectory, a moderate-level desister trajectory and a no-problem trajectory (Nagin & Tremblay, 1999). Previous studies have suggested a strong environmental effect in the development of these trajectories, implicating a possible epigenetic component mediating these effects; the high physical aggression trajectory group were more likely to be boys, from low income families, from families where the mother had not completed high school and who reported using hostile/ineffective parenting strategies (Côté, Vaillancourt, LeBlanc, Nagin, & Tremblay, 2006). We asked the question of whether these different tra-jectories were associated with different DNA methylation patterns in IL-1β and rRNA genes. We also looked at the genes encoding ribosomal RNA (rRNA). rRNA is a basic building block of the ribosome, the protein syn-thesis machinery of the cell. The human genome contains a few hundred copies of the genes encoding rRNA, but only a fraction of these genes are active. The fraction of the rRNA genes that are expressed in a cell at a given point in time determines the overall protein synthesis capacity of the cell. DNA methylation of rRNA genes determines which fraction of rRNA gene copies would be expressed (Brown & Szyf, 2007; Chen & Pikaard, 1997; Santoro & Grummt, 2001; Swisshelm, Disteche, Thorvaldsen, Nelson, & Salk, 1990). Thus, differences in methylation of rRNA genes would predict differences in the capacity to launch protein synthesis effort in response to immediate challenges, which requires extensive DNA synthesis. We therefore determined whether differences in aggression trajectories are associated with a change in methylation of rRNA genes.

It was unknown whether any potential differences in DNA methylation between the aggression trajectories would be limited to a specific cell type or whether they would be detectable in whole blood. We therefore isolated whole blood as well as T cells, B cells and monocytes. DNA was prepared from the cells from eight subjects per trajectory. All subjects were 27 years of age to rule out age-related differences in DNA methylation. DNA was subjected to sodium bisulfite treatment and PCR amplification of the converted DNA with either rRNA- or IL-β-specific primers. This method converts all the unmethylated cytosines to uridines, which upon amplification are converted to thymidines, whereas methylated cytosines are unconverted. Thus, a sequence difference is generated between methylated cytosines and unmethylated cytosines that could be determined by standard sequencing techniques. Ten to fifteen clones were sequenced per subject. Our preliminary data indicate the emergence of a difference in methylation of both rRNA genes and IL-β between the chronic aggressive trajectory and the high desisters, a trajectory showing reduced aggression with age (Figure 3.12). There is a trend for higher methylation in both genes in the subjects from the chronic trajectory. It is still early to define the significance of these differences and more subjects need to be studied and analysed. Additional random trials need to be performed to validate these methylation events as biomarkers of aggression. In addition, if these differences in methylation are found to be true, future mechanistic studies need to be performed to determine the biological significance of these differences. It is critical to determine whether the changes in methylation reflect variations in expression of the cytokine IL-1β and whether DNA methylation plays a causal role in the putative changes in expression. Once this is validated, it will be important to determine the link between the differences in cytokine expression and the behavioural pathology. Establishing such a link between the immune system and aggressive behaviour has obvious implications beyond the study of aggressive behaviour.

Summary

Recent data from the rat maternal-care model charts a pathway leading from the behaviour of the mother to long-term programming of gene expression in the offspring. This pathway involves the firing of neurotransmitter receptors in response to the behaviour, signalling pathways that activate sequence-specific transcription factors such as NGFI-A. NGFI-A interacts with its recognition element in the GR exon 1_7 promoter and recruits the histone acetyltransferase CBP to the gene. This results in acetylation of chromatin and recruitment of DNA demethylases such as MBD2 leading to demethylation and stable activation of this gene. These data point to a thought-provoking notion that epigenetic processes play a role in shaping human behaviour in response to different levels of social adversity early in life and later during adulthood. Preliminary data examining a few genes suggests that differences in epigenetic programming do exist between individuals, and that these variations might associate with different trajectories of aggressive behaviours. The rapid development of high-throughput sequencing techniques will enable, in the future, the unbiased mapping of epigenomes and identification of candidate genes that exhibit epigenetic differences among individuals. The possibility that epigenetic mechanisms might be playing a role in generating inter-individual differences in behaviour has tremendous potential in providing mechanisms for the age-old question of the relationship of nurture and nature. Moreover

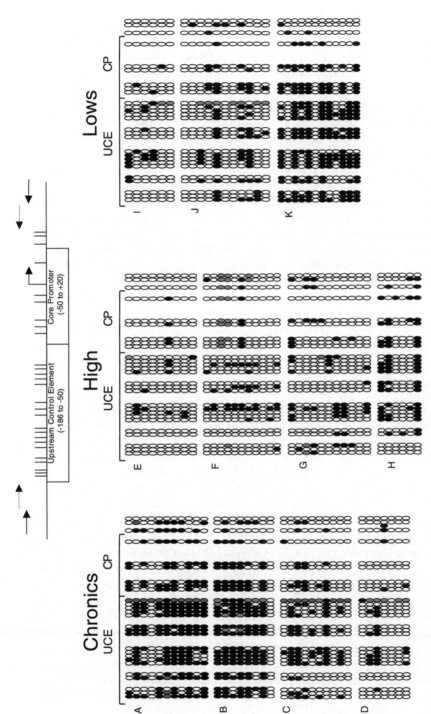

Figure 3.12 Bisulfite analysis of rRNA promoters in DNA from total blood in subjects from different groups of aggressive behaviour (chronic problem trajectory, high level near-desister trajectory and low aggression trajectory). Each line is a different clone and each circle indicates a CG site. A dark circle indicates methylation.

this approach carries additional promise for improving our ability to understand, predict and treat behavioural abnormalities.

Note

1 These studies were supported by a grant from the Canadian Institutes for Health
   Research (CIHR) to MJM and MS and from the National Cancer Institute of
   Canada to MS. MJM is supported by a CIHR Senior Scientist award and the project
   was supported by a Distinguished Investigator Award to MJM from the National
   Alliance for Research on Schizophrenia and Affective Disorders (NARSAD).

References

Barreto, G., Schafer, A., Marhold, J., Stach, D., Swaminathan, S. K., Handa, V., et al.
   (2007). Gadd45a promotes epigenetic gene activation by repair-mediated DNA
   demethylation. *Nature, 445*, 671–675.

Baylin, S. B., Esteller, M., Rountree, M. R., Bachman, K. E., Schuebel, K., & Herman,
   J. G. (2001). Aberrant patterns of DNA methylation, chromatin formation and
   gene expression in cancer. *Human Molecular Genetics, 10*, 687–692.

Beck, S., Olek, A., & Walter, J. (1999). From genomics to epigenomics: A loftier view
   of life. *Nature Biotechnology, 17*, 1144.

Bergmann, A., & Lane, M. E. (2003). Hidden targets of microRNAs for growth
   control. *Trends in Biochemical Science, 28*, 461–463.

Bhattacharya, S. K., Ramchandani, S., Cervoni, N., & Szyf, M. (1999). A mammalian
   protein with specific demethylase activity for mCpG DNA [see comments]. *Nature,
   397*, 579–583.

Bourc'his, D., Xu, G. L., Lin, C. S., Bollman, B., & Bestor, T. H. (2001). Dnmt3L and
   the establishment of maternal genomic imprints. *Science, 294*, 2536–2539.

Brown, S. E., & Szyf, M. (2007). Epigenetic programming of the rRNA promoter by
   MBD3. *Molecular and Cellular Biology, 27*, 4938–4952.

Bruniquel, D., & Schwartz, R. H. (2003). Selective, stable demethylation of the
   interleukin-2 gene enhances transcription by an active process. *Nature Immunology,
   4*, 235–240.

Bultman, S. J., Gebuhr, T. C., & Magnuson, T. (2005). A Brg1 mutation that uncouples
   ATPase activity from chromatin remodeling reveals an essential role for SWI/SNF-
   related complexes in beta-globin expression and erythroid development. *Genes and
   Development, 19*, 2849–2861.

Caspi, A., Sugden, K., Moffitt, T. E., Taylor, A., Craig, I. W., Harrington, H., et al.
   (2003). Influence of life stress on depression: Moderation by a polymorphism in
   the 5-HTT gene. *Science, 301*, 386–389.

Cervoni, N., Detich, N., Seo, S. B., Chakravarti, D., & Szyf, M. (2002). The oncopro-
   tein Set/TAF-1beta, an inhibitor of histone acetyltransferase, inhibits active
   demethylation of DNA, integrating DNA methylation and transcriptional silencing. *Journal of Biological Chemistry, 277*, 25026–25031.

Cervoni, N., & Szyf, M. (2001). Demethy lase activity is directed by histone acetylation. *Journal of Biological Chemistry, 276*, 40778–40787.

Chen, Z. J., & Pikaard, C. S. (1997). Epigenetic silencing of RNA polymerase I
   transcription: A role for DNA methylation and histone modification in nucleolar
   dominance. *Genes and Development, 11*, 2124–2136.

Cheng, X., Kumar, S., Posfai, J., Pflugrath, J. W., & Roberts, R. J. (1993). Crystal structure of the HhaI DNA methyltransferase complexed with S-adenosyl-L-methionine. *Cell, 74*, 299–307.

Comb, M., & Goodman, H. M. (1990). CpG methylation inhibits proenkephalin gene expression and binding of the transcription factor AP-2. *Nucleic Acids Research, 18*, 3975–3982.

Côté, S. M., Vaillancourt, T., LeBlanc, J. C., Nagin, D. S., & Tremblay, R. E. (2006). The development of physical aggression from toddlerhood to pre-adolescence: A nation wide longitudinal study of Canadian children. *Journal of Abnormal Child Psychology, 34*, 71–85.

D'Alessio, A. C., & Szyf, M. (2006). Epigenetic tete-a-tete: The bilateral relationship between chromatin modifications and DNA methylation. *Biochemistry and Cell Biology, 84*, 463–476.

Detich, N., Bovenzi, V., & Szyf, M. (2003b). Valproate induces replication-independent active DNA demethylation. *Journal of Biological Chemistry, 278*, 27586–27592.

Detich, N., Hamm, S., Just, G., Knox, J. D., & Szyf, M. (2003a). The methyl donor S-adenosylmethionine inhibits active demethylation of DNA: A candidate novel mechanism for the pharmacological effects of S-adenosylmethionine. *Journal of Biological Chemistry, 278*, 20812–20820.

Detich, N., Theberge, J., & Szyf, M. (2002). Promoter-specific activation and demethylation by MBD2/demethylase. *Journal of Biological Chemistry, 277*, 35791–35794.

Di Croce, L., Raker, V. A., Corsaro, M., Fazi, F., Fanelli, M., et al. (2002). Methyltransferase recruitment and DNA hypermethylation of target promoters by an oncogenic transcription factor. *Science, 295*, 1079–1082.

Eckhardt, F., Lewin, J., Cortese, R., Rakyan, V. K., Attwood, J., Burger, M., et al. (2006). DNA methylation profiling of human chromosomes 6, 20 and 22. *Nature Genetics, 38*, 1378–1385.

Falek, P. R., Ben-Sasson, S. Z., & Ariel, M. (2000). Correlation between DNA methylation and murine IFN-gamma and IL-4 expression. *Cytokine, 12*, 198–206.

Finch, J. T., Lutter, L. C., Rhodes, D., Brown, R. S., Rushton, B., Levitt, M., & Klug, A. (1977). Structure of nucleosome core particles of chromatin. *Nature, 269*, 29–36.

Fitzpatrick, D. R., Shirley, K. M., & Kelso, A. (1999). Cutting edge: Stable epigenetic inheritance of regional IFN-gamma promoter demethylation in CD44highCD8+ T lymphocytes. *Journal of Immunology, 162*, 5053–5057.

Francis, D., Diorio, J., Liu, D., & Meaney, M. J. (1999). Nongenomic transmission across generations of maternal behavior and stress responses in the rat. *Science, 286*, 1155–1158.

Fujita, N., Takebayashi, S., Okumura, K., Kudo, S., Chiba, T., Saya, H., & Nakao, M. (1999). Methylation-mediated transcriptional silencing in euchromatin by methyl-CpG binding protein MBD1 isoforms. *Molecular and Cellular Biology, 19*, 6415–6426.

Fuks, F., Burgers, W. A., Brehm, A., Hughes-Davies, L., & Kouzarides, T. (2000). DNA methyltransferase Dnmt1 associates with histone deacetylase activity. *Nature Genetics, 24*, 88–91.

Fuks, F., Hurd, P. J., Wolf, D., Nan, X., Bird, A. P., & Kouzarides, T. (2003). The methyl-CpG-binding protein MeCP2 links DNA methylation to histone methylation. *Journal of Biological Chemistry, 278*, 4035–4040.

Gillespie, N. A., Whitfield, J. B., Williams, B., Heath, A. C., & Martin, N. G. (2005).

The relationship between stressful life events, the serotonin transporter (5-HTTLPR) genotype and major depression. *Psychological Medicine, 35*, 101–111.

Gonzalez-Zulueta, M., Bender, C. M., Yang, A. S, Nguyen, T., Beart, R. W., Van Tornout, J. M., & Jones, P. A. (1995). Methylation of the 5′ CpG island of the p16/CDKN2 tumor suppressor gene in normal and transformed human tissues correlates with gene silencing. *Cancer Research, 55*, 4531–4535.

Goto, K., Numata, M., Komura, J. I., Ono, T., Bestor, T. H., & Kondo, H. (1994). Expression of DNA methyltransferase gene in mature and immature neurons as well as proliferating cells in mice. *Differentiation, 56*, 39–44.

Groudine, M., Eisenman, R., Gelinas, R., & Weintraub, H. (1983). Developmental aspects of chromatin structure and gene expression. *Progress in Clinical Biological Research, 134*, 159–182.

Grunstein, M. (1997). Histone acetylation in chromatin structure and transcription. *Nature, 389*, 349–352.

Hendrich, B., & Bird, A. (1998). Identification and characterization of a family of mammalian methyl-CpG binding proteins. *Molecular and Cellular Biology, 18*, 6538–6547.

Henikoff, S., McKittrick, E., & Ahmad, K. (2004). Epigenetics, histone H3 variants, and the inheritance of chromatin states. *Cold Spring Harbor Symposia on Quantitative Biology, 69*, 235–243.

Inamdar, N. M., Ehrlich, K. C, & Ehrlich, M. (1991). CpG methylation inhibits binding of several sequence-specific DNA-binding proteins from pea, wheat, soybean and cauliflower. *Plant and Molecular Biology, 17*, 111–123.

Jackson, J. P., Lindroth, A. M., Cao, X., & Jacobsen, S. E. (2002). Control of CpNpG DNA methylation by the KRYPTONITE histone H3 methyltransferase. *Nature, 416*, 556–560.

Jenuwein, T. (2001). Re-SET-ting heterochromatin by histone methyltransferases. *Trends in Cell Biology, 11*, 266–273.

Jenuwein, T., & Allis, C. D. (2001). Translating the histone code. *Science, 293*, 1074–1080.

Jost, J. P. (1993). Nuclear extracts of chicken embryos promote an active demethylation of DNA by excision repair of 5-methyldeoxycytidine. *Proceedings of the National Academy of Sciences of the USA, 90*, 4684–4688.

Kersh, E. N., Fitzpatrick, D. R., Murali-Krishna, K., Shires, J., Speck, S. H., Boss, J. M., & Ahmed, R. (2006). Rapid demethylation of the IFN-{gamma} gene occurs in memory but not naive CD8 T cells. *Journal of Immunology, 176*, 4083–4093.

Kovacs, E. J., Oppenheim, J. J., Carter, D. B., & Young, H. A. (1987). Enhanced interleukin-1 production by human monocyte cell lines following treatment with 5-azacytidine. *Journal of Leukocyte Biology, 41*, 40–46.

Kramer, O. H., Gottlicher, M., & Heinzel, T. (2001). Histone deacetylase as a therapeutic target. *Trends in Endocrinology and Metabolism, 12*, 294–300.

Kuo, M. H., & Allis, C. D. (1998). Roles of histone acetyltransferases and deacetylases in gene regulation. *Bioessays, 20*, 615–626.

Lachner, M., O'Carroll, D., Rea, S., Mechtler, K., & Jenuwein, T. (2001). Methylation of histone H3 lysine 9 creates a binding site for HP1 proteins. *Nature, 410*, 116–120.

Laplante, P., Diorio, J., & Meaney, M. J. (2002). Serotonin regulates hippocampal glucocorticoid receptor expression via a 5-HT7 receptor. *Brain Research and Developmental Brain Research, 139*, 199–203.

Lee, D. Y., Hayes, J. J., Pruss, D., & Wolffe, A. P. (1993). A positive role for histone acetylation in transcription factor access to nucleosomal DNA. *Cell*, *72*, 73–84.

Li, E., Bestor, T. H., & Jaenisch, R. (1992). Targeted mutation of the DNA methyltransferase gene results in embryonic lethality. *Cell*, *69*, 915–926.

Lichtenstein, M., Keini, G., Cedar, H., & Bergman, Y. (1994). B cell-specific demethylation: a novel role for the intronic kappa chain enhancer sequence. *Cell*, *76*, 913–923.

Liu, D., Diorio, J., Tannenbaum, B., Caldji, C., Francis, D., Freedman, A., et al. (1997). Maternal care, hippocampal glucocorticoid receptors, and hypothalamic-pituitary-adrenal responses to stress. *Science*, *277*, 1659–1662.

Lucarelli, M., Fuso, A., Strom, R., & Scarpa, S. (2001). The dynamics of myogenin site-specific demethylation is strongly correlated with its expression and with muscle differentiation. *Journal of Biological Chemistry*, *276*, 7500–7506.

Marks, P. A., Sheffery, M., & Rifkind, R. A. (1985). Modulation of gene expression during terminal cell differentiation. *Progress in Clinical Biological Research*, *191*, 185–203.

McCormick, J. A., Lyons, V., Jacobson, M. D., Noble, J., Diorio, J., Nyirenda, M., et al. (2000). 5'-Heterogeneity of glucocorticoid receptor messenger RNA is tissue specific: Differential regulation of variant transcripts by early-life events. *Molecular Endocrinology*, *14*, 506–517.

Meaney, M. J., Aitken, D. H., & Sapolsky, R. M. (1987). Thyroid hormones influence the development of hippocampal glucocorticoid receptors in the rat: A mechanism for the effects of postnatal handling on the development of the adrenocortical stress response. *Neuroendocrinology*, *45*, 278–283.

Meaney, M. J., Diorio, J., Francis, D., Weaver, S., Yau, J., Chapman, K., & Seckl, J. R. (2000). Postnatal handling increases the expression of cAMP-inducible transcription factors in the rat hippocampus: The effects of thyroid hormones and serotonin. *Journal of Neuroscience*, *20*, 3926–3935.

Meaney, M. J., & Szyf, M. (2005). Maternal care as a model for experience-dependent chromatin plasticity? *Trends in Neuroscience*, *28*, 456–463.

Milutinovic, S., D'Alessio, A. C., Detich, N., & Szyf, M. (2006). Valproate induces widespread epigenetic reprogramming which involves demethylation of specific genes. *Carcinogenesis*, *28*, 560–571.

Momparler, R. L. (2005). Epigenetic therapy of cancer with 5-aza-2'-deoxycytidine (decitabine). *Seminars in Oncology*, *32*, 443–451.

Nagin, D., & Tremblay, R. E. (1999). Trajectories of boys' physical aggression, opposition, and hyperactivity on the path to physically violent and nonviolent juvenile delinquency. *Child Development*, *70*, 1181–1196.

Nan, X., Campoy, F. J., & Bird, A. (1997). MeCP2 is a transcriptional repressor with abundant binding sites in genomic chromatin. *Cell*, *88*, 471–481.

Neel, J. V., & Falls, H. F. (1951). The rate of mutation of the gene responsible for retinoblastoma in man. *Science*, *114*, 419–422.

Ng, H. H., Zhang, Y., Hendrich, B., Johnson, C. A., Turner, B. M., Erdjument-Bromage, H., et al. (1999). MBD2 is a transcriptional repressor belonging to the MeCP1 histone deacetylase complex. *Nature Genetics*, *23*, 58–61.

Northrop, J. K., Thomas, R. M., Wells, A. D., & Shen, H. (2006). Epigenetic remodeling of the IL-2 and IFN-gamma loci in memory CD8 T cells is influenced by CD4 T cells. *Journal of Immunology*, *177*, 1062–1069.

Ogryzko, V. V., Schiltz, R. L., Russanova, V., Howard, B. H., & Nakatani, Y. (1996).

The transcriptional coactivators p300 and CBP are histone acetyltransferases. *Cell*, *87*, 953–959.

Okano, M., Bell, D. W., Haber, D. A., & Li, E. (1999). DNA methyltransferases DNMT3a and DNMT3b are essential for de novo methylation and mammalian development. *Cell*, *99*, 247–257.

Okano, M., Xie, S., & Li, E. (1998). Cloning and characterization of a family of novel mammalian DNA (cytosine-5) methyltransferases [letter]. *Nature Genetics*, *19*, 219–220.

Perry, M., & Chalkley, R. (1982). Histone acetylation increases the solubility of chromatin and occurs sequentially over most of the chromatin. A novel model for the biological role of histone acetylation. *Journal of Biological Chemistry*, *257*, 7336–7347.

Ramain, P., Bourouis, M., Dretzen, G., Richards, G., Sobkowiak, A., & Bellard, M. (1986). Changes in the chromatin structure of Drosophila glue genes accompany developmental cessation of transcription in wild type and transformed strains. *Cell*, *45*, 545–553.

Ramchandani, S., Bhattacharya, S. K., Cervoni, N., & Szyf, M. (1999). DNA methylation is a reversible biological signal. *Proceedings of the National Academy of Sciences of the USA*, *96*, 6107–6112.

Razin, A. (1998). CpG methylation, chromatin structure and gene silencing-a three-way connection. *EMBO Journal*, *17*, 4905–4908.

Razin, A., & Cedar, H. (1977). Distribution of 5-methylcytosine in chromatin. *Proceedings of the National Academy of Sciences of the USA*, *74*, 2725–2728.

Razin, A., & Riggs, A. D. (1980). DNA methylation and gene function. *Science*, *210*, 604–610.

Razin, A., & Szyf, M. (1984). DNA methylation patterns. Formation and function. *Biochimica et Biophysica Acta*, *782*, 331–342.

Reid, T. R., Merigan, T. C., & Basham, T. Y. (1992). Resistance to interferon-alpha in a mouse B-Cell lymphoma involves DNA methylation. *Journal of Interferon Research*, *12*, 131–137.

Rountree, M. R., Bachman, K. E., & Baylin, S. B. (2000). DNMT1 binds HDAC2 and a new co-repressor, DMAP1, to form a complex at replication foci. *Nature Genetics*, *25*, 269–277.

Santoro, R., & Grummt, I. (2001). Molecular mechanisms mediating methylation-dependent silencing of ribosomal gene transcription. *Molecular Cell*, *8*, 719–725.

Sarma, K., & Reinberg, D. (2005). Histone variants meet their match. *Nature Reviews in Molecular Cell Biology*, *6*, 139–149.

Shi, Y., Lan, F., Matson, C., Mulligan, P., Whetstine, J. R., Cole, P. A., et al. (2004). Histone demethylation mediated by the nuclear amine oxidase homolog LSD1. *Cell*, *119*, 941–953.

Shilatifard, A. (2006). Chromatin modifications by methylation and ubiquitination: Implications in the regulation of gene expression. *Annual Review of Biochemistry*, *75*, 243–269.

Simonini, M. V., Camargo, L. M., Dong, E., Maloku, E., Veldic, M., Costa, E., & Guidotti, A. (2006). The benzamide MS-275 is a potent, long-lasting brain region-selective inhibitor of histone deacetylases. *Proceedings of the National Academy of Sciences of the USA*, *103*, 1587–1592.

Sparkes, R. S., Murphree, A. L., Lingua, R. W., Sparkes, M. C., Field, L. L., Funderburk, S. J., & Benedict, W. F. (1983). Gene for hereditary retinoblastoma assigned to human chromosome 13 by linkage to esterase D. *Science, 219,* 971–973.

Swisshelm, K., Disteche, C. M., Thorvaldsen, J., Nelson, A., & Salk, D. (1990). Age-related increase in methylation of ribosomal genes and inactivation of chromosome-specific rRNA gene clusters in mouse. *Mutation Research, 237,* 131–146.

Szyf, M. (1994). DNA methylation properties: consequences for pharmacology. *Trends in Pharmacological Science, 15,* 233–238.

Szyf, M. (2001). Towards a pharmacology of DNA methylation. *Trends in Pharmacological Science, 22,* 350–354.

Takao, T., Culp, S. G., Newton, R. C., & De Souza, E. B. (1992). Type I interleukin-1 receptors in the mouse brain-endocrine-immune axis labelled with [125I]recombinant human interleukin-1 receptor antagonist. *Journal of Neuroimmunology, 41,* 51–60.

Takao, T., Culp, S. G., & De Souza, E. B. (1993). Reciprocal modulation of interleukin-1 beta (IL-1 beta) and IL-1 receptors by lipopolysaccharide (endotoxin) treatment in the mouse brain-endocrine-immune axis. *Endocrinology, 132,* 1497–1504.

Takao, T., Tracey, D. E., Mitchell, W. M., & De Souza, E. B. (1990). Interleukin-1 receptors in mouse brain: characterization and neuronal localization. *Endocrinology, 127,* 3070–3078.

Tremolizzo, L., Carboni, G., Ruzicka, W. B., Mitchell, C. P., Sugaya, I., Tueting, P., et al. (2002). An epigenetic mouse model for molecular and behavioral neuropathologies related to schizophrenia vulnerability. *Proceedings of the National Academy of Sciences of the USA, 99,* 17095–17100.

Tsukada, Y., Fang, J., Erdjument-Bromage, H., Warren, M. E., Borchers C. H., Tempst, P., & Zhang, Y. (2006). Histone demethylation by a family of JmjC domain-containing proteins. *Nature, 439,* 811–816.

Varga-Weisz, P. D., & Becker, P. B. (2006). Regulation of higher-order chromatin structures by nucleosome-remodelling factors. *Current Opinion in Genetics and Development, 16,* 151–156.

Veldic, M., Guidotti, A., Maloku, E., Davis, J. M., & Costa, E. (2005). In psychosis, cortical interneurons overexpress DNA-methyltransferase 1. *Proceedings of the National Academy of Sciences of the USA, 102,* 2152–2157.

Vilain, A., Apiou, F., Dutrillaux, B., & Malfoy, B. (1998). Assignment of candidate DNA methyltransferase gene (DNMT2) to human chromosome band 10p15.1 by in situ hybridization. *Cytogenetics and Cell Genetics, 82,* 120.

Vire, E., Brenner, C., Deplus, R., Blanchon, L., Fraga, M., Didelot, C., et al. (2005). The Polycomb group protein EZH2 directly controls DNA methylation. *Nature, 439,* 871–874.

Vo, N., Klein, M. E., Varlamova, O., Keller, D. M., Yamamoto, T., Goodman, R. H., & Impey, S. (2005). A cAMP-response element binding protein-induced microRNA regulates neuronal morphogenesis. *Proceedings of the National Academy of Sciences of the USA, 102,* 16426–16431.

Wade, P. A., Pruss, D., & Wolffe, A. P. (1997). Histone acetylation: chromatin in action. *Trends in Biochemical Science, 22,* 128–132.

Weaver, I. C., Cervoni, N., Champagne, F. A., D'Alessio, A. C., Sharma, S., Seckl, J. R., et al. (2004a). Epigenetic programming by maternal behavior. *Nature Neuroscience, 7,* 847–854.

Weaver, I. C., Champagne, F. A., Brown, S. E., Dymov, S., Sharma, S., Meaney, M. J., & Szyf, M. (2005). Reversal of maternal programming of stress responses in adult offspring through methyl supplementation: altering epigenetic marking later in life. *Journal of Neuroscience, 25*, 11045–11054.

Weaver, I. C., D'Alessio, A. C., Brown, S. E., Hellstrom, I. C., Dymov, S., Sharma, S., et al. (2007). The transcription factor nerve growth factor-inducible protein a mediates epigenetic programming: Altering epigenetic marks by immediate-early genes. *Journal of Neuroscience, 27*, 1756–1768.

Weaver, I. C., Diorio, J., Seckl, J. R., Szyf, M., & Meaney, M. J. (2004b). Early environmental regulation of hippocampal glucocorticoid receptor gene expression: Characterization of intracellular mediators and potential genomic target sites. *Annals of the New York Academy of Sciences, 1024*, 182–212.

Weaver, I. C., Meaney, M. J., & Szyf, M. (2006). Maternal care effects on the hippocampal transcriptome and anxiety-mediated behaviors in the offspring that are reversible in adulthood. *Proceedings of the National Academy of Sciences of the USA, 103*, 3480–3485.

Weidle, U. H., & Grossmann, A. (2000). Inhibition of histone deacetylases: A new strategy to target epigenetic modifications for anticancer treatment. *Anticancer Research, 20*, 1471–1485.

Wolffe, A. P. (1996). Histone deacetylase: a regulator of transcription. *Science, 272*, 371–372.

Yoshida, M., Kijima, M., Akita, M., & Beppu, T. (1990). Potent and specific inhibition of mammalian histone deacetylase both in vivo and in vitro by trichostatin A. *Journal Biological Chemistry, 265*, 17174–17179.

Zhang, B., Pan, X., Cobb, G. P., & Anderson, T. A. (2007). microRNAs as oncogenes and tumor suppressors. *Developmental Biology, 302*, 1–12.

Zhu, B., Zheng, Y., Hess, D., Angliker, H., Schwarz, S., Siegmann, M., et al. (2000). 5-Methylcytosine-DNA glycosylase activity is present in a cloned G/T mismatch DNA glycosylase associated with the chicken embryo DNA demethylation complex. *Proceedings of the National Academy of Sciences of the USA, 97*, 5135–5139.

4 Maternal smoking, genes and adolescent brain and body
The Saguenay Youth Study

T. Paus, Z. Pausova, M. Abrahamowicz,
J. Almerigi, N. Arbour, M. Bernard, D. Gaudet,
P. Hanzalek, P. Hamet, A. C. Evans, M. Kramer,
L. Laberge, S. Leal, G. Leonard, J. Lerner,
R. M. Lerner, J. Mathieu, M. Perron, B. Pike,
A. Pitiot, L. Richer, J. R. Séguin, C. Syme,
R. E. Tremblay, S. Veillette and K. Watkins

Background

Prevalence of maternal cigarette smoking during pregnancy

The prevalence of cigarette smoking in pregnant women varies widely in different countries (Ebrahim, Decoufle, & Palakathodi, 2000; Kendrick & Merritt, 1996). In the United States, for example, the average prevalence was 16.3% in 1984 and decreased to 11.8% in 1994 (Ebrahim, Decoufle, & Palakthodi, 2000). In England, maternal smoking during pregnancy is less common (10%, The Stationery Office, 2002). In Canada, 25% of women aged 15 years and above are current smokers; of these, 58% smoked during their most recent pregnancy (Health Canada, 1995). In the National Longitudinal Study of Children and Youth (Canada), 23.7% of mothers reported smoking cigarettes during pregnancy (Connor & McIntyre, 1998); the highest prevalence of prenatal exposure to maternal cigarette smoking (PEMCS) was found during teenage pregnancies (50%). In Quebec, we found that 25% of expectant mothers smoked cigarettes throughout pregnancy and that 24% reported smoking daily 5 months after giving birth; these findings are based on a population sample of 2300 mothers who gave birth during 1997–1998 (Japel, Tremblay & McDuff, 2000).

It is important to note that the prevalence rates of cigarette smoking in general and of cigarette smoking during pregnancy in particular are not uniform across different groups of women. The strongest predictor of smoking both before and during pregnancy is a woman's socio-economic status (SES); for example, a prospective study of 589 pre-adolescent children found that 52% of their low-SES mothers smoked cigarettes during pregnancy (Cornelius, Leech, Goldschmidt, & Day, 2000). Tobacco smoking is particularly frequent in young mothers; in Canada, 40–50% of teen mothers reported that they smoked during their pregnancy (Paquette & Morrisson, 1999). Similar relationships were observed in the Saguenay-Lac-Saint-Jean (SLSJ) region; we found that prevalence of tobacco use is negatively correlated with the level of schooling and with household income (Institute de la Statistique du Quebec, 2001). The following rates of cigarette smoking in women were found: 39.0% of women with the lowest level of education (1st quintile) vs. 23.6% of women with the highest level of education (5th quintile); 47.2% of women with the lowest income vs. 27.4% of women with the highest income. Finally, several factors have been identified as predictors of the likelihood of quitting smoking during pregnancy; these include again a woman's SES, lower smoking level, having a partner who does not smoke and not consuming alcohol (Severson, Andrews, Lichtenstein, Wall, & Zoref, 1995).

Cigarette smoking, the foetus and the foetal–placental unit

The impact of maternal smoking on the developing foetus is complex. First of all, tobacco smoke may affect the foetus in several ways (Lockhart et al., 1996): (a) inhaled nicotine induces vasoconstriction of the uteroplacental vasculature, leading to uteroplacental underperfusion and, in turn, decreased flow of nutrients and oxygen to the foetus, (b) increased levels of carboxy-haemoglobin reduce tissue oxygenation of the foetus, (c) nicotine suppresses the mother's appetite, leading to reduced energy intake by the mother and hence reduced energy supply to the foetus, and (d) nicotine causes alterations in the cellular growth and activity of the central and peripheral nervous systems (Slotkin, 1998). Second, tobacco smoking is frequently associated with epiphenomena, such as risky behaviours, co-abuse of other substances, poor prenatal care and low socio-economic status (Slotkin, 1998), which themselves may exert adverse effects on the developing foetus. Third, cigarette smoking after birth may also influence the early postnatal environment and maternal behaviour, such as the duration of breastfeeding (Eriksen, 1996; Hill & Aldag, 1996). Finally, inter-individual variability in genetic background is likely to modify the response of the foetus to tobacco smoke, i.e., gene–environment interactions (Pausova, Tremblay, & Hamet, 1999). Perhaps the most dramatic example of gene–environment interaction is the finding of a 1200 g difference in the birth weight of babies born to the cigarette-smoking mothers with different variants of enzymes that metabolize polycyclic aromatic hydrocarbons in tobacco smoke (Wang et al., 2002). As reviewed below, PEMCS is a leading cause of intrauterine growth retardation (IUGR) in developed countries (Kramer, 2000). Cigarette smoking during pregnancy has been associated with a number of adverse outcomes related to the child's mental and cardiovascular and metabolic health.

PEMCS and behaviour

In human subjects, there is growing evidence that PEMCS is associated with cognitive sequelae and increased incidence of psychiatric disorders in childhood and adolescence. In a prospective cohort study, Fried and colleagues (Fried, 1995) observed systematic differences between children born to "heavy smokers" (> 20 cigarettes/day) compared with non-smoking mothers, in several cognitive domains, including processing of auditory stimuli, attention, and language comprehension. Some of these effects were seen as early as 3–6 days after birth and persisted until the last follow-up visit carried out during pre-adolescence. Other (Lassen & Oei, 1998; Obel, Henriksen, Hedegaard, Secher, & Ostergaard, 1998; Olds, Henderson, & Tatelbaum, 1994) but not all (MacArthur, Knox, & Lancashire, 2001) investigators have also observed similar effects. Several studies revealed an increased incidence of externalizing disorders in general (Breslau & Chilcoat, 2000), and attention deficit hyperactivity (Milberger, Biederman, Faraone, & Jones, 1998) and conduct (Wakschlag, Lahey, Loeber, Green, Gordon, & Leventhal, 1997; Weissman, Wickramaratne, & Kandel, 2000) disorders in particular. Some studies also observed an association between PEMCS and criminal behaviour in adulthood (Brennan, Grekin, & Mednick, 1999; Räsänen, Hakko, Isohanni, Hodgins, Järvelin, & Tiihonen, 1999), with the association being specific to violent as opposed to non-violent criminality. Thus, PEMCS has been associated with higher rates of aggression in children and adults (Orlebeke, Knol, & Verhulst, 1999; Räsänen et al., 1999). Furthermore, PEMCS may increase the probability of experimenting with cigarette smoking in childhood (Cornelius et al., 2000) and of developing cigarette-smoking addiction in adolescence (Kandel & Udry, 1999; Weissman et al., 2000).

PEMCS and the brain

The effect of PEMCS on the human brain is largely unknown. A recent study demonstrated subtle differences in the expression of nicotinic and muscarinic acetylcholine receptors in the brains of 5- to 12-week-old foetuses exposed and not exposed to maternal cigarette smoking (Falk, Nordberg, Seiger, Kjaeldgaard, & Hellstrom-Lindahl, 2005). Several lines of *indirect* evidence suggest detrimental effects of PEMCS on brain growth and development. Kallen (2000) analysed the Swedish Medical Birth Registry (1983–1996: 1,362,169 infants) and found significant negative correlation between PEMCS and head circumference at birth. Maternal cigarette smoking was found to increase the relative risk of periventricular-intraventricular haemorrhage in premature babies (Bada et al., 1990). As pointed out above, a higher incidence of attention deficit hyperactivity disorder (ADHD) is found in children with PEMCS. Several magnetic resonance (MR) studies of ADHD revealed a smaller corpus callosum in this group compared with controls (Baumgardner et al., 1996; Giedd et al., 1994; Hynd, Semrud-Clikeman,

Lorys, Novey, Eliopulos, & Lyytinen, 1991; Semrud-Clikeman et al., 1994), suggesting abnormalities in the number of inter-hemispheric fibres and/or their myelination. It is also interesting to note that corpus callosum abnormalities, ranging from complete callosal agenesis to a hypoplastic corpus callosum, are found rather frequently in offspring exposed *in utero* to various teratogens, including alcohol (Bookstein, Sampson, Streissguth, & Connor, 2001; Riley, Mattson, Sowell, Jernigan, Sobel, & Jones, 1995; Roebuck, Mattson, & Riley, 1998; Sowell, Mattson, Thompson, Jernigan, Riley, & Toga, 2001; Swayze et al., 1997), cocaine (Dominguez, Aguirre Vila-Coro, Slopis, & Bohan, 1991; Ojima, Abiru, Matsumoto, & Fukui, 1996), anti-epileptic drugs (Lindhout, Omtzigt, & Cornel, 1992) and corticosteroids (Huang, Harper, Evans, Newnham, & Dunlop, 2001). Neuro-anatomical studies of experimental animals exposed prenatally to nicotine facilitate interpretation of the human studies by controlling for some of the confounding variables and by allowing investigators to examine possible neural effects at the microscopic level. These studies showed nicotine-induced acute and chronic changes in cholinergic, catecholaminergic and other neurotransmitter systems (Lichtensteiger, Ribary, Schlumpf, Odermatt, & Widmer, 1988; Slotkin, 1998). In terms of brain structure, Roy and Sabherwal (1994, 1998) observed a significant reduction in brain weight, cortical thickness in the somatosensory cortex, neural density in layer V of the somatosensory cortex and the neural area of the dentate gyrus, CA1 and CA3 regions of the hippocampus. Using a whole-embryo culture, Roy, Andrews, Seidler and Slotkin (1998) were able to demonstrate a direct effect of nicotine on neuroepithelium; they found evidence of cytoplasmic vacuolation, enlargement of intercellular spaces and an increased incidence of apoptotic cells. The above effects may be mediated by the direct effect of nicotine on cell proliferation, survival and migration (Levitt, 1998; Slotkin, 1998). As pointed out by Levitt (1998), "the convergence of neurotransmitter, growth factor and hormone activity on similar intracellular signalling systems suggests the potential for significant interactions among molecular components that regulate [neural] development".

PEMCS and the offspring's metabolic health

Despite being associated with "low" body weight at birth, PEMCS has been recently implicated in the development of obesity in later life. The British National Child Development Study, involving all births in England, Wales and Scotland between 3 March and 9 March 1958, reported that PEMCS significantly increases the risk of obesity beginning in adolescence (Power & Jefferis, 2002), and diabetes mellitus in adulthood (Montgomery & Ekbom, 2002). In this prospective cohort study (Power & Jefferis, 2002), the impact of PEMCS increased with age and remained robust even after adjustment for known confounding factors, such as SES at birth, during childhood and in adulthood, infant feeding, current diet and physical activity. In addition, cross-sectional data obtained on German children aged 5–6 years during the obligatory school-entry health examination suggest that the impact of PEMCS on obesity may be emerging as early as in childhood (Toschke, Montgomery, Pfeiffer, & Von Kries, 2003; Von Kries, Toschke, Koletzko, & Slikker, 2002). This early emergence has been also observed in a prospective, population-based cohort study from Norway and Sweden in which women were followed up throughout pregnancy and their children from birth until 5 years of age (Wideroe, Vik, Jacobsen, & Bakketeig, 2003). In addition to the early emergence, the study showed that adjusting for maternal diet, breastfeeding, maternal obesity and SES does not affect the association between PEMCS and childhood obesity. It also showed that the associated risk of obesity is independent of intrauterine growth retardation and, thus, may be attributed to specific effects of cigarette smoke (Wideroe et al., 2003).

PEMCS and the offspring's cardiovascular health

Recent clinical and epidemiological studies suggest that PEMCS may play a role in the development of hypertension in later life (Blake et al, 2000; Morley, Payne, & Lucas, 1995; Williams & Poulton, 1999). It has been shown that blood pressure (BP) is significantly higher in neonates born to smoking mothers than in neonates born to non-smoking mothers (Beratis, Pangoulias, & Varvarigou, 1996; O'Sullivan, Kearney, & Crowley, 1996), with a significant positive correlation observed between the number of cigarettes smoked during pregnancy and the BP of the newborn (Beratis et al., 1996). Prospective cohort studies have demonstrated that BP is also higher in children and adolescents with PEMCS as compared with the controls (Blake et al., 2000). Multivariate analyses suggest that the relationship between PEMCS and BP is independent of SES. Furthermore, pathway analyses indicate that the relationship may be mediated in part by mechanisms that are independent of those involving the impact of PEMCS on birth weight (Morley et al., 1995). In experimental animals, prenatal exposure to nicotine has been related to elevated basal BP in adolescence (Pausova, Paus, Sedova, & Berube, 2003).

Design

In order to evaluate long-term consequences of PEMCS in adolescence and to assess how such an adverse intrauterine environment interacts with the individual's genetic background, the design of the Saguenay Youth Study has the following features: (a) a family-based (sibship) design where only children with one or more siblings and with both biological parents are included; (b) a cross-sectional design with participants' age ranging from 12 to 18 years, and an equal proportion of exposed ($n = 500$) and non-exposed ($n = 500$) adolescents of both sexes (1:1 male-to-female ratio); (c) a retrospective-cohort design where *in utero* exposure is assessed retrospectively, while the acquisition of the majority of phenotypes in the offspring is carried out in a prospective fashion; (d) quantitative assessment of brain/behaviour and cardiovascular/metabolic phenotypes; and (e) acquisition of DNA samples from the adolescent participants and their biological parents. Figure 4.1 provides a flow diagram of the recruitment and data collection.

Setting and participants

The sibships are being recruited from a relatively geographically isolated population with a known founder effect (Grompe, St-Louis, Demers, Al-Dhalimy, Leclerc, & Tanguay, 1994) living in the Saguenay-Lac-Saint-Jean (SLSJ) region of Quebec, Canada.

History of the SLSJ population

The initial settlement of the SLSJ region occurred between 1838 and 1911. From a total of 28,656 settlers who moved there during that time, 75% originated from the neighbouring Charlevoix region (Gradie, Jorde, & Bouchard, 1988). The settling of the Charlevoix region itself started in 1675 when 599 founders of mostly French descent moved to this region from the Quebec City area (Roy, Bouchard, & Declos, 1991). Due to relatively high birth rates and low immigration into the SLSJ region, today the population represents one of the largest population isolates in North America, with almost 300,000 inhabitants. As a consequence of the SLSJ population history, the prevalence of several recessive disorders is higher in the SLSJ region than in other populations (De Braekeleer, 1991), and a limited allelic diversity exists among patients with these disorders. For example, a single homozygous

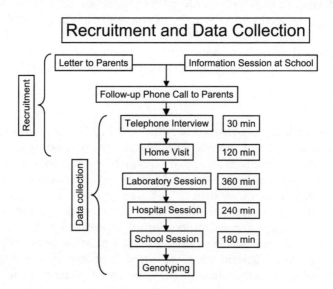

Figure 4.1 Overview of recruitment and data collection.

mutation was identified in 80% of patients with hereditary tyrosinaemia type I (Grompe et al., 1994), and only three mutations were found in 94% of patients with cystic fibrosis (De Braekeleer et al., 1998). These studies clearly indicate that genetic heterogeneity, i.e., the number of gene variants contributing to a trait in question, is reduced in the SLSJ population. This feature is critical for the success of genetic studies of complex traits, as it increases their power and, hence, the likelihood of identifying the genes. Moreover, population isolates usually have good genealogical records. A combined use of such records and linkage/association analyses may again increase the power of these analyses and the probability of identifying genes (Pausova et al., 2003, 2005). For the SLSJ population, extensive computerized genealogical records exist in the BALSAC population register maintained at the Inter-university Institute for Population Research. The register contains ascending genealogies going back as far as the 16th century; they have been constructed on the basis of parish records of baptisms, marriages and deaths of approximately 1,500,000 individuals (Roy et al., 1991).

The SLSJ population at present

According to the 2001 census, the region has a population of 278,279 inhabitants. In 2001, there were 19,114 French-speaking students in 24 secondary schools (20 public and 4 private). A large part of the SLSJ population (60%) is living in the Chicoutimi-Jonquière urban area. There are four school boards in the region, two in Saguenay and two in the Lac-Saint-Jean region. According to the 2001 census, there were 80,325 families living in the region. More than half (51,660) of all families have children living at home: 46.5% of families have one child; 38.1% have two children; 15.4% have three or more children.

Selection criteria

The following selection criteria are used for the exposed subjects: age 12–18 years; one or more siblings in the same age group; maternal and paternal grand-parents of French-Canadian ancestry; and positive history of maternal cigarette smoking (> 1 cigarette/day in the second trimester of pregnancy). The main exclusion criteria are: positive history of alcohol abuse during pregnancy; positive medical history for meningitis, malignancy and heart disease requiring heart surgery; severe mental illness (e.g., autism, schizophrenia) or mental retardation (IQ < 70); and MRI contraindications such as metal in the body (braces, metal plates, pins, non-removable body piercing), pacemaker, pregnancy and claustrophobia. The non-exposed subjects are matched to the exposed ones based on the level of maternal education as a proxy of SES and also on the school attended. Other inclusion and exclusion criteria are identical except in the case of mothers of non-exposed offspring where we require negative history of maternal cigarette smoking during pregnancy and during the 12-month period preceding the pregnancy. The full list of exclusion–inclusion criteria is presented in Table 4.1.

Recruitment

Potential subjects are recruited through regional high schools. A representative of the Groupe ÉCOBES (Groupe d'Étude des Conditions de Vie et des Besoins de la Population) first approaches local school boards and school principals to solicit their cooperation. The Groupe ÉCOBES is based in the College of Jonquière and has a long tradition of conducting psychoeducational research in the region. Each recruitment stage is centred at a particular high school; the number of students in each school varies between 600 and 1900. Following a briefing of the teachers, the team visits individual classrooms and presents the project using a series of posters depicting the different components of the study (e.g., MRI, psychological and cardiovascular testing). Before the visit, we mail a letter to all parents of students attending the visited school; the letter contains an information brochure, a letter from the principal, a consent form for a telephone interview and a self-addressed and stamped response card. We ask the parents to mail the response card back to the team and indicate whether or not they are interested in participating in the project, how many children aged 12–18 years they have and to provide the home phone number for a follow-up call by a research nurse. During the follow-up call to the interested families, the nurse verifies basic eligibility for the project (number of children and their age), solicits consent to a telephone interview and, if agreed, proceeds with the interview. Given the nature of the interview (see below), the respondent should be the children's biological mother whenever possible. The telephone interview is carried out on a laptop computer using software written for the project, providing the nurse with the script and allowing her to record all responses on line; the software navigates the nurse through the interview by skipping "not-applicable" questions. The interview covers the following areas: demographics of the parents (French-Canadian origin, age, level of education), pregnancy (smoking, drinking, drug use, medical complications) and medical history of the children and parents. If the nurse deems the family eligible, she sets up an appointment for a home visit; this can be done immediately only for the exposed subjects, while non-exposed subjects are called back once selected by matching to the exposed subjects from the same school. The home visit concludes the recruitment phase; it begins with the signing of the consent (parents) and assent (adolescents) forms.

Measurements

Data collection begins with the telephone interview, continues with a home visit, neuropsychological testing in the laboratory, a hospital visit for the cardiovascular & metabolic phenotyping and magnetic resonance imaging

Table 4.1 Exclusion and inclusion criteria

	Criteria	Instrument	Actions
Demographics	1. Both biological parents are French-Canadians (two generations)	A07f	Inclusion
	2. Both parents are available for providing a blood sample	A07f	Inclusion
	3. There are two siblings in the eligible age range (12–18 years)	A07f	Inclusion
	4. Child, parent or grand-parent is adopted	A07f	Exclusion
Pregnancy and birth	1. Exposed: Prenatal exposure to maternal cigarette smoking (1 cigarette or more per day) during the 2nd trimester	A07f	Inclusion
	2. Non-exposed: No maternal cigarette smoking during the following two periods: • 12 months before the pregnancy • during pregnancy • during breastfeeding	A07f	Inclusion
	3. Use of alcohol by the mother during pregnancy	B02f	Exclusion (> 210 ml alcohol/week, e.g., 14 bottles of beer, 9 glasses of wine, 7 glasses of hard liquor)
	4. Diabetes of the mother during pregnancy (onset before pregnancy, treated by insulin)	A07f	Exclusion
	5. Premature birth (< 35 weeks) and/ or detached placenta	A07f	Exclusion
	6. Multiple births (e.g., twins)	A07f	Exclusion
	7. Hyperbilirubinaemia requiring transfusion	A07f	Exclusion
Child's medical history	1. Type 1 diabetes	A07f	Exclusion
	2. Systemic rheumatological disorders (e.g., complications of strep throat, such as glomerulonephritis or endocarditis)	A07f	Exclusion
	3. Malignant tumours requiring chemotherapy (e.g., leukaemia)	A07f	Exclusion
	4. Congenital heart defects or heart surgery	A07f	Exclusion
	5. Aneurysm		Exclusion

(*Continued overleaf*)

Table 4.1 Continued

	Criteria	Instrument	Actions
Neurological conditions	1. Epilepsy 2. Bacterial infection of CNS 3. Brain tumour	A07f	Exclusion
	4. Head trauma with loss of consciousness > 30 minutes	A07f	Exclusion
	5. Muscular dystrophy, myotonic dystrophy	A07f	Exclusion
Developmental conditions	1. Nutritional and metabolic diseases (e.g., failure to thrive, phenylketonuria) 2. Major neurodevelopmental disorders (e.g., autism)	A07f	Exclusion
	3. Hearing deficit (requiring hearing aid)	A07f	Exclusion
	4. Vision problems (strabismus, visual deficit not correctible)	A07f	Exclusion
Mental health and abilities	1. Treatment for schizophrenia, bipolar disorder	A07f	Exclusion
	2. IQ < 70	WISC	Exclusion
	3. Reading ability (< 2 SD)	Woodcock-Johnson	Exclusion
	4. Special education (special classes)	A07f	Exclusion
MR contraindications	1. Metal implants	A07f	Exclusion
	2. Electronic implants (e.g., pacemakers)	A07f	Exclusion
	3. Severe claustrophobia	A07f	Exclusion

Notes: A07f, telephone interview; B02f, medical questionnaire; WISC, Wechsler Intelligence Scale for Children; CNS, central nervous system; IQ, intelligence quotient.

(MRI), and it concludes with a school visit (Figure 4.1); note that hospital visits always take place on Saturdays. In this section, we will describe the various instruments by types of datasets rather than by place/time of their collection, which are indicated in the overview of all instruments (Table 4.2).

Questionnaires

Demographics and measures of socio-economic status

Table 4.3A provides a summary of datasets acquired in these domains, together with the instruments used for their collection. Note that a large number of SES measures, as well as stressful life events, are recorded for the following four periods of each child's life: birth, 3 years, 10 years and present.

Table 4.2 Instruments

Instrument	Duration (min)	Code name	Tool	Data entry
1. Screening				
Telephone interview	20	A07f	Interview software	Computer upload
2. Home visit				
Medical and SES questionnaire	40	B02f	Questionnaire	Manual
Consent – mother	10	B04f	Form	Filed but not entered
Consent – father	10	B11f	Form	Filed but not entered
Assent	10	B05f	Form	Filed but not entered
Family environment	40	B09f	Questionnaire	Scanner (OMR software)
Mental health and anti-social behaviour: mother	20	B10f	Questionnaire	Scanner (OMR software)
Mental health and anti-social behaviour: father	20	B12f	Questionnaire	Scanner (OMR software)
Positive youth development	20	B08f	Questionnaire	Scanner (OMR software)
Handedness: father and his relatives	20	B15f	Form	Manual (web-based GUI)
Handedness: mother and her relatives	20	B17f	Form	Manual (web-based GUI)
Healthy lifestyle	20	J02f	Questionnaire	Scanner (OMR software)
Blood sample (parents)	10			
Session duration (min): mother	140			
Session duration (min): father	60			
Session duration (min): adolescent	50			
3. Laboratory (neuropsychology)				
Handedness: adolescent	5	E01f	MNI	Manual (web-based GUI)
Wechsler Intelligence Scale-III	60	Standard Form	WISC	Manual (web-based GUI)
Academic abilities: maths, maths fluency, reading comprehension and spelling subscales of Woodcock-Johnson	45	E30f E31f E32f E33f	W-J	Manual (web-based GUI)
Long-term memory: Children's Memory Scale	5	E12f	CMS	Manual (web-based GUI)

(Continued overleaf)

Table 4.2 Continued

Instrument	Duration (min)	Code name	Tool	Data entry
Short-term memory: digit span	5		Form	Manual (web-based GUI)
Working memory: self-ordered pointing (cuffed)	3	E25f	Npsych PC (NeuroCog Battery SW)/Finometer	Computer upload
Sustained attention: Ruff 2–7	7	E08f	Form	Manual (web-based GUI)
Resistence to interference: Stroop	3	E28f	Form	Manual (web-based GUI)
Divergent thinking: word fluency	7	E29f	Form	Manual (web-based GUI)
Fine motor skills: grooved pegboard	7	E10f	Form/Hardware	Manual (web-based GUI)
Motor speed: tapping	5	E40f	Test	Manual (web-based GUI)
Transcallosal interaction: bimanual coordination	15	E41f	Npsych PC (MeasurEnd SW)	Computer upload
Temporal processing of sound: frequency-modulation threshold	10	E36f	Npsych PC (Oxford SW)	Computer upload
Phonological learning	20	E37f	Npsych PC (Oxford SW)	Computer upload
Awareness of self-generated movement: delayed auditory feedback	12	E43f	Npsych PC (CoolEdit)	Computer upload
Body image perception	15	E38f	Npsych PC (Presentation)	Computer upload
Imitation: runner observation (cuffed)	10	E24f	Npsych PC (Presentation)/Finometer	Computer upload
Perception of facial expressions: Pollak faces (cuffed)	10	E26f	Npsych PC (Superlab)/Finometer	Computer upload

Task	Min	Code	Equipment/Software	Method
Sensitivity to gains and losses: Newman's Card Playing (cuffed)	5	E25f	Npsych PC (NeuroCog Battery SW)/Finometer	Computer upload
Sensitivity to failure: Repeated Failure Test (cuffed) Anagrams	15	E23f	Npsych PC (Superlab, CoolEdit/Finometer)	Computer upload
Number sense	7	E35f	Npsych PC (Superlab)	Computer upload
Session duration (min): adolescent	271			
4. Hospital (magnetic resonance imaging)				
Brain T1W MRI	16	H04f	Philips 1.0T scanner	CD upload
Brain T2W/PDW MRI	14	H05f	Philips 1.0T scanner	CD upload
Brain MT MRI	12	H06f	Philips 1.0T scanner	CD upload
Abdominal MRI	5	H07f	Philips 1.0T scanner	CD upload
Phantoms (living and ACR)		H13f	Philips 1.0T scanner	CD upload
Radiologist report		M06f	Form	Manual
Session duration (min): adolescent	47			
5. Hospital (questionnaires)				
Food recall	30	J03f	Questionnaire	Scanner (OMR software)
Psychiatric diagnosis likelihood (DPS)	20	P05f	Questionnaire	
Session duration (min): adolescent	50			
6. Hospital (cardiovascular reactivity)				
Posture test	30	N06f	Form (p1 + 4)	Manual
Maths stress test	20	N06f	Form (p6)	Scanner (OMR software)
Salivary cortisol	1	N05f	Salivette	Manual
Session duration (min): adolescent	51			

(Continued overleaf)

Table 4.2 Continued

Instrument	Duration (min)	Code name	Tool	Data entry
7. Hospital (body composition)				
Anthropometry: body height, weight, circumferences and skinfolds	10	N06f	Form (p2+W+H)	Manual
Bioimpedance/body composition	20	N06f	Form (p3)/Xitron	Manual/CD upload
Session duration (min): adolescent	30			
8. School (questionnaires, blood sample)				
Personality: NEO-PI	50	P04f	Questionnaire	Scanner (OMR software)
Adolescent behaviour	25	J04f	Questionnaire	Scanner (OMR software)
Adolescent school experience and friends	25	P06f	Questionnaire	Scanner (OMR software)
Blood sample	5			
Quest-appreciation	10	P07f	Questionnaire	Scanner (OMR software)
Session duration (min): adolescent	115			
9. Other				
Medical chart		Q02f	Form	Manual (web-based GUI)
Total duration (min): adolescent	614			

Notes: SES, socio-economic status; OMR, optical mark reading; GUI, graphical user interface; MNI, Montreal Neurological Institute; W-J, Woodcock-Johnson; WISC, Wechsler Intelligence Scale for Children; CMS, Children's Memory Scale; Npsych PC, neuropsychological personal computer; SW, software; MRI, magnetic resonance imaging; ACR, American College of Radiology; CD, compact disk; MT, magnetization transfer.

Table 4.3 Questionnaires

Domains/scales	Respondent	Instrument (code name)	Source
A. Demographics			
Eligibility	Mother	Telephone interview (A07f)	SYS
Parents' date of birth, education level	Mother	Telephone interview (A07f)	SYS
Family structure at birth, 3 yr, 10 yr and now	Mother	Medical and SES questionnaire (B02f)	SYS
Primary caregiver (birth to 4 yr)	Mother	Medical and SES questionnaire (B02f)	SYS
Height and weight of the parents	Mother	Medical and SES questionnaire (B02f)	SYS
Place and date of birth of parents	Mother	Medical and SES questionnaire (B02f)	SYS
Parental employment status	Mother	Medical and SES questionnaire (B02f)	SYS
Family income	Mother	Medical and SES questionnaire (B02f)	SYS
Type of residence	Mother	Medical and SES questionnaire (B02f)	SYS
Stressful events	Mother/ father	Family environment (B09f)	SYS
Parental education	Mother/ father	Family environment (B09f)	SYS
Handedness of the mother and her relatives	Mother	Handedness: mother and her relatives (B17f)	MNI
Handedness of the father and his relatives	Father	Handedness: father and his relatives (B15f)	MNI
Handedness of the adolescent	Adolescent	Handedness: adolescent (E01f)	MNI
B. Medical and psychiatric history			
Child's medical history	Mother	Telephone interview (A07f)	SYS
MR contraindications	Mother	Telephone interview (A07f)	SYS
Pregnancies, stillbirths, abortions, IVF	Mother	Medical and SES questionnaire (B02f)	SYS
Pregnancy and birth	Mother	Medical and SES questionnaire (B02f)	SYS
Breastfeeding	Mother	Medical and SES questionnaire (B02f)	SYS
Child's medical and psychiatric history	Mother	Medical and SES questionnaire (B02f)	SYS
Family (1st degree relatives) medical history	Mother	Medical and SES questionnaire (B02f)	SYS
Mother's depression	Mother	Mental health and anti-social behaviour (B10f)	GRIP-A
Mother's anxiety	Mother	Mental Health and anti-social behaviour (B10f)	GRIP-B
Father's depression	Father	Mental Health and anti-social behaviour (B12f)	GRIP-A

(Continued overleaf)

76 *Paus et al.*

Table 4.3 Continued

Domains/scales	Respondent	Instrument (code name)	Source
Father's anxiety	Father	Mental health and anti-social behaviour (B12f)	GRIP-B
Hyperactivity	Adolescent	Adolescent behaviour (J04f)	GRIP-C
Inattention	Adolescent	Adolescent behaviour (J04f)	GRIP-C
Anxiety	Adolescent	Adolescent behaviour (J04f)	GRIP-C
Depression and suicide	Adolescent	Adolescent behaviour (J04f)	GRIP-A
Social phobia	Adolescent	Psychiatric diagnosis likelihood (P05f)	DPS
Simple anxiety disorder	Adolescent	Psychiatric diagnosis likelihood (P05f)	DPS
Agoraphobia	Adolescent	Psychiatric diagnosis likelihood (P05f)	DPS
Panic	Adolescent	Psychiatric diagnosis likelihood (P05f)	DPS
Generalized anxiety disorder	Adolescent	Psychiatric diagnosis likelihood (P05f)	DPS
Specific phobia	Adolescent	Psychiatric diagnosis likelihood	DPS
Obsessive compulsive disorder	Adolescent	Psychiatric diagnosis likelihood (P05f)	DPS
Eating disorder	Adolescent	Psychiatric diagnosis likelihood (P05f)	DPS
Elimination disorder	Adolescent	Psychiatric diagnosis likelihood (P05f)	DPS
Major depressive disorder	Adolescent	Psychiatric diagnosis likelihood (P05f)	DPS
Mania	Adolescent	Psychiatric diagnosis likelihood (P05f)	DPS
Schizophrenia	Adolescent	Psychiatric diagnosis likelihood (P05f)	DPS
Attention deficit hyperactivity disorder	Adolescent	Psychiatric diagnosis likelihood (P05f)	DPS
Oppositional defiant disorder	Adolescent	Psychiatric diagnosis likelihood (P05f)	DPS
Conduct disorder	Adolescent	Psychiatric diagnosis likelihood (P05f)	DPS
Alcohol	Adolescent	Psychiatric diagnosis likelihood (P05f)	DPS
Marijuana dependence	Adolescent	Psychiatric diagnosis likelihood (P05f)	DPS
Other substances abused	Adolescent	Psychiatric diagnosis likelihood	DPS
Concussion	Adolescent	Healthy lifestyle (J02f)	D. Goodman

C. Cigarettes, alcohol and drugs

Maternal cigarette smoking (past, present, pregnancy)	Mother	Telephone interview (A07f)	SYS
Maternal cigarette smoking during pregnancy	Physician	Obstetric chart	QMH
Second-hand smoke during pregnancy	Mother	Medical and SES questionnaire (B02f)	SYS
Father's cigarette smoking	Father	Mental health and anti-social behaviour (B12f)	GRIP-D
Adolescent drugs, alcohol, sexual abuse	Mother/father	Family environment (B09f)	SYS
Mother's alcohol and drug use	Mother	Mental health and anti-social behaviour (B10f)	GRIP-D
Father's alcohol and drug use	Father	Mental Health and anti-social behaviour (B12f)	GRIP-D
Cigarette smoking	Adolescent	Adolescent behaviour (J04f)	GRIP-E
Drugs and alcohol	Adolescent	Adolescent behaviour (J04f)	GRIP-F

D. Anti-social behaviour

Mother's anti-social behaviour	Mother	Mental health and anti-social behaviour (B10f)	GRIP-G
Father's anti-social behaviour	Father	Mental health and anti-social behaviour (B12f)	GRIP-G
Physical aggression	Adolescent	Adolescent behaviour (J04f)	GRIP-C
Indirect aggression	Adolescent	Adolescent behaviour (J04f)	GRIP-H
Fighting	Adolescent	Adolescent behaviour (J04f)	GRIP-I
Stealing	Adolescent	Adolescent behaviour (J04f)	GRIP-I
Vandalism	Adolescent	Adolescent behaviour (J04f)	GRIP-I
Friends and problems	Adolescent	School experience and friends (P06f)	ÉCOBES-A
Acceptance of societal phenomena (illegal activities)	Adolescent	School experience and friends (P06f)	ÉCOBES-B

E. Lifestyle

Physical activity (sports)	Adolescent	Healthy lifestyle (J02f)	Sante Quebec
Nutrition (food frequency)	Adolescent	Healthy lifestyle (J02f)	Sante Quebec
Sleep	Adolescent	Healthy lifestyle (J02f)	J. Carrier
Sexuality	Adolescent	Adolescent behaviour (J04f)	GRIP-J
School experience	Adolescent	School experience and friends (P06f)	ÉCOBES-C
Extracurricular activities	Adolescent	School experience and friends (P06f)	ÉCOBES-D

(*Continued overleaf*)

78   *Paus et al.*

Table 4.3 Continued

Domains/scales	Respondent	Instrument (code name)	Source
Drop-out attitudes	Adolescent	School experience and friends (P06f)	ÉCOBES-E
Teachers	Adolescent	School experience and friends (P06f)	ÉCOBES-F
School performance	Adolescent	School experience and friends (P06f)	ÉCOBES-G
Working while studying	Adolescent	School experience and friends (P06f)	Statistics Canada
Academic and vocational aspirations	Adolescent	School Experience and friends (P06f)	ÉCOBES-H

F. Self-attributes and personality

Industry (Rosenthal)	Adolescent	Positive youth development (B08f)	4-H PYD-A
Identity (Rosenthal)	Adolescent	Positive youth development (B08f)	4-H PYD-A
Intimacy (Rosenthal)	Adolescent	Positive youth development (B08f)	4-H PYD-A
Elective selection (SOC)	Adolescent	Positive youth development (B08f)	4-H PYD-B
Optimization (SOC)	Adolescent	Positive youth development (B08f)	4-H PYD-B
Compensation (SOC)	Adolescent	Positive youth development (B08f)	4-H PYD-B
Depression (CES-D)	Adolescent	Positive youth development (B08f)	4-H PYD-C
Academic competence (Harter)	Adolescent	Positive youth development (B08f)	4-H PYD-D
Social competence (Harter)	Adolescent	Positive youth development (B08f)	4-H PYD-D
Physical competence (Harter)	Adolescent	Positive youth development (B08f)	4-H PYD-D
Physical appearance (Harter)	Adolescent	Positive youth development (B08f)	4-H PYD-D
Conduct behaviour (Harter)	Adolescent	Positive youth development (B08f)	4-H PYD-D
Self-worth (Harter)	Adolescent	Positive youth development (B08f)	4-H PYD-D
Connection to community	Adolescent	Positive youth development (B08f)	4-H PYD-E
Connection to family	Adolescent	Positive youth development (B08f)	4-H PYD-E
Connection to peers	Adolescent	Positive youth development (B08f)	4-H PYD-F
Connection to school	Adolescent	Positive youth development (B08f)	4-H PYD-E
Maternal warmth	Adolescent	Positive youth development (B08f)	4-H PYD-G

Paternal warmth	Adolescent	Positive youth development (B08f)	4-H PYD-G
School engagement	Adolescent	Positive youth development (B08f)	4-H PYD-H
Risk avoidance	Adolescent	Positive youth development (B08f)	4-H PYD-E
Interpersonal skills	Adolescent	Positive youth development (B08f)	4-H PYD-E
Adult mentors	Adolescent	Positive youth development (B08f)	4-H PYD-E
Parental monitoring	Adolescent	Positive youth development (B08f)	4-H PYD-I
Personal values	Adolescent	Positive youth development (B08f)	4-H PYD-J
Positive identity	Adolescent	Positive youth development (B08f)	4-H PYD-K
Social conscience	Adolescent	Positive youth development (B08f)	4-H PYD-E
Social responsibility	Adolescent	Positive youth development (B08f)	4-H PYD-L
Values diversity	Adolescent	Positive youth development (B08f)	4-H PYD-E
Sympathy	Adolescent	Positive youth development (B08f)	4-H PYD-M
Puberty Development Scale	Adolescent	Positive youth development (B08f)	4-H PYD-N
Confidence (Revised Mean Scale)	Adolescent	Positive youth development (B08f)	4-H PYD-J
Competence (Revised Mean Scale)	Adolescent	Positive youth development (B08f)	4-H PYD-J
Character (Revised Mean Scale)	Adolescent	Positive youth development (B08f)	4-H PYD-J
Caring (Standardized Mean of Eisenberg Scale)	Adolescent	Positive youth development (B08f)	4-H PYD-J
Connection (5Cs – Revised Mean Scale)	Adolescent	Positive youth development (B08f)	4-H PYD-J
Positive Youth Development (Mean of 5Cs)	Adolescent	Positive youth development (B08f)	4-H PYD-J
Pro-social behaviour	Adolescent	Adolescent behaviour (J04f)	GRIP-C
Neuroticism	Adolescent	Personality (P04f)	NEO PI-R
Extroversion	Adolescent	Personality (P04f)	NEO PI-R
Openness	Adolescent	Personality (P04f)	NEO PI-R
Agreeableness	Adolescent	Personality (P04f)	NEO PI-R
Conscientiousness	Adolescent	Personality (P04f)	NEO PI-R
Body esteem	Adolescent	Healthy lifestyle (J02f)	Mendelson
Body image	Adolescent	Healthy lifestyle (J02f)	Sante Quebec
Peer influence	Adolescent	School experience and friends (P06f)	RPI

(*Sources to table overleaf*)

Table 4.3 Continued

Sources: SYS: Saguenay Youth Study, developed by the project team; MNI: Neuropsychology Unit, Montreal Neurological Institute and Hospital, McGill University, Montreal, Quebec, Canada; GRIP: Groupe de Recherche sur l'Inadaptation Psychosociale chez l'Enfant, University of Montreal, Montreal, Quebec, Canada; DPS: DISC Predictive Scales (Lucas et al., 2001; adapted by J. J. Breton, Riviere-des-Prairies Hospital, Montreal, Quebec, Canada); D. Goodman: Simon Fraser University, Vancouver, BC, Canada; ECOBES: Le Groupe d'Étude des Conditions de Vie et des BeSoins de la Population, Cegep Jonquiere, Quebec, Canada; J. Carrier: University of Montreal, Montreal, Quebec, Canada; 4-H PYD: 4-H Study of Positive Youth Development (Richard Lerner and colleagues, Tufts University, MA, USA); RPI: Resistance to Peer Influence Scale (Steinberg, 2002); Sante Quebec: Questionnaire aux Adolescentes et Adolescents; Statistics Canada: Youth In Transition Survey, 2000; Mendelson: Mendelson, Mendelson, & White (2001).

GRIP-A: Based on Radloff, 1977; GRIP-B: Based on Séguin, Freeston, Tarabulsy, Zoccolillo, Tremblay, & Carbonneau, 2000; GRIP-C: Based on Behar & Stringfield, 1974; Offord et al., 1987; Ontario Child Health Study and Child Behavior Checklist (Achenbach, 1999); Rutter, 1967; Weir & Duveen, 1981; GRIP-D: Based on Enquête Nationale sur la Santé de la Population; GRIP-E: Based on Loiselle, 2000; GRIP-F: Based on Selzer, 1971; GRIP-G: Based on Robins, Helzer, Croughan, & Ratcliff, 1981; Zoccolillo, Price, Ji, & Hwu, 1999; GRIP-H: Based on Vaillancourt, Brendgen, Boivin, & Tremblay, 2003; GRIP-I: Based on LeBlanc & Tremblay, 1988; GRIP-J: Based on Malo & Tremblay, 1995.

ÉCOBES-A: Based on Le Blanc, 1996; ÉCOBES-B: Based on Galland, 1994; ÉCOBES-C: Based on Ntamakiliro, Monnard, & Gurtner, 2000; ÉCOBES-D: Based on Janosz, Lacroix, & Rondeau, 1999; ÉCOBES-E: Based on Janosz et al., 1999; ÉCOBES-F: Based on Larose & Boivin, 1998; ÉCOBES-G: Based on Rosenberg, Schooler, Schoenbach, & Rosenberg, 1995; Ntamakiliro et al., 2000; ÉCOBES-H: Based on Bélanger & Rocher, 1972.

4-H PYD-A: Based on Erikson Psychological Stage Inventory (Rosenthal, Gurbey, & Moore, 1981); 4-H PYD-B: Based on Selection, Optimization and Compensation (SOC) Questionnaire (Freund & Bates, 2002); 4-H PYD-C: Based on Radloff, 1977; 4-H PYD-D: Based on the Self-Perception Profile for Children (Harter, 1983); 4-H PYD-E: Based on Theokas et al., 2005; 4-H PYD-F: Based on Peer Support Scale of Teen Assessment Project Survey Question Bank (Small & Rodgers, 1995); 4-H PYD-G: Based on the Child's Report of Parenting Behaviors Inventory (Schludermann & Schludermann, 1970); 4-H PYD-H: Based on School Engagement Scale of Profiles of Student Life: Attitudes and Behaviours (Benson, Leffert, Scales, & Blyth, 1998; Leffert, Benson, Scales, Sharma, Drake, & Blyth, 1998; Scales, Benson, Leffert, & Blyth, 2000); 4-H PYD-I: Based on Parental Monitoring Scale (Small & Kerns, 1993); 4-H PYD-J: Based on Lerner et al., 2005; 4-H PYD-K: Based on Target Based Beliefs Scale (Buchanan & Holmbeck, 1998); 4-H PYD-L: Based on Social Responsibility Scale of Teen Assessment Project Survey Question Bank (Small & Rodgers, 1995); 4-H PYD-M: Based on Sympathy Scale (Eisenberg, Fabes, Murphy, Karbon, Smith, & Maszk, 1996); 4-H PYD-N: Based on Puberty Development Scale (Petersen, Crockett, Richards, & Boxer, 1988).

Medical and psychiatric history

Table 4.3B summarizes measures collected in this domain. In addition to the medical history of each child from conception to present (pregnancy, delivery, breastfeeding, concussions, etc.), we also collect data on the parental mental, cardiovascular and metabolic health (depression, anxiety, hypertension, dyslipidaemia and diabetes mellitus) and, in the adolescents, evaluate the likelihood of psychiatric diagnosis with DISC Predictive Scales.

Cigarettes, alcohol and drugs

Table 4.3C shows that several instruments are used to collect information about the use of cigarettes, alcohol and illegal substances by the adolescent, as well as his/her mother and father. Maternal reports of the use of these substances during pregnancy are checked against medical records. *In utero* exposure to second-hand cigarette smoke is also documented. As seen in Table 4.3D, anti-social behaviour is documented extensively in both adolescents (self-report and parental report) and their parents (maternal and paternal self-report). Lifestyle measures provide information about the adolescents' engagement in physical activities, their eating habits, sleep pattern, sexuality, extracurricular activities, attitudes towards school, as well as their academic/vocational aspirations (Table 4.3E). A number of self-attributes and personality traits (Table 4.3F) are evaluated using two instruments, namely the 5C (Competence, Connection, Character, Confidence and Caring/ Compassion) questionnaire and the NEO-Personality Inventory (Costa & McCrae, 1992). In addition, we employ two body-esteem and body-image instruments and a resistance to peer-pressure questionnaire.

Neuropsychological assessment

This assessment (Table 4.2, Section 3) consists of two types of tests: standardized psychological instruments and domain-specific tests. Testing is carried out by trained psychometricians supervised by experienced neuropsychologists. Total testing time is 6 hours, divided into two 3-hour blocks separated by a lunch break. In order to characterize the two groups of subjects and collect clinically relevant information, we administer several standardized tests, including the WISC-III (except Mazes), Woodcock-Johnson Achievement subtests (reading comprehension and arithmetic and a spelling test) and Children's Memory Scale (Dot Locations and Stories). As we argued previously (Paus, Collins, Evans, Leonard, Pike, & Zijdenbos, 2001), non-standardized "experimental tests are more likely to capture 'building blocks' rather than a 'composite' of a given behaviour; in turn, the 'building blocks' are more likely to be linked to a single neural system and as such, be more readily detectable [with MRI] during brain development". For this reason, we have included an extensive battery of domain-specific tests based on neuropsychological and cognitive-neuroscience research. The following domains are assessed: (a) executive functions, including working memory (self-ordered pointing; Petrides & Milner, 1982), word fluency (phonetic and semantic) and resistance to interference (Stroop test; Stroop, 1935), (b) phonological skills and frequency-modulation (FM) auditory threshold (Talcott et al., 2000), delayed auditory feedback and phonological learning, (c) fine motor skills (Grooved Pegboard, Simple Tapping) and motor coordination (bimanual coordination; Stephan et al., 1999), (d) number sense (Gallistel & Gelman, 2000) and (e) emotion and motivation (Pollak faces; Pollak & Kistler, 2002), repeated failure test and card playing task (Newman, Patterson, & Kosson, 1987).

Magnetic resonance imaging of the brain, abdominal fat and the kidneys

MRI data are collected on a Philips 1.0-T superconducting magnet.

Structural MRI of the brain

High-resolution anatomical MR images are acquired using the following three sequences: T1-weighted images (T1W; 3D RF-spoiled gradient echo scan with 140–160 slices, 1-mm isotropic resolution, TR = 25 ms, TE = 5 ms, flip angle = 30°), T2-weighted images (T2W; 2D multi-slice fast spin echo scan with 140–160 2-mm contiguous slices with a 1-mm in-plane resolution, TR = 3300 ms, TE effective = 11 ms) and proton-density weighted images (PDW; same as for T2 scan, but with TE effective = 105 ms).

Magnetization transfer (MT) imaging (Wolff & Balaban, 1989) is a quantitative MRI technique that provides information on the macromolecular content and structure of tissue; it has been shown to reveal subtle white matter abnormalities that are undetected by conventional MRI, in diseases such as multiple sclerosis (Dousset et al., 1992; Gass et al., 1994; Pike et al., 2000). In the context of this study, MT data should provide a more sensitive and accurate measure of myelination as compared with white matter (WM) density maps obtained via the methods discussed below. MT data are acquired using a dual acquisition (3D RF-spoiled gradient echo scan with approximately 50 slices of 3-mm thickness and 1-mm in-plane resolution, TR = 41 ms, TE = 7.9 ms, flip angle = 20°) with and without an MT saturation pulse (Gaussian RF pulse of 7.68 ms duration, 1.5 kHz off resonance and 500° effective pulse angle). Magnetization transfer ratio (MTR) images are calculated as the percentage signal change between the two acquisitions (Pike, 1996).

MRI of abdominal fat

Imaging of adipose tissue using MRI is relatively straightforward, as the T1 relaxation time of adipose tissue is much shorter than that of most other tissues (Snijder et al., 2002). Thus, in the present project, the MR images of abdominal fat are acquired with a heavily T1-weighted, single breath-hold, multi-slice (10 axial slices of 10-mm thickness) spin-echo (TR/TE = 200 ms/20 ms) measurement that is centred on the L4–L5 region (see Figure 4.3).

Kidney MRI

The kidneys can be well visualized on T1-weighted MRI acquisitions provided that respiratory motion can be controlled for. Therefore, anatomical MR images of the kidneys are obtained with a multi-slice T1-weighted gradient recalled echo acquisition (3D Gradient Echo, TR/TE = 4 ms/1.9 ms; flip angle = 10°), collected within a single breath-hold. Approximately 27 coronal slices of 3-mm thickness and 3-mm in-plane resolution are acquired.

Computational analysis of high-resolution structural brain MR images

This analysis is used to assess differences in brain structure between exposed and non-exposed adolescents, as well as to identify more general effects of age and sex, structure–function relationships and genetic/familial influences on brain structure. A typical image-processing "pipeline" (Figure 4.2) begins with the linear registration of a T1W image from the acquisition ("native") space to standardized stereotaxic space, namely that of the average MNI-305 atlas (Evans, Collins, Mills, Brown, Kelly, & Peters, 1993), aligned with Talairach and Tournoux space (Talairach & Tournoux, 1988). We use as a registration target the average brain computed from our population (Guimond, Meunier, & Thirion, 2000) and aligned = gend with the average MNI-305 atlas. Note that there is a negligible difference in the overall brain size between adolescent brains and those of young adults (23.4 ± 4.1 years) who constitute the MNI-305 atlas. The next step involves brain-tissue classification into grey matter (GM), white matter (WM) and cerebrospinal fluid (CSF); an automatic classification is achieved by combining information from different types of MR images, namely T1W, T2W and PDW acquisitions (Cocosco, Zijdenbos, & Evans, 2003; Zijdenbos, Forghani, & Evans, 2002). The tissue-classification step yields three sets of binary 3D images (i.e., GM, WM and CSF). Each of the binary images can be smoothed to generate probabilistic "density" images. These maps are used in voxel-wise analyses of age- or group-related differences in GM or WM density (see Ashburner & Friston, 2000, for methodological overview). Another important processing step is a non-linear registration of the subject's image to a template brain; local differences between the subject and the template are captured in a deformation field. The template brain contains information about anatomical boundaries; this anatomical information can be "projected" onto each subject's brain using the corresponding deformation field and fine-tuned by combining it with the tissue-classification map (Collins, Neelin, Peters, & Evans, 1994; Collins, Holmes, Peters, & Evans, 1995). In this way, the pipeline provides automatic estimates of regional volumes. Another

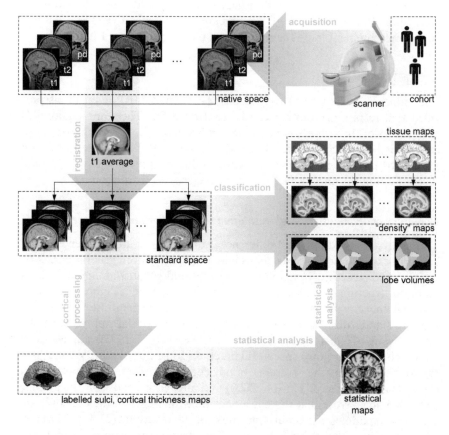

Figure 4.2 Acquisition and analysis of brain magnetic resonance images: t1, t2, pd, T1-weighted, T2-weighted and proton-density-weighted images, respectively.

voxel-wise approach has been developed to quantify individual differences in the 3D anatomy of the cerebral cortex. These include estimates of the cortical thickness (Fischl & Dale, 2000; Lerch & Evans, 2004; MacDonald, Kabani, Avis, & Evans, 2000) and the quantification of individual differences in the position, depth and length of the cerebral sulci (Le Goualher, Procyk, Collins, Venugopal, Barillot, & Evans, 1999; Mangin et al., 2004).

Computational analysis of fat and kidneys

Fat is well contrasted on T1W images and therefore amenable to semi-automated or automated segmentation (Figure 4.3). To this end, we developed a histogram-based classification algorithm where the combination of local intensity measures and geometrical constraints enabled the segmentation and volumetric measurements of subcutaneous and intra-abdominal

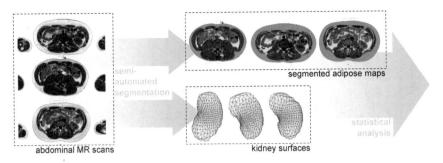

Figure 4.3 Acquisition and analysis of abdominal magnetic resonance images.

(visceral) adipose tissues. We are also developing deformable-model-based techniques for the automated segmentation of the kidneys to provide an overall volume of each kidney, and semi-automated classification approaches to partition the kidney into the cortex and medulla to calculate cortex/medulla ratio.

Blood pressure and heart rate measurements at rest and in response to postural and mental challenges

The protocol to obtain BP and heart rate (HR) measurements at rest and in response to postural and mental challenges is carried out in a hospital setting and lasts 55 minutes (Figure 4.4). It includes posture and mental stress tests. The former consists of three consecutive 10-minute periods during which the subjects are supine, standing and sitting. The mental-stress test involves a sequence of 23 simple arithmetic problems presented each for 5 seconds, except for the first three problems that are each presented for 10 seconds. The problems are simple addition or subtraction equations followed by multiplication or division equations; the level of difficulty increases progressively during the test to ensure some failure for most subjects (McAdoo, Weinberg, Miller, Fineberg, & Grim, 1990). All answers are recorded.

During the cardiovascular protocol (Figure 4.4), BP and HR are measured (a) with an automated blood pressure monitor (Omron) at two time points when the subjects are resting in a sitting position and (b) with a Finometer™ (Finapres Medical Systems, Arnhem, The Netherlands) continuously, i.e., beat-to-beat, throughout the entire protocol. The Finometer is a non-invasive haemodynamic cardiovascular monitor based on the measurement of finger arterial pressure (Penaz, Voigt, & Teichmann, 1976). Using Beatscope software (Finapres Medical Systems, Arnhem, The Netherlands), the Finometer provides the following parameters at each beat: upstroke, systolic, diastolic and mean blood pressure, heart rate, inter-beat interval, stroke volume, cardiac output, ventricular ejection time, peripheral resistance, aortic impedance and aortic compliance. During the entire protocol, respiration rate is

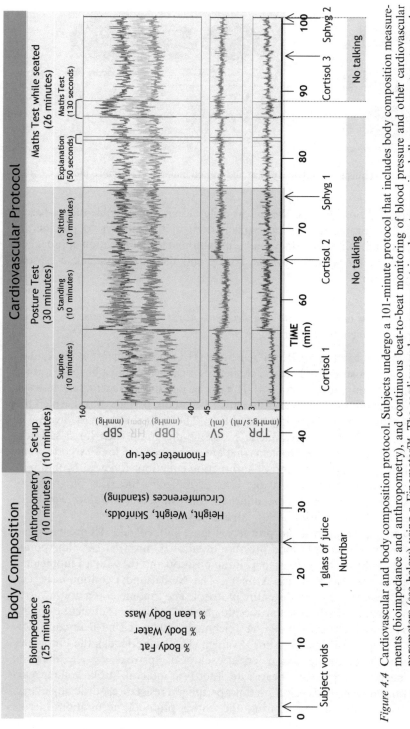

Figure 4.4 Cardiovascular and body composition protocol. Subjects undergo a 101-minute protocol that includes body composition measurements (bioimpedance and anthropometry), and continuous beat-to-beat monitoring of blood pressure and other cardiovascular parameters (see below) using a Finometer™. The cardiovascular component involves two main challenges: a posture test and a maths stress-test. SBP, systolic blood pressure; DBP, diastolic blood pressure; HR, heart rate; SV, stroke volume; TPR, total peripheral resistance; Sphyg 1, 2, additional measurements of blood pressure using a sphygmomanometer; Cortisol 1, 2, 3, samples of saliva obtained for cortisol measurements.

recorded with a sensor (Model 1132 Pneumotrace II Respiration Transducer, UFI, Morro Bay, CA, USA). In addition, salivary cortisol is measured at rest and in response to a change in posture and to mental stress (Roy, Kirschbaum, & Steptoe, 2001).

Power spectral analysis of continuous BP and HR data is used to evaluate the relative contributions of the sympathetic and parasympathetic nervous systems during posture and mental stress tests (Malpas, 2002; Parati et al., 1994; Persson et al., 2001). This analysis provides a means of separating sources of variance that can be distinguished in the frequency domain. Typically, fluctuations in the high-frequency (HF) band of the spectrum (0.15–0.40 Hz) reflect respiratory sinus arrhythmia and a vagal (parasympathetic) signal (Critchley et al., 2003). A low-frequency (LF) band (0.04–0.15 Hz) includes a signal of about 0.10 Hz, attributed to oscillations in the vasomotor (sympathetic) system; lower frequencies in this band (< 0.04 Hz) are thought to represent homeostatic processes (Mulder, 1988). The LF/HF ratio provides an index of autonomic balance; high and low values of this ratio indicate sympathetic nervous system and parasympathetic nervous system dominance, respectively.

Assessments of the quantity and distribution of body fat, energy intake and energy expenditure

The quantity and distribution of body fat is measured with anthropometry, bioelectrical impedance and MRI (described above). Anthropometry measurements include body weight, height, six circumferences (upper arm, waist, hips, proximal thigh, middle thigh and distal thigh) and five skinfolds (triceps, biceps, subscapular, suprailiac muscles and at the mid-thigh) (Pausova et al., 2000, 2001). Bioelectrical impedance measurements of total body fat, water and fat-free mass are obtained with a multi-frequency bio-impedance spectrum analysis. The analysis is carried out with the 4000B bio-impedance spectrum analyser (Xitron Technologies, Inc., San Diego, CA, USA). The analyser uses the measurement of whole body electrical impedance (Z) and its components: resistance (R) and reactance (Xc). These parameters are obtained with a four-electrode system attached to both the wrists and ankles when a small alternating current is passed through the body (Pausova et al., 2000).

Energy intake and expenditure are assessed with a 24-hour food recall interview, and food-frequency and physical activity questionnaires. The 24-hour food recall, conducted by a trained nutritionist, is employed to collect quantitative and qualitative information on foods and drinks that the subject has consumed during the past 24 hours. Volume models are used to estimate the size of food portions. This information is then used to compute calorie and nutrient (carbohydrates, fat, protein, vitamins and minerals) diet content with the Canadian Nutrient Data File (Health Canada, 2001) and the USDA Recipe File. The 24-hour food recall is complemented by a food-frequency questionnaire used by Santé Québec in its survey of Quebec children aged 6–16 years. A physical activity questionnaire evaluates the frequency with which they perform certain physical activities; the questions cover the number of physical activity sessions in a given week, as well as the number of days in a week where at least one physical activity session takes place. The scores are calculated by adding up the checkmarks to arrive at the number of "activity days" or the number of "activity sessions", including or excluding physical education classes.

Biochemical analyses of a fasting blood sample

In all adolescents, a fasting blood sample is drawn between 8 am and 9 am. This sample is used to evaluate (a) glucose and lipid metabolism (glucose, insulin, total cholesterol, LDL-cholesterol, HDL-cholesterol, triglycerides, free fatty acids, glycerol and apolipoproteins A, B, C and E), (b) pro-inflammatory and pro-thrombotic states (C-reactive protein and PAI-I), (c) the hypothalamic-pituitary-adrenal axis and sympathico-adrenal system (cortisol, epinephrine and norepinephrine), (d) sexual maturation (total and bio-available testosterone, oestradiol and leptin) and (e) current cigarette smoking (cotinine). The sample is also used for DNA extraction.

Web-based project management system

Various components of the project are carried out at different geographical locations. Thus, recruitment and phenotyping are done by four different groups operating in two cities in the SLSJ region (Chicoutimi and Jonquière). Overall coordination of the project and data analyses takes place in three countries (Canada, United Kingdom and United States). In order to manage smooth communication across the various project sites, we have implemented a number of web-based tools. The entire procedure manual is available on a password-protected web site. The manual contains a detailed version of the study flowchart (Table 4.2) and electronic versions (Word, PDF) of all instruments (e.g., consent and assent forms, questionnaires, instructions on how to administer various tests, data-entry forms, follow-up forms, etc.); a total of 107 individual documents are available in this electronic procedures manual.

The key element for the management of recruitment, screening and scheduling is the field module. This is a web-based system, developed with MySQL/ PHP programming tools; it allows a research nurse to track a subject through the different stages of the study, from recruitment to study completion. When the team receives the response card from an interested family, the family name and the telephone number are entered into the field module, and the family is assigned automatically an identification code (FAM9999). To ensure confidentiality, nominal information is restricted to local access (nurse) and is not accessible through the web. In order to proceed with the screening of families, this information is transferred electronically to the telephone interview software installed on stand-alone personal computers employed by research nurses.

The software guides the nurse through a structured interview with the parent; the generic text is tailored to each particular family by inserting automatically family-specific text (e.g., children's names) and skipping irrelevant questions based on the recorded answers. The first data-collection step in the interview identifies all biological children of the mother and their biological father. At this point, a six-digit identification code is assigned automatically to each family member; this code is combined with the family identification number assigned in the field module (see above). This combination of the family and subject identification numbers (e.g., FAM9999_888888) is carried together throughout the study. Information recorded during the telephone interview, together with the family and subject identification codes, is transferred electronically back to the field module. At this point, all nominal information is stripped away and denominalized data are released to the web-based part of the field module that is accessible to all members of the research team. From this point on, the field module is used to schedule home and hospital visits, neuropsychological testing and the school session; a list of participants ready to proceed with a particular phase of the study is available at all times and updated daily. At any point, different members of the phenotyping team are able to check which subjects have been scheduled for testing in their domain on a given day/week. Overall statistics are available to track the number of participants who have completed the various components of the study all the way to the disbursement of the subject fees and mailing of a neuropsychological report to the families. Tracking of data and data entry is an integral component of the system; this is described below.

Data entry, data transfer and quality control

The project database is a relational database developed with MySQL/PHP programming tools. Each participant (i.e., biological mother, biological father and all their biological children) is identified using a unique six-digit code assigned automatically by the telephone-interview software (see above); this subject code is always linked with a (biological) family code assigned automatically in the field module (see above). This combination of the family and subject identification (ID) number (e.g., FAM9999_888888) is entered on all paper forms (e.g., questionnaires and testing forms) and in the subject field of the various computer-based instruments (e.g., Finometer, MRI, neuropsychological tests). Given the variety of instruments, there are several modes of data entry (Table 4.2). Web-based manual data entry is employed for the majority of standardized neuropsychological tests and some other data-entry forms. Individual data-entry modules are available on a password-protected data-entry web site; write or read-only access is assigned per instrument to individual personnel. Graphical user interface (GUI) is designed (PHP/Java script) to mirror the actual layout of a given form; this facilitates data entry and reduces possible errors due to spatial incompatibilities between the GUI and the hardcopy. Each data-entry form begins with the subject identification; the operator is requested to enter both subject and family ID and the computer validates whether the combination of the two numbers (e.g., FAM9999 and 888888) is correct. This system minimizes the possibility of entering data under an incorrect ID number (e.g., FAM9999_898888). In addition to data entry, this module allows investigators to view and export (in text format) all entered data. Most of the questionnaires are entered using the Remark Office Optical Mark Recognition (OMR) software (www.PrincipiaProducts.com; Paoli, Pennsylvania, USA). This software is "designed to collect data from optical marks (bubbles, checkboxes) and bar-codes on plain paper forms. The software works in conjunction with an image scanner to collect the data" (Remark Office OMR, Version 5.5 for Windows, User's Guide, May 2002). The output forms generated by the Remark Office OMR software are uploaded to the project database, raw data are stored in questionnaire-specific tables and relevant scales are calculated and stored.

Magnetic resonance images are stored at the MR console in DICOM (Digital Imaging and Communication in Medicine; http://medical.nema.org) format (12 bits) and copied onto a compact disk. Using a secure file transfer protocol, DICOM images are then transferred into a dedicated MR database and converted into MINC (Medical Imaging NetCDF; http://www.bic.mni.mcgill.ca/software/minc/) format; this data format and an associated set of image-analysis tools and libraries represent the main platform used for an automatic analysis of MR images described above. All other electronic files collected using various computer programs (e.g., computer-based neuropsychological tests) or specialized hardware (e.g., Finometer, Bioimpedance) are stored in their proprietary format, copied onto a compact disk and uploaded to the project database using, again, a secure file transfer protocol. Using the data-tracking feature of the field module, a project coordinator is able to monitor the progress of data collection and check completion of data entry and transfer against the report of phenotyping completion for a given subject. In this way, missing datasets can be immediately traced and recovered. Finally, quality control is performed at different levels and includes certification of psychometricians (at start and once every year), a review of MR scans and all image-processing steps using a web-based interface, validation of data-entry fields using a range check at the data entry and upload levels, identification of outliers and cross-correlation of related questions in various questionnaires.

Statistical analyses

Here we highlight only the main principles that will guide statistical analyses of the entire dataset. These analyses will rely on the Generalized Estimating Equations (GEE) extension of the multiple linear regression for clustered data (Liang & Zeger, 1986). This methodology will allow us to account for:

(a) quantitative (continuous) measurement scales of primary and intermediary variables; (b) potential imbalances between exposed and non-exposed subjects in the distribution of characteristics related to the variables, such as duration of breastfeeding and second-hand smoke; and (c) a likely correlation between the variables within sib-pairs. Point (a) calls for statistical analyses designed for continuous, normally distributed data, such as linear regression analysis. Point (b) requires multivariable linear regression methods that will adjust the estimated PEMCS effect for potential confounding factors. Point (c) requires the GEE extension of the conventional multiple linear regression to account for the dependence of observations within sib-pairs. In GEE, we will assume the exchangeable covariance structure of the residuals, with just two observations per cluster, i.e., a pair of siblings (Jennrich & Schluchter, 1986).

The sample size of 500 sib-pairs (50% "exposed" and 50% "non-exposed") has been fixed on the basis of power calculations for genome-wide scan. Here, we focus on estimating the statistical power for testing our hypotheses, given this sample size. Specifically, we assessed the power to detect the "main effect" of PEMCS on the "primary outcome" and "intermediary/mechanistic" variables, and the ability of specific genes to modify this effect. The power of the latter, i.e., gene–exposure interactions, depends on (a) the impact of "exposure" (PEMCS) on the outcome, (b) the strength of the interaction, (c) the prevalence of the interacting gene and (d) the prevalence of exposure (which is fixed at 50% here) (Wang & Zhao, 2003). None of the published studies on the power testing of gene–exposure interactions deals with our specific context (GEE analyses of quantitative variables, while accounting for all the design parameters (a)–(d) (Garcia-Closas & Lubin, 1999; Gauderman, 2002; Gauderman, 2004; Hwang, Beaty, Liang, Coresh, & Khoury, 1994), therefore we have directly evaluated the power by a comprehensive simulation study (Leffondre, Abrahamowicz, & Siemiatycki, 2003) under a range of plausible assumptions. These simulations indicate that we will have adequate to excellent power to detect any, even very weak, impact of PEMCS on the "primary outcome" and "intermediary/mechanistic" variables, and also very good power to detect moderate interactions (increasing a strong PEMCS effect in the presence of a gene with the prevalence of 15–30%) and strong to very strong interactions (increasing a weak PEMCS effect by a factor of three to four in the presence of a less prevalent gene: 10–15%). The power will exceed 80% as long as the difference between "exposed" and "non-exposed" subjects in the mean values of the "primary outcome" and "intermediary/mechanistic" variables will correspond to at least 17% of the within-group standard deviation (SD). This implies that PEMCS explains as little as 3% of the total variance, which is considered a very small effect (Cohen, 1988). For example, if the SD for the body mass index (BMI) is 3 kg/m^2, then we have adequate power to detect an average increase of only $0.17 \times 3 = 0.51$ kg/m^2 in the PEMCS group. The power approaches 100% for any increase greater than 25% of SD.

Findings

As of October 2006, we have collected full datasets in 408 adolescents and 198 sets of their biological parents. In this section, we provide information on ascertainment, demographics of the exposed and non-exposed adolescents and their parents, and the initial data on cigarette smoking in adolescents and their parents.

Ascertainment

Between November 2003 and October 2006, the research team has approached a total of 9833 students. Table 4.4A provides statistics on the different stages of the recruitment. An overall response rate (i.e., number of returned response cards) was 19% and varied between 38% (School 1) and 6% (School 5); recruitment in School 8 was still in progress at the time of this evaluation. Of the number of returned response cards, 64% of families agreed to being contacted by the research nurse. Based on the telephone interview ($n = 768$), 37% of families were excluded for a variety of reasons: cigarette smoking 12 months before but not during pregnancy ($n = 104$), one of the two adolescents not interested ($n = 73$), child not of eligible age ($n = 75$), MR contraindications (braces: $n = 59$), other than French-Canadian origin ($n = 46$), medical reasons ($n = 42$; most common were heart abnormalities: 12, epilepsy: 6 and diabetes: 4), one parent not available ($n = 30$), twins ($n = 28$), premature birth ($n = 14$) and placental detachment/rupture ($n = 5$).

In the total of 423 eligible families, there were 229 (26%) exposed and 657 (73%) non-exposed adolescents eligible for the study. Note that the ratio of the exposed and non-exposed adolescents is similar to the population average

Table 4.4A Ascertainment (adolescents)

Students (number)	9833
Letter to parents (number)	9541
All response cards (number [%])	1806 [19]
Positive response cards (number [%])	1148 [64]
Positive response cards with two or more children (number [%])	826 [46]
Telephone interview (number)	767
Excluded families (number [%])	283 [37]
Eligible families (number [%])	423 [55]
Eligible adolescents (number)	896
Eligible adolescents (number [%]): exposed	229 [26]
Eligible adolescents (number [%]): non-exposed	657 [73]
Phenotyped (number)	408
Enrolled adolescents (number [%]): exposed	199 [49]
Enrolled adolescents (number [%]): non-exposed	209 [51]

of maternal cigarette smoking during pregnancy established in this region previously (Japel et al., 2000). Based on the information gathered during the telephone interview, we are able to compare the education level (elementary school, high school not completed, high school completed, college, university) across the different schools (Table 4.4B). Note that the schools differ significantly in the level of education attained by the mothers of their students; for example, more than 50% of mothers in School 2 (private school) attended a university, as compared with only 8% of mothers in Schools 6, 7 and 8. We then compared level of education of the mothers of exposed (n = 229) and non-exposed (n = 657) adolescents across all schools, with the following results: non-exposed (high school not completed, 5%; high school completed, 30%; college, 33%; university, 32%) and exposed (high school not completed, 15%; high school completed, 54%; college, 23%; university, 8%). As expected, there were highly significant (χ^2 = 38.2, p < .001) differences in the level of education attained by the mothers of exposed and non-exposed adolescents eligible for the study.

From the pool of all eligible families, we have matched (maternal education, school attended) 199 exposed and 209 non-exposed adolescents belonging to a total of 198 families. These subjects and families have completed the entire protocol and are considered below.

The exposure status and the number of cigarettes smoked during each pregnancy rely on information provided by the mother during the telephone interview; note that the research nurse first asks about cigarette smoking in general and only then about smoking during each of the pregnancies. For all subjects born in the two main hospitals in the region (Chicoutimi, 159 adolescents; Jonquiere, 140 adolescents), we have ventured to verify the mother's report by extracting relevant antenatal information from the medical chart completed during pregnancy (1st trimester, 73%; 2nd trimester, 7%; 3rd trimester, 20%). We were able to obtain relevant information in a total of 260 adolescents (87%), with an equal distribution across the exposed and non-exposed adolescents. To assess the overall agreement between the exposure

Table 4.4B Maternal education (all eligible subjects)

School	Elementary school (%)	High school: not completed (%)	High school: completed (%)	College (%)	University (%)	All mothers (n)
School 1	0	7	35	36	22	105
School 2	0	0	12	34	54	59
School 3	0	4	32	32	31	102
School 4	0	7	45	25	23	44
School 5	0	9	43	35	13	23
School 6	0	23	43	26	9	47
School 7	0	12	60	20	8	25
School 8	0	8	54	31	8	13

status ascertained antenatally from the medical records and by the maternal report during the telephone interview, we calculated Kappa statistics (range: −1 to +1) and found that, with a value of .69 ± .04, it indicates a "good" strength of agreement (Landis & Koch, 1977; good agreement: > .6 to ≤ .8). We observed the following discrepancies between the two sources of information. In the non-exposed group ($n = 126$), the medical records indicated that 120 mothers (95%) reported absence of smoking, 2 (1.5%) reported smoking and 4 (3%) said that they quit smoking. In the exposed group, the medical records indicated that 96 mothers (72%) reported smoking, 24 (18%) reported absence of smoking and 14 (10%) said that they quit smoking. Clearly, we see under-reporting of smoking in the medical records, as compared with the information volunteered by the mothers during the telephone interview 12–18 years later. This will be addressed in more detail below. In the subgroup that reported smoking in both the medical records and the telephone interview, and provided the number of cigarettes smoked per day on both occasions ($n = 88$), we found a moderate correlation in the number of cigarettes between the two time points ($r^2 = .11$, $p = .002$).

Demographics

The exposed and non-exposed groups do not differ in their mean age and sex distribution. All subjects are of French-Canadian origin and live within the region (98,709 km²). The two groups do not differ in the different measures of socio-economic status, including the level of maternal education (used for matching non-exposed adolescents to the exposed ones), level of employment of both parents and household income (Table 4.5A).

Pregnancy/parturition and medical and psychiatric history

Table 4.5B provides an overview of this domain. Duration of pregnancy did not differ between the two groups, but note that pregnancy shorter than 35 weeks was exclusionary. As expected, birth weight of the exposed offspring was lower compared to the non-exposed offspring by 291 g, or 8.5% ($p < .0001$; effect size defined as Cohen's $d = 0.6$). When comparing the difference between exposed and non-exposed subjects, the effect of exposure was similar in males ($d = 0.57$) and females ($d = 0.61$). In the exposed males, we observed a small but significant dose effect in that the number of cigarettes smoked during the 2nd trimester of pregnancy correlated negatively with the birth weight ($r^2 = .05$, $F(1,90) = 4.6$, $p = .04$). This was not the case in the exposed female subjects. Exposed adolescents were less likely to have been breastfed ($\chi^2 = 25.7$, $p < .0001$); when breastfed though, there were no group differences in the total duration of breastfeeding. Exposed adolescents were given other liquids ($F(1,400) = 5.6$, $p = .02$, $d = 0.23$) and other solids ($F(1,398) = 3.99$, $p = .05$, $d = 0.19$) a bit earlier than the non-exposed adolescents. The two groups were also comparable in the overall frequency of

Table 4.5 Results

	Non-exposed	Exposed	Mixed
	A. Demographics		
Ado: Age (M±SD [n])	14.5±1.87 [209]	14.7±1.86 [199]	N/A
Ado: Sex (F:M)	103:106	107:92	N/A
Female Ado: Menstruation (% menstruating)	84% (83/99)	83% (87/105)	N/A
Female Ado: Menarche (years; M±SD; [n])	11.8±1.4 [83]	12.1±1.4 [87]	N/A
Puberty (Tanner stage; M±SD; [n])	3.75±0.9 [191]	3.86±0.85 [173]	N/A
Sibship size (M±SD [n])	2.2±0.45 [89]	2.1±0.39 [82]	2.2±0.4 [24]
Mother: Age (M±SD [n])	42.01±3.65 [89]	41.6±3.6 [82]	41.7±3.8 [24]
Father: Age (M±SD [n])	44.8±3.8 [88]	43.96±3.3 [82]	44.4±4.5 [24]
A07f: Mother: Edu (M±SD [n])	3.3±0.9 [78]	3.3±0.8 [67]	3.7±0.9 [20]
A07f: Father: Edu (M±SD [n])	3.6±0.9 [74]	3.3±0.8 [66]	3.5±0.96 [19]
B09f: Mother: Edu (M±SD [n])	4.7±1.5 [82]	4.5±1.45[71]	5.5±1.4 [19]
B09f: Father: Edu (M±SD [n])	5.3±1.7 [77]	4.7±1.6 [66]	5.1±1.4 [19]
Mother: Employment (M±SD [n])	2.5±1.8 [86]	2.7±1.9 [81]	2.3±2.1 [24]
Father: Employment (M±SD [n])	1.6±1.6 [83]	1.7±1.6 [75]	1.3±1.3 [23]
Household income (in thousands CAD; M±SD [n])	54.9±21.4 [87]	51.7±25.4 [81]	59.2±18.5 [24]
Perceived economic situation (M±SD [n])	1.9±0.6 [84]	1.9±0.6 [75]	1.7±0.5 [23]
Number of children in household (M±SD [n])	2.46±0.7 [84]	2.3±0.6 [75]	2.4±0.8 [23]
Number of persons in household (M±SD [n])	4.57±0.9 [84]	4.3±0.8 [74]	4.5±1.03 [23]
	B. Pregnancy/birth and medical/psychiatric history		
Number of pregnancies (M±SD [n])	3.3±1.2 [89]	3.2±1.4 [81]	3.58±1.5 [24]
Number of spontaneous abortion /stillbirths (M±SD [n])	0.48±0.8 [89]	0.54±0.9 [81]	0.79±1.14 [24]
Pregnancy duration (weeks; M±SD [n])	39.1±1.6 [206]	39.2±1.5 [198]	N/A
Pregnancy/birth complications (M±SD [n])	0.28±0.5 [208]	0.26±0.5 [195]	N/A
Birth weight (g; M±SEM)	3530±468 [205][a]	3239±486 [195][a]	N/A
Breastfeeding: Frequency of yes [total n]	116 [206][a]	61 [195][a]	N/A
Breastfeeding: Total duration (age in weeks; M±SD [n])	18.6±16.3 [116]	15.2±12.3 [61]	N/A
Breastfeeding: First other milk (age in weeks; M±SD [n])	13.8±12.5 [116]	11.3±8.7 [61]	N/A
Breastfeeding: First other liquid (age in weeks; M±SD [n])	12.6±9.3 [208][a]	10.45±8.6 [193][a]	N/A
Breastfeeding: First solids (age in weeks; M±SD [n])	14.02±9.7 [208][a]	12.2±8.5 [191][a]	N/A

(*Continued overleaf*)

Table 4.5 Continued

	Non-exposed	Exposed	Mixed
Child's medical history: Positive answers (M±SD [n])	0.09±0.3 [208]	0.1±0.32 [195]	N/A
Ado: History of head trauma (frequency)	27/200	19/191	N/A
Ado: Psychiatric symptoms (sum of DPS symptoms)	15.5±11.5 [201][a]	18.8±12.8 [188][a]	N/A
Family's medical history, mother's side:			
Positive answers (M±SD [n])	3.7±2.01 [88]	3.2±2.2 [81]	3.04±2.2 [24]
Family's medical history, father's side:			
Positive answers (M±SD [n])	3.98±2.3 [88]	3.3±2.2 [81]	3.5±2.00 [24]
Mother's depression (M±SD [n])	16.25±4.0 [84]	17.1±4.0 [77]	17.04±5.4 [23]
Mother's anxiety (M±SD [n])	19.3±5.98 [84]	19.1±4.9 [77]	18.3±4.1 [23]
Father's depression (M±SD [n])	16.5±4.1 [82]	15.8±4.3 [73]	16.7±5.6 [23]
Father's anxiety (M±SD [n])	18.1±5.9 [82]	17.3±4.96 [73]	17.7±5.4 [23]
C. Anti-social behaviour			
Mother's anti-social behaviour in adolescence (M±SD [n])	0.13±0.4 [84][a]	0.36±0.6 [77][a]	0.17±0.4 [23][a]
Mother's anti-social behaviour in adulthood (M±SD [n])	0.05±0.26 [84]	0.05±0.28 [77]	0.04±0.21 [23]
Father's anti-social behaviour in adolescence (M±SD [n])	0.39±0.86 [82]	0.7±0.9 [73]	0.4±0.9 [23]
Father's anti-social behaviour in adulthood (M±SD [n])	0.16±0.46 [82]	0.24±0.6 [73]	0.13±0.46 [23]
Ado: Physical aggression (M±SD [n])	3.34±0.9 [200]	3.3±0.9 [181]	N/A
Ado: Indirect aggression (M±SD [n])	6.3±1.6 [200]	6.3±1.5 [181]	N/A
Ado: Fighting (M±Sd [n])	5.2±0.8 [200]	5.2±0.8 [181]	N/A
Ado: Stealing (M±SD [n])	4.6±1.4 [200]	4.7±1.4 [181]	N/A
Ado: Vandalism (M±SD [n])	2.1±0.4 [200]	2.2±0.6 [181]	N/A
D. Cigarette smoking			
Mother: Cig smoking during pregnancy (no. cig/day in 2nd trimester; M±SD [n])	0 [209]	11±6.7 [199]	N/A
Mother: Cig smoking during breastfeeding (no. cig/day; M±SD [n])	0	7.5±7.5 [65]	N/A
Mother: Age of onset for cig smoking (years; M±SD [n])	12.4±5.2 [35][a]	14.3±2.5 [59][a]	15.4±2.9 [14][a]
Mother: Negative life long history of cig smoking (no. of mothers [n])	45 [88][a]	0 [82][a]	0 [23][a]
Mother: Cig smoking at present (no. of mothers [n])	8 [88][a]	48 [82][a]	5 [23][a]

Mother: Cig smoking at present (no. cig/day; M±SD [n])	7±4.2 [8][a]	16.8±7.98 [48][a]	12.4±3.6 [5][a]
Father: Cig smoking at present, frequency (Yes [total n])	17 [82][a]	32 [73][a]	3 [23][a]
Father: Cig smoking at present (no. cig/day; M±SD [n])	8.4±9.8 [17][a]	20.5±10.8 [32][a]	11.7±7.6 [3][a]
Father: Cig smoking during pregnancy, frequency (Yes [total n])	52 [193][a]	102 [178][a]	N/A
Father: Cig smoking during pregnancy (no. cig/day; M±SD [n])	17±6.3 [52][a]	20±7.4 [102][a]	N/A
Father: Age of onset for cig smoking (years, M±SD [n])	15.9±2.6 [47]	14.9±2.8 [57]	15.1±2.7 [15]
Father: Negative life long history of cig smoking (no. cig/day; M±SD [n])	33 [82][a]	14 [73][a]	8 [23][a]
Ado: Negative life history of cig smoking (no. Ado/n)	140/200	115/178	N/A
Ado: Cig smoking at present (no. Ado/n)	23 [200]	30 [178]	N/A
Ado: Cig smoking over last 30 days (No cig/day; M±SD [n])	2.1±0.9 [16][a]	2.5±0.8 [28][a]	N/A
Ado: Age of onset for cig smoking (years; M±SD [n])	12.2±2.1 [60]	12.5±2.4 [64]	N/A

Notes: Ado, adolescents; M, mean; SD, standard deviation; F, female; M, male; CAD, Canadian dollars; Exposed, all children exposed to maternal cigarette smoking during pregnancy; Non-exposed, no children exposed; Mixed, some children exposed, some non-exposed.
[a] Statistically significant differences between the groups (see results for details).

positive answers to various questions related to the children's medical history.

As for the mental health of the parents at the time of the home visit, we found no significant group differences on the scales of depression and anxiety reported by the mothers and fathers in the Mental Health and Anti-social Behaviour questionnaire. We have observed no differences in the current anti-social behaviour (Table 4.5C) of the mothers and fathers, but we found a slightly higher score on the scale of anti-social behaviour during adolescence in mothers of exposed vs. non-exposed adolescents ($F(3,188) = 2.95$, $p = .03$, $d = 0.38$).

Cigarette smoking

Table 4.5D provides a summary of our findings in this domain. By definition, mothers of exposed adolescents smoked during pregnancy while the mothers of non-exposed subjects did not. As a group, the mothers reported smoking an average of 11 ± 6.7 cigarettes per day during the 2nd trimester (range: 1–42; quartiles: 1–6, 7–10, 11–15, > 15 cigarettes per day). A significant number of mothers of non-exposed adolescents never smoked in their life (51%). On the other hand, many more mothers of exposed (vs. non-exposed) adolescents smoke at present ($c^2 = 52.2, p < .0001$). When smoking, the number of cigarettes smoked per day at present is higher in the mothers of exposed vs. mothers of non-exposed adolescents ($F(3,61) = 5.6, p = .002, d = 1.23$) and, in the mothers of exposed subjects, it is similar to the number of cigarettes smoked during pregnancy ($r^2 = .47, p < .0001$).

Given the under-reporting of smoking during pregnancy in the medical records, we decided to compare the subgroups of mothers of exposed adolescents. Based on their statements during the visit to their obstetricians, we classified them into the following three groups: Smoking ($n = 96$), Not Smoking ($n = 24$) and Quit Smoking ($n = 14$). The three groups differ in the following respects. The number of cigarettes smoked during the 2nd trimester (as reported during the telephone interview) is different ($F(2,133) = 3.6$, $p = .03$), with the following means ± SD: Smoking, 12.3 ± 6.9; Not Smoking, 9.4 ± 7.2; and Quit Smoking, 8.2 ± 3.3 cigarettes per day. On the other hand, the three subgroups do not differ from each other in the proportion of current smokers (Smoking, 46%; Not Smoking, 50%; Quit Smoking, 70%; as compared with mothers of non-exposed adolescents, 6%) or in the number of cigarettes smoked per day at present (Smoking, 8.1 ± 0.8; Not Smoking, 8.2 ± 1.5; Quit Smoking, 9.2 ± 1.97; as compared with mothers of non-exposed adolescents, 0.42 ± 0.7 cigarettes per day). Finally, we observed a trend towards differences across the three subgroups of mothers in their rate of current depressive symptoms ($F(2,128) = 1.6, p = .2$; Smoking, 16.9 ± 3.8; Not Smoking, 17.9 ± 4.3; Quit Smoking, 18.9 ± 5.2; as compared with the mothers of non-exposed adolescents, 16.3 ± 4.2) and their anti-social behaviour during adolescence ($F(2,128) = 1.3, p = .3$; Smoking, 0.37 ± 0.05; Not Smoking, 0.23 ± 0.11; Quit Smoking, 0.14 ± 0.14; as compared with the mothers of non-exposed adolescents, 0.11 ± 0.05).

A significantly higher number of fathers of non-exposed (vs. exposed) adolescents never smoked in their life ($\chi^2 = 12.1, p = .01$). On the other hand, fathers of exposed (vs. non-exposed) adolescents are more likely to smoke at present ($\chi^2 = 13.7, p = .003$), and smoke more cigarettes per day ($F(3,53) = 5.5, p = .002, d = 1.12$). Furthermore, they were also more likely to smoke during their partner's pregnancy ($\chi^2 = 35.2, p < .001$) and, when smoking, smoked more cigarettes per day ($F(1,153) = 6.2, p = .01, d = 0.41$).

In the adolescents, the initial findings suggest group differences in cigarette smoking in that there is a trend towards a higher number of exposed (vs. non-exposed) adolescents smoking at present ($\chi^2 = 2.2, p = .1$), with the difference approaching significance in males ($\chi^2 = 3.3, p = .07$) but not females. Similarly, there is a trend towards a higher number of cigarettes smoked by the exposed (vs. non-exposed) adolescents during the last 30 days ($F(1,43) = 1.96$, $p = .2, d = 0.44$), with the difference being significant in males ($F(1,21) = 11.4$, $p = .003, d = 1.4$) but not in females.

Discussion

The main purpose of this chapter is the description of the Saguenay Youth Study. Nonetheless, the few initial findings mentioned here are largely consistent with the existing literature. For example, birth weight of offspring born to mothers who smoked during pregnancy, as compared with the non-exposed control group, is lower by 8.5% (291 g). Note, however, that we have not adjusted our data using any of the possible confounding variables and/or corrected for within-sibling similarity; this will be done in the upcoming detailed reports of our findings. For the same reason, we should not over-interpret the initial observations of possibly higher levels of cigarette smoking in the male adolescents exposed (vs. non-exposed) prenatally to maternal cigarette smoking; note that these offspring are also exposed to a greater extent to paternal cigarette smoking at present.

One of the possible limitations of the Saguenay Youth Study is the retrospective nature of our questionnaire-based assessments of perinatal events, most importantly the exposure to maternal cigarette smoking during pregnancy. But, as concluded by Rice, Harold and Thapar (2006) in their recent paper on the reliability of maternal reports of various perinatal events, "mothers can provide accurate reports in comparison to information from medical records". In their study, which compared medical records with questionnaire-based maternal reports obtained 4–9 years later, Kappa statistics varied between "very good" for smoking during pregnancy (Kappa = .81) and "poor" for alcohol during pregnancy (Kappa = .17). For the birth weight, the correlation between the two time points was excellent ($r = 0.99$). In our study, Kappa statistics for smoking during pregnancy were comparable to the Rice et al. (2006) findings (Kappa = .69); after excluding the mothers who claimed that they quit smoking when talking to their physicians ($n = 18$), Kappa increased to .79 ($n = 242$). Mothers who claimed that they were not smoking or quit smoking when interviewed by their physician during pregnancy, but who reported smoking during pregnancy when interviewed by our research nurse 12–18 years later, did not differ from other mothers of the exposed adolescents in variables such as the maternal age, maternal education, current smoking status and the number of cigarettes smoked at present, or their anti-social behaviour during adolescence. They did report fewer cigarettes smoked during pregnancy; whether this is a true reflection of their intention to smoke less during pregnancy or a reporting bias remains unclear. Importantly, the birth weight of their children was not different from the birth weight of the children born to mothers who reported smoking at both time points; it was lower than that of the non-exposed adolescents. Overall, we conclude that information about the exposure status obtained by a research nurse 12–18 years after pregnancy is reliable and, given the similarities between the mothers of exposed adolescents with the different smoking status in the medical records, we believe that our assessment is probably more accurate than that based on the medical records.

Nonetheless, we will be able to analyse our data with and without adolescents born to the mothers who provided discordant information about cigarette smoking during pregnancy at the two time points.

We will now discuss several general features of the Saguenay Youth Study, focusing on the following aspects of its design: quantitative assessment of multiple complex traits in seemingly unrelated domains (e.g., brain anatomy and cardiovascular reactivity), genetic strategies, an adolescent population and involvement of several disparate disciplines (e.g., sociology and anatomy). We will discuss these features, pointing out their respective strengths and weaknesses, as well as practical issues related to their implementation.

The study has been designed to investigate consequences of prenatal exposure to maternal cigarette smoking in four major domains, namely brain structure, brain function, cardiovascular health and metabolic health. Quantitative assessment of multiple phenotypes in these domains occurs in several sessions and takes, on average, 7 hours per adolescent. Each adolescent spends an additional 4 hours completing various self-report measures. What are the advantages and disadvantages of such an extensive phenotyping effort? The single most important advantage of this strategy is the opportunity to evaluate interactions between different systems of the human body in the same group of individuals. For example, do certain personality traits affect cardiovascular reactivity? Can we identify brain regions that differ in their morphological features in relation to cardiovascular reactivity and/or personality? Furthermore, quantification of multiple phenotypes will facilitate the identification of variables that mediate or moderate a particular effect. For example, is the hypothesized difference between exposed and non-exposed adolescents in the quantity of body fat mediated or moderated by birth weight? Finally, the use of questionnaire-based measures of family environment and various events that occurred in the individual's life will allow us to evaluate possible effects of confounding variables such as second-hand smoke, socio-economic disadvantage, current nutrition and breastfeeding and child-rearing practices. There is, however, a cost of collecting such a large dataset. This includes the burden put on the participants, and the time and funds needed to complete the project. Our initial experience suggests that most families who committed to the participation found the load acceptable; following the home visit, only eight subjects did not complete the entire protocol.

Inclusion of the genetic component in the Saguenay Youth Study is motivated conceptually by the emerging view in which the expression of a given phenotype is determined by a combination of environmental and genetic factors (Caspi et al., 2003; Pausova et al., 1999; Rice et al., 2007; Thapar et al., 2005; Wang et al., 2002). Identifying genes that modulate individuals' response to prenatal exposure to maternal cigarette smoking should also provide the initial pointers vis-à-vis possible molecular pathways, and hence possible mechanisms, mediating such effects. The family-based design involving sibships (full phenotyping and genotyping) and their parents (partial phenotyping and full genotyping) will allow us to carry out genome-wide linkage and association analyses, and identify regions of the genome not necessarily predicted by previous knowledge. At the same time, candidate-gene studies can also be used to test specific hypotheses. The reduced genetic heterogeneity of a geographically isolated population should increase the power of these analyses, as the number of genes involved in determining individual complex traits is expected to be lower in this population than in multi-ethnic populations (e.g., Montreal metropolitan area). The overall advantage of the genetic approach is the control of yet another variable – the genome – that may explain some of the variance in the studied phenotypes. Disadvantages of this approach, other than its additional cost, include organizational demands associated with the siting of the study in a specific geographical location and a selective recruitment (siblings only).

The full phenotype is being acquired in adolescents 12–18 years of age. Adolescence is a highly dynamic period of human development during which the children's brains and bodies adopt adult roles. It is also a time when adolescents begin to make their own choices affecting their health: sexual behaviour, eating habits, physical activity, consumption of alcohol, cigarette smoking and the use of recreational drugs, to name but a few. What are the factors determining such choices? The relatively comprehensive design of the Saguenay Youth Study and its large sample size ($n = 1000$) should provide a suitable platform for predicting variance in a particular phenotype, such as blood pressure, cardiovascular reactivity and school performance, using multiple independent variables capturing the individual's environment and life habits, his/her genetic background and the state of other organs (e.g., fat metabolism, brain morphology). The structure and function of the adolescent's organs are less likely to be affected by a disease process that requires treatment, a situation quite common in adults; this minimizes possible confounding effects of medication. Furthermore, recent epidemiological studies suggest that processes underlying the development of common disorders may be emerging as early as in adolescence. Some of them have been attributed to the increasing incidence of obesity in this age category. Obesity is a major risk factor for metabolic syndrome, which is a cluster of metabolic, cardiovascular and inflammatory abnormalities that contribute to the development of disorders such as diabetes mellitus, hypertension, stroke and ischaemic heart disease. In a recent American study of 4- to 20-year-old obese individuals (Weiss et al., 2004), it has been estimated that almost 50% of obese children and adolescents fulfil the criteria of having metabolic syndrome. Moreover, they showed that each component of the syndrome worsens with increasing adiposity and that these associations are independent of age, gender and pubertal status. They estimated that for each half-unit increase in BMI, the risk of metabolic syndrome increases by 1.55% (Weiss et al., 2004). Thus, considering that the prevalence of cigarette smoking during pregnancy is still high and that PEMCS may be an important risk factor for obesity and associated metabolic and cardiovascular disorders, *in utero* exposure to maternal cigarette

102 Paus et al.

smoking may represent a major public health problem in adolescence, a critical period during which meaningful prevention strategies are still possible.

The comprehensive design of the Saguenay Youth Study requires input from many disparate disciplines, such as medicine, computer science, bio-informatics and statistics, physics, psychology and sociology. Although the different conceptual background of investigators working in the respective fields often hampers the initial communication and the setting of common goals, the richness of the various approaches and tools benefits the pro-gramme at the end. To succeed, individual investigators must be willing to adapt their approaches to fit the overall design. For example, questionnaires must be designed in a way that maximizes collection of quantitative data based on an individual (e.g., a composite index of academic achievement) rather than a group (e.g., frequency of individuals with a particular grade in maths), or MR acquisition protocols must be robust to allow for a consistent collection of images over a long period of time (e.g., 5 years) at the expense, perhaps, of fine-tuning the acquisition as new sequences are developed. As the data become available, the biggest challenge is faced by colleagues working at the interface between data processing (bioinformatics, computer science, statistics) and their biological interpretation (genetics, psychology, sociology, medicine). In our view, this challenge can be best met by having a core group of investigators working in the same physical location for an extended period of time.

Overall, we hope that the above description of the Saguenay Youth Study will be helpful to colleagues interested in similar studies of environmental and genetic factors influencing human health.

Acknowledgements

This project is supported by the Canadian Institutes of Health Research (to TP and ZP, who are equal contributors to this chapter and co-directors of the Saguenay Youth Study), the Heart and Stroke Foundation of Quebec (ZP) and the Canadian Foundation for Innovation (ZP). We thank the fol-lowing individuals for their contributions in designing the protocol and acquiring and analysing the data: MR technicians (Sylvie Masson, Suzanne Castonguay, Julien Grandisson, Marie-Josée Morin), cardio nurses (Jessica Blackburn, Mélanie Gagné, Jeannine Landry, Lisa Pageau, Réjean Savard, Jacynthe Tremblay), psychometricians (Chantale Belleau, Mélanie Drolet, Catherine Harvey, Stéphane Jean, Mélanie Tremblay), ÉCOBES team (Julie Auclair, Marie-Ève Blackburn, Marie-Ève Bouchard, Annie Houde, Catherine Lavoie), nutritionists (Caroline Benoit and Henriette Langlais), laboratory technicians (Denise Morin and Nadio Mior), Dr Michel Bérubé, Julie Bérubé, Celine Bourdon, Rosanne Aleong, Dr Jennifer Barrett, Candice Cartier, Valerie Legge, Helena Jelicic and Dale Einarson.

References

Achenbach, T. M. (1999). The Child Behavior Checklist and related instruments. In M. E. Maruish (Ed.), *The use of psychological testing for treatment planning and outcomes assessment* (2nd ed., pp. 429–466). Mahwah, NJ: Lawrence Erlbaum Associates, Inc.

Ashburner, J., & Friston, K. J. (2000). Voxel-based morphometry – the methods. *Neuroimage, 11*, 805–821.

Bada, H. S., Korones, S. B., Perry, E. H., Arheart, K. L., Pourcyrous, M., Runyan, J. W. 3rd, et al. (1990). Frequent handling in the neonatal intensive care unit and intraventricular hemorrhage. *Journal of Pediatrics, 117*(1 Pt 1), 126–131.

Baumgardner, T. L., Singer, H. S., Denckla, M. B., Rubin, M. A., Abrams, M. T., Colli, M. J., & Reiss, A. L. (1996). Corpus callosum morphology in children with Tourette syndrome and attention deficit hyperactivity disorder. *Neurology, 47*(2), 477–482.

Behar, L., & Stringfield, S. (1974). A behavior rating scale for the preschool child. *Developmental Psychology, 10*, 601–640.

Bélanger, P. W., & Rocher, G. (1972). Le projet de recherche: Étude des aspirations scolaires et des orientations professionnelles des étudiants (ASOPE). *L'Orientation Professionnelle, 8*, 114–127.

Benson, P. L., Leffert, N., Scales, P. C., & Blyth, D. A. (1998). Beyond the "village" rhetoric: Creating healthy communities for children and adolescents. *Applied Developmental Science, 2*, 138–159.

Beratis, N. G., Panagoulias, D., & Varvarigou, A. (1996). Increased blood pressure in neonates and infants whose mothers smoked during pregnancy. *Journal of Pediatrics, 128*, 806–812.

Blake, K. V., Gurrin, L. C., Evans, S. F., Beilin, L. J., Landau, L. I., Stanley, F. J., & Newnham, J. P. (2000). Maternal cigarette smoking during pregnancy, low birth weight and subsequent blood pressure in early childhood. *Early Human Development, 57*, 137–147.

Bookstein, F. L., Sampson, P. D., Streissguth, A. P., & Connor, P. D. (2001). Geometric morphometrics of corpus callosum and subcortical structures in the fetal-alcohol-affected brain. *Teratology, 64*(1), 4–32.

Brennan, P. A., Grekin, E. R., & Mednick, S. A. (1999). Maternal smoking during pregnancy and adult male criminal outcomes. *Archives of General Psychiatry, 56*, 215–219.

Breslau, N., & Chilcoat, H. D. (2000). Psychiatric sequelae of low birth weight at 11 years of age. *Biological Psychiatry, 47*, 1005–1011.

Buchanan, C. M., & Holmbeck, G. N. (1998). Measuring beliefs about adolescent personality and behavior. *Journal of Youth and Adolescence, 27*, 607–627.

Caspi, A., Sugden, K., Moffitt, T. E., Taylor, A., Craig, I. W., Harrington, H., et al. (2003). Influence of life stress on depression: moderation by a polymorphism in the 5-HTT gene. *Science, 301*, 386–389.

Cocosco, C. A., Zijdenbos, A. P., & Evans, A. C. (2003). A fully automatic and robust MRI tissue classification method. *Medical Imaging Analysis, 7*, 513–527.

Cohen, J. (1988). *Statistical power analysis for the behavioral sciences.* Hillsdale, NJ: Lawrence Erlbaum Associates, Inc.

Collins, D. L., Holmes, C. J., Peters, T. M., & Evans, A. C. (1995). Automatic 3D model-based neuroanatomical segmentation. *Human Brain Mapping, 3*, 190–208.

Collins, D. L., Neelin, P., Peters, T. M., & Evans, A. C. (1994). Automatic 3D intersubject registration of MR volumetric data in standardized Talairach space. *Journal of Computer-Assisted Tomography, 18*, 192–205.

Connor, S. K., & McIntyre, L. (1998). *How tobacco and alcohol affect newborn children.* http://www.hrdc-drhc.gc.ca/arb/nlscy-elnej/w-98-34es-e.pdf.

Cornelius, M. D., Leech, S. L., Goldschmidt, L., & Day, N. L. (2000). Prenatal tobacco exposure: Is it a risk factor for early tobacco experimentation? *Nicotine and Tobacco Research, 2*, 45–52.

Costa, P. T. Jr., & McCrae, R. M. (1992). *NEO Personality Inventory-Revised (NEO PI-R).* Odessa: Psychological Assessment Resources, Inc.

Critchley, H. D., Mathias, C. J., Josephs, O., O'Doherty, J., Zanini, S., Dewar, B. K., et al. (2003). Human cingulate cortex and autonomic control: Converging neuroimaging and clinical evidence. *Brain, 126*, 2139–2152.

De Braekeleer, M. (1991). Hereditary disorders in Saguenay-Lac-St-Jean (Quebec, Canada). *Human Heredity, 41*, 141–146.

De Braekeleer, M., Mari, C., Verlingue, C., Allard, C., Leblanc, J. P., Simard, F., et al. (1998). Complete identification of cystic fibrosis transmembrane conductance regulator mutations in the CF population of Saguenay-Lac-Saint-Jean (Quebec, Canada). *Clinical Genetics, 53*, 44–46.

Dominguez, R., Aguirre Vila-Coro, A., Slopis, J. M., & Bohan, T. P. (1991). Brain and ocular abnormalities in infants with in utero exposure to cocaine and other street drugs. *American Journal of Diseases of Children, 145*(6), 688–695.

Dousset, V., Grossman, R. I., Ramer, K. N., Schnall, M. D., Young, L. H., Gonzales-Scarano, F., et al. (1992). Experimental allergic encephalomyelitis and multiple sclerosis: Lesion characterization with magnetization transfer imaging. *Radiology, 182*(2), 483–491.

Ebrahim, S. H., Decoufle, P., & Palakathodi, A. S. (2000). Combined tobacco and alcohol use by pregnant and reproductive-aged women in the United States. *Obstetrics and Gynecology, 96*, 767–771.

Eisenberg, N., Fabes, R. A., Murphy, B. C., Karbon, M., Smith, M., & Maszk, P. (1996). The relations of children's dispositional empathy-related responding to their emotionality. *Developmental Psychology, 32*, 195–209.

Enquête Nationale sur la Santé de la Population (National Population Health Survey). http://www.statcan.ca/english/concepts/nphs/nphs1.htm; http://www.phac-aspc.gc.ca/dca-dea/7-18yrs-ans/hbschealth_e.html

Eriksen, W. (1996). Breastfeeding, smoking and the presence of the child's father in the household. *Acta Paediatrica, 85*, 1272–1277.

Evans, A. C., Collins, D. L., Mills, S. R., Brown, E. D., Kelly, R. L., & Peters, T. M. (1993). 3D statistical neuroanatomical models from 305 MRI volumes. In *Proceedings of the IEEE-Nuclear Science Symposium and Medical Imaging Conference* (pp. 1813–1817). Piscataway, NJ: Institute of Electrical and Electronics Engineers.

Falk, L., Nordberg, A., Seiger, A., Kjaeldgaard, A., & Hellstrom-Lindahl, E. (2005). Smoking during early pregnancy affects the expression pattern of both nicotinic and muscarinic acetylcholine receptors in human first trimester brainstem and cerebellum. *Neuroscience, 132*, 389–397.

Fischl, B., & Dale, A. M. (2000). Measuring the thickness of the human cerebral cortex from magnetic resonance images. *Proceedings of the National Academy of Sciences of the USA, 97*, 11050–11055.

Freund, A. M., & Bates, P. B. (2002). Life-management strategies of selection, optimization and compensation: Measurement by self-report and construct validity. *Journal of Personality and Social Psychology, 82*, 642–662.

Fried, P. A. (1995). Prenatal exposure to marihuana and tobacco during infancy, early and middle childhood: Effects and an attempt at synthesis. *Archives of Toxicology Supplement, 17*, 233–260.

Galland, O. (1994). Âge et valeurs. In H. Riffault (Ed.), *Les valeurs des Français* (pp. 251–296). Paris: Presses Universitaires de France.

Gallistel, C. R., & Gelman, I. I. (2000). Non-verbal numerical cognition: From reals to integers. *Trends in Cognitive Science, 4*(2), 59–65.

Garcia-Closas, M., & Lubin, J. (1999). Power and sample size calculations in case-control studies of gene–environment interactions: Comments on different approaches. *American Journal of Epidemiology, 149*, 689–692.

Gass, A., Barker, G. J., Kidd, D., Thorpe, J. W., MacManus, D., Brennan, A., et al. (1994). Correlation of magnetization transfer ratio with clinical disability in multiple sclerosis. *Annals of Neurology, 36*(1), 62–67.

Gauderman, W. (2002). Sample size requirements for matched case-control studies of gene–environment interaction. *Statistics in Medicine, 21*, 35–50.

Gauderman, W. (2004). Sample size requirements for matched case-control studies of gene–gene interaction. *American Journal of Epidemiology, 155*, 478–484.

Giedd, J. N., Castellanos, F. X., Casey, B. J., Kozuch, P., King, A. C., Hamburger, S. D., & Rapoport, J. L. (1994). Quantitative morphology of the corpus callosum in attention deficit hyperactivity disorder. *American Journal of Psychiatry, 151*(5), 665–669.

Gradie, M. I., Jorde, L. B., & Bouchard, G. (1988). Genetic structure of the Saguenay, 1852–1911: Evidence from migration and isonymy matrices. *American Journal of Physical Anthropology, 77*, 321–333.

Grompe, M., St-Louis, M., Demers, S., Al-Dhalimy, M., Leclerc, B., & Tanguay, R. (2004). A single mutation in the fumaryl acetoacetate hydrolase gene in French Canadians with hereditary tyrosinemia type I. *New England Journal of Medicine, 331*, 353–357.

Guimond, J., Meunier, A., & Thirion, J.-P. (2000). Average brain models: A convergence study. *Computer Vision and Image Understanding, 77*, 192–210.

Harter, S. (1983). *Supplementary description of the Self-Perception Profile for Children: Revision of the Perceived Competence Scale for Children.* Unpublished manuscript, University of Denver, CO.

Health Canada (1995). *Fact Sheet 4. Smoking behaviour of women – November 1994.* Survey on Smoking in Canada, Cycle 3 Ottawa: Health Canada.

Health Canada (2001). http://www.hc-sc.gc.ca/fn-an/nutrition/fiche-nutri-data/

Hill, P. D., & Aldag, J. C. (1960). Smoking and breastfeeding status. *Research in Nursing Health, 19*, 125–132.

Huang, W. L., Harper, C. G., Evans, S. F., Newnham, J. P., & Dunlop, S. A. (2001). Repeated prenatal corticosteroid administration delays myelination of the corpus callosum in fetal sheep. *International Journal of Developmental Neuroscience, 19*(4), 415–425.

Hwang, S., Beaty, T., Liang, K., Coresh, J., & Khoury, M. (1994). Minimum sample size estimation to detect gene–environment interaction in case-control designs. *American Journal of Epidemiology, 140*, 1029–1037.

Hynd, G. W., Semrud-Clikeman, M., Lorys, A. R., Novey, E. S., Eliopulos, D., &

Lyytinen, H. (1991). Corpus callosum morphology in attention deficit-hyperactivity disorder: Morphometric analysis of MRI. *Journal of Learning Disability*, *24*(3), 141–146.

Institute de la Statistique du Québec (2001). *L'enquête sociale et de santé 1998*. Division Santé Québec, Collection la santé et le bien-être. Sainte-Foy: Publications du Québec.

Janosz, M., Lacroix, M., & Rondeau, N. (1999). *A decisional balance measure for assessing school disengagement in adolescence*. Presented at the biennal meeting of the Society for Research in Child Development (SRCD), Albuquerque, NM.

Japel, C., Tremblay, R. E., & McDuff, P. (2000). Parent's health and social adjustment, Part I – Lifestyle habits and health status. In *Longitudinal Study of Child Development in Québec (ÉLDEQ 1998–2002)* (Vol. 1, No. 9). Québec: Institute de la Statistique du Québec.

Jennrich, R., & Schluchter, M. (1986). Unbalanced repeated-measures models with structured covariance matrices. *Biometrics*, *42*, 805–820.

Kallen, K. (2000). Maternal smoking during pregnancy and infant head circumference at birth. *Early Human Development*, *58*(3), 197–204.

Kandel, D. B., & Udry, J. R. (1999). Prenatal effects of maternal smoking on daughters' smoking: nicotine or testosterone exposure? *American Journal of Public Health*, *89*(9), 1377–1383.

Kendrick, J. S., & Merritt, R. K. (1996). Women and smoking: An update for the 1990s. *American Journal of Obstetric Gynecology*, *175*, 528–535.

Kramer, M. S. (2000). Invited commentary: association between restricted fetal growth and adult chronic disease: Is it causal? Is it important? *American Journal of Epidemiology*, *152*, 605–608.

LeBlanc, M. (1996). *MASPAQ: Mesures de l'adaptation sociale et personnelle pour les adolescents québécois. Manuel et guide d'utilisation 3ᵉ édition*. Montréal: École de Psychoéducation, Groupe de Recherche sur les Adolescents en Difficulté, Université de Montréal.

LeBlanc, M., & Tremblay, R. E. (1988). A study of factors associated with the stability of hidden delinquency. *International Journal of Adolescence and Youth*, *1*, 269–292.

Landis, J. R., & Koch, G. G. (1977). The measurement of observer agreement for categorical data. *Biometrics*, *33*, 159–174.

Larose, S., & Boivin, M. (1998). Attachment to parents, social support expectations, and socioemotional adjustment during the high school–college transition. *Journal of Research on Adolescence*, *8*, 1–27.

Lassen, K., & Oei, T. P. (1998). Effects of maternal cigarette smoking during pregnancy on long-term physical and cognitive parameters of child development. *Addictive Behaviors*, *23*(5), 635–653.

Leffert, N., Benson, P. L., Scales, P. C., Sharma, A. R., Drake, D. R., & Blyth, D. A. (1998). Developmental assets: Measurement and prediction of risk behaviors among adolescents. *Applied Developmental Science*, *2*, 209–230.

Leffondre, K., Abrahamowicz, M., & Siemiatycki, J. (2003). Evaluation of Cox's model and logistic regression for matched case-control data with time-dependent covariates: A simulation study. *Statistics in Medicine*, *22*, 3781–3794.

Le Goualher, G., Procyk, E., Collins, D. L., Venugopal, R., Barillot, C., & Evans, A. C. (1999). Automated extraction and variability analysis of sulcal neuroanatomy. *IEEE Transactions on Medical Imaging*, *18*, 206–217.

Lerch, J., & Evans, A. C. (2004). Cortical thickness analysis examined through power analysis and a population simulation. *Neuroimage, 24*(1), 163–173.

Lerner, R. M., Lerner, J. V., Almerigi, J., Theokas, C., Phelps, E., Gestsdottir, S., et al. (2005). Positive youth development, participation in community youth development programs and contributions of fifth grade adolescents: Findings from the first wave of the 4-h study of positive youth development. *Special Issue of the Journal of Early Adolescence, 25*(1).

Levitt, P. (1998). Prenatal effects of drugs of abuse on brain development. *Drug and Alcohol Dependency, 51*(1–2), 109–125.

Liang, K., & Zeger, S. (1986). Longitudinal data analysis using generalized linear models. *Biometrics, 73*, 13–22.

Lichtensteiger, W., Ribary, U., Schlumpf, M., Odermatt, B., & Widmer, H. R. (1988). Prenatal adverse effects of nicotine on the developing brain. *Progress in Brain Research, 73*, 137–157.

Lindhout, D., Omtzigt, J. G., & Cornel, M. C. (1992). Spectrum of neural-tube defects in 34 infants prenatally exposed to antiepileptic drugs. *Neurology, 42*(4, Suppl. 5), 111–118.

Lockhart, D. J., Dong, H., Byrne, M. C., Follettie, M. T., Gallo, M. V. C. M. S., Mittmann, M., et al. (1996). Expression monitoring by hybridization to high-density oligonucleotide arrays. *Nature Biotechnology, 14*, 1675–1680.

Loiselle, J. (2000). *Enquête québécoise sur le tabagisme chez les élèves du secondaire (Rep. No. 1)*. Québec, QC, Canada: Institute de la Statistique du Québec.

Lucas, C. P., Zhang, H., Fisher, P. W., Shaffer, D., Regier, D. A., Narrow, W. E., et al. (2001). The DISC Predictive Scales (DPS): Efficiently screening for diagnoses. *Journal of the American Academy of Child and Adolescent Psychiatry, 40*, 443–449.

MacArthur, C., Knox, E. G., & Lancashire, R. J. (2001). Effects at age nine of maternal smoking in pregnancy: Experimental and observational findings. *BJOG: an International Journal of Obstetrics and Gynaecology, 108*(1), 67–73.

MacDonald, D., Kabani, N., Avis, D., & Evans, A. C. (2000). Automated extraction of inner and outer surfaces of cerebral cortex from MRI. *Neuroimage, 11*, 564–574.

Malo, J., & Tremblay, R. E. (1995). Rates of precocity of sexual intercourse among adolescents of disadvantaged sections of the population. *Contraception Fertilite Sexualite, 23*, 545–551.

Malpas, S. C. (2002). Neural influences on cardiovascular variability: Possibilities and pitfalls. *American Journal of Physiology, Heart Circulation Physiology, 282*, H6–H20.

Mangin, J. F., Riviere, D., Cachia, A., Duchesnay, E., Cointepas, Y., Papadopoulos-Orfanos, D., et al. (2004). A framework to study the cortical folding patterns. *Neuroimage, 23*(Suppl. 1), S129–S138.

McAdoo, W. G., Weinberger, M. H., Miller, J. Z., Fineberg, N. S., & Grim, C. E. (1990). Race and gender influence hemodynamic responses to psychological and physical stimuli. *Journal of Hypertension, 8*(10), 961–967.

Mendelson, B. K., Mendelson, M. J., & White, D. R. (2001). Body-esteem scale for adolescents and adults. *Journal of Personality Assessment, 76*, 90–106.

Milberger, S., Biederman, J., Faraone, S. V., & Jones, J. (1998). Further evidence of an association between maternal smoking during pregnancy and attention deficit hyperactivity disorder: Findings from a high-risk sample of siblings. *Journal of Clinical Child Psychology, 27*(3), 352–358.

108   *Paus et al.*

Montgomery, S. M., & Ekbom, A. (2002). Smoking during pregnancy and diabetes mellitus in a British longitudinal birth cohort. *British Medical Journal, 324,* 26–27.

Morley, R., Payne, C. L., & Lucas, A. (1995). Maternal smoking and blood pressure in 7.5 to 8 year old offspring. *Archives of Disease in Childhood, 72,* 120–124.

Mulder, L. J. M. (1988). *Assessment of cardiovascular reactivity by means of spectral analysis.* Dissertation. Groningen: Rijksuniversiteit Groningen.

Newman, J. P., Patterson, C. M., & Kosson, D. S. (1987). Response perseveration in psychopaths. *Journal of Abnormal Psychology, 96,* 145–148.

Ntamakiliro, L., Monnard, I., & Gurtner, J.-L. (2000). Mesure de la motivation scolaire des adolescents: Construction et validation de trois échelles complémentaires. *L'Orientation Scolaire et Professionnelle, 29*(4), 673–693.

Obel, C., Henriksen, T. B., Hedegaard, M., Secher, N. J., & Ostergaard, J. (1998). Smoking during pregnancy and babbling abilities of the 8-month-old infant. *Paediatric and Perinatal Epidemiology, 12*(1), 37–48.

Offord, D. R., Boyle, M. H., Szatmari, P., Rae-Grant, N. I., Links, P. S., Cadman, D. T., et al. (1987). Ontario Child Health Study. II. Six-month prevalence of disorder and rates of service utilization. *Archives of General Psychiatry, 44,* 832–836.

Ojima, K., Abiru, H., Matsumoto, H., & Fukui, Y. (1996). Effects of postnatal exposure to cocaine on the development of the rat corpus callosum. *Reproductive Toxicology, 10*(3), 221–225.

Olds, D. L., Henderson, C. R. Jr., & Tatelbaum. R. (1994). Intellectual impairment in children of women who smoke cigarettes during pregnancy. *Pediatrics, 93*(2), 221–227.

Orlebeke, J. F., Knol, D. L., & Verhulst, F. C. (1999). Child behavior problems increased by maternal smoking during pregnancy. *Archives of Environmental Health, 54,* 15–19.

O'Sullivan, M. J., Kearney, P. J., & Crowley, M. J. (1996). The influence of some perinatal variables on neonatal blood pressure. *Acta Paediatrica, 85,* 849–853.

Paquette, D., & Morrisson, D. (1999). *Un profil descriptif de 100 mères adolescentes: étude préliminaire dans le cadre du projet la Mère veille.* [A descriptive profile of 100 adolescent mothers: Preliminary study]. Montréal: Institute de Recherche pour le Développement Social des Jeunes.

Parati, G., Ravogli, A., Frattola, A., Groppelli, A., Ulian, L., Santucciu, C., & Mancia, G. (1994). Blood pressure variability: Clinical implications and effects of antihypertensive treatment. *Journal of Hypertension, 12,* S35–S40.

Paus, T., Collins, D. L., Evans, A. C., Leonard, G., Pike, B., & Zijdenbos, A. (2001). Maturation of white matter in the human brain: A review of magnetic-resonance studies. *Brain Research Bulletin, 54,* 255–266.

Pausova, Z., Deslauriers, B., Gaudet, D., Tremblay, J., Kotchen, T. A., Larochelle, P., et al. (2000). Role of tumor necrosis factor-alpha gene locus in obesity and obesity-associated hypertension in French Canadians. *Hypertension, 36*(1), 14–19.

Pausova, Z., Gaudet, D., Gossard, F., Bernard, M., Kaldunski, M. L., Jomphe, M., et al. (2005). Genome-wide scan for linkage to obesity-associated hypertension in French Canadians. *Hypertension, 46,* 1280–1285.

Pausova, Z., Gossard, F., Gaudet, D., Tremblay, J., Kotchen, T. A., Cowley, A. W., & Hamet, P. (2001). Heritability estimates of obesity measures in siblings with and without hypertension. *Hyptertension, 38*(1), 41–47.

Pausova, Z., Paus, T., Sedova, L., & Berube, J. (2003). Prenatal exposure to nicotine modifies kidney weight and blood pressure in genetically susceptible rats: A case of gene–environment interaction. *Kidney International, 64*, 829–835.

Pausova, Z., Tremblay, J., & Hamet, P. (1999). Gene–environment interactions in hypertension. *Current Hypertension Reports, 1*, 42–50.

Penaz, J., Voigt, A., & Teichmann, W. (1976). Contribution to the continuous indirect blood pressure measurement. *Zeitschrift fuer die Gesamte Innere Medizin, 31*, 1030–1033.

Persson, P. B., DiRenzo, M., Castiglioni, P., Pagani, M., Honzikova, N., Akselrod, S., & Parati, G. (2001). Time versus frequency domain techniques for assessing baroreflex sensitivity. *Journal of Hypertension, 19*, 1699–1705.

Petersen, A. C., Crockett, L., Richards, M., & Boxer, A. (1988). A self-report measure of pubertal status: Reliability, validity, and initial norms. *Journal of Youth and Adolescence, 17*, 117–133.

Petrides, M., & Milner, B. (1982). Deficits on subject-ordered tasks after frontal- and temporal-lobe lesions in man. *Neuropsychologia, 20*, 249–262.

Pike, G. B. (1996). Pulsed magnetization transfer contrast in gradient echo imaging: A two-pool analytic description of signal response. *Magnetic Resonance in Medicine, 36*(1), 95–103.

Pike, G. B., De Stefano, N., Narayanan, S., Worsley, K. J., Pelletier, D., Francis, G. S., et al. (2000). Multiple sclerosis: Magnetization transfer MR imaging of white matter before lesion appearance on T2-weighted images. *Radiology, 215*(3), 824–30.

Pollak, S. D., & Kistler, D. J. (2002). Early experience is associated with the development of categorical representations for facial expressions of emotion. *Proceedings of the National Academy of Science of the USA, 99*, 9072–9076.

Power, C., & Jefferis, B. (2002). Fetal environment and subsequent obesity: A study of maternal smoking. *International Journal of Epidemiology, 31*, 413–419.

Radloff, L. S. (1977). The CES-D scale: A self-report depression scale for research in general population. *Applied Psychological Measurement, 1*, 385–401.

Räsänen, P., Hakko, H., Isohanni, M., Hodgins, S., Järvelin, M. R., & Tiihonen, J. (1999). Maternal smoking during pregnancy and risk of criminal behavior among adult male offspring in the Northern Finland 1966 Birth Cohort. *American Journal of Psychiatry, 156*, 857–862.

Rice, F., Harold, G. T., & Thapar, A. (2006). The effect of birth-weight with genetic susceptibility on depressive symptoms in childhood and adolescence. *European Child and Adolescent Psychiatry, 15*, 383–391.

Rice, F., Lewis, A., Harold, G., van den Bree, M., Boivin, J., Hay, D. F., et al. (2007). Agreement between maternal report and antenatal records for a range of pre and peri-natal factors: The influence of maternal and child characteristics. *Early Human Development, 83*(8), 497–504.

Riley, E. P., Mattson, S. N., Sowell, E. R., Jernigan, T. L., Sobel, D. F., & Jones, K. L. (1995). Abnormalities of the corpus callosum in children prenatally exposed to alcohol. *Alcoholism: Clinical and Experimental Research, 19*(5), 1198–1202.

Robins, L. N., Helzer, J. E., Croughan, J., & Ratcliff, K. S. (1981). National Institute of Mental Health Diagnostic Interview Schedule. Its history, characteristics, and validity. *Archives of General Psychiatry, 38*, 381–389.

Roebuck, T. M., Mattson, S. N., & Riley, E. P. (1998). A review of the neuroanatomical findings in children with fetal alcohol syndrome or prenatal exposure to alcohol. *Alcoholism: Clinical and Experimental Research, 22*(2), 339–344.

Rosenberg, M., Schooler, C., Schoenbach, C., & Rosenberg, F. (1995). Global self-esteem and specific self-esteem: Different concepts, different outcomes. *American Sociological Review, 60*(1), 141–156.

Rosenthal, D., Gurbey, R., & Moore, S. (1981). From trust to intimacy: A new inventory for examining Erikson's stages of psychosocial development. *Journal of Youth and Adolescence, 10*, 525–535.

Roy, M. P., Kirschbaum, C., & Steptoe, A. (2001). Psychological, cardiovascular, and metabolic correlates of individual differences in cortisol stress recovery in young men. *Psychoneuroendocrinology, 26*, 375–391.

Roy, R., Bouchard, G., & Declos, M. (1991). La premiere generation de Saguenayens. In G. Bouchard & M. De Braekeleer (Eds.), *Histoire d'un genome* (pp. 164–186). Quebec: Presses de l'Universite du Quebec.

Roy, T. S., Andrews, J. E., Seidler, F. J., & Slotkin, T. A. (1998). Nicotine evokes cell death in embryonic rat brain during neurulation. *Journal of Pharmacology and Experimental Therapeutics, 287*(3), 1136–1144.

Roy, T. S., & Sabherwal, U. (1994). Effects of prenatal nicotine exposure on the morphogenesis of somatosensory cortex. *Neurotoxicology and Teratology, 16*(4), 411–421.

Roy, T. S., & Sabherwal, U. (1998). Effects of gestational nicotine exposure on hippocampal morphology. *Neurotoxicology and Teratology, 20*(4), 465–473.

Rutter, M. (1967). A children's behaviour questionnaire for completion by teachers: Preliminary findings. *Journal of Child Psychology and Psychiatry, 8*, 1–11.

Scales, P. C., Benson, P. L., Leffert, N., & Blyth, D. A. (2000). Contribution of developmental assets to the prediction of thriving among adolescents. *Applied Developmental Science, 4*, 27–46.

Schludermann, E., & Schludermann, S. (1970). Replicability of factors in children's reports of parent behavior (CRPBI). *Journal of Psychology, 76*, 239–249.

Séguin, J. R., Freeston, M. H., Tarabulsy, G. M., Zoccolillo, M., Tremblay, R. E., & Carbonneau, R. (2000, June). *Développement des comportements anxieux au préscolaire: De nouvelles mesures et influences familiales.* Presented at the annual meeting of Québec's Mental Health Network, Montréal, Canada.

Selzer, M. L. (1971). Michigan alcoholism screening test – quest for a new diagnostic instrument. *American Journal of Psychiatry, 127*, 1653.

Semrud-Clikeman, M., Filipek, P. A., Biederman, J., Steingard, R., Kennedy, D., Renshaw, P., & Bekken, K. (1994). Attention-deficit hyperactivity disorder: Magnetic resonance imaging morphometric analysis of the corpus callosum. *Journal of the American Academy of Child and Adolescent Psychiatry, 33*(6), 875–881.

Severson, H. H., Andrews, J. A., Lichtenstein, E., Wall, M., & Zoref, L. (1995). Predictors of smoking during and after pregnancy: A survey of mothers of newborns. *Preventive Medicine, 24*(1), 23–28.

Slotkin, T. A. (1998). Fetal nicotine or cocaine exposure: Which one is worse? *Journal of Pharmacology and Experimental Therapeutics, 85*, 931–945.

Small, S. A., & Kerns, D. (1993). Unwanted sexual activity among peers during early and middle adolescence: Incidence and risk factors. *Journal of Marriage and the Family, 55*, 941–952.

Small, S. A., & Rodgers, K. B. (1995). *Teen Assesment Project (TAP) Survey Question Bank.* Madison, WI: University of Wisconsin-Madison.

Snijder, M. B., Visser, M., Dekker, J. M., Seidell, J. C., Fuerst, T., Tylavsky, F., et al. (2002). The prediction of visceral fat by dual-energy X-ray absorptiometry in the elderly: A comparison with computed tomography and antropometry. *International Journal of Obesity*, *26*, 984–993.

Sowell, E. R., Mattson, S. N., Thompson, P. M., Jernigan, T. L., Riley, E. P., & Toga, A. W. (2001). Mapping callosal morphology and cognitive correlates: Effects of heavy prenatal alcohol exposure. *Neurology*, *57*, 235–244.

Statistics Canada (2000). *Youth In Transition Survey (YITS)*. http://www.pisa.gc.ca/t-00-5e.pdf

Steinberg, L. (2002). *Resistance to Peer Pressure (RPI) Scale. Instrument developed for the MacArthur Juvenile Adjudicative Competence Study*. Unpublished measure available from the author, Department of Psychology, Temple University.

Stephan, K. M., Binkofski, F., Halsband, U., Dohle, C., Wunderlich, G., Schnitzler, A., et al. (1999). The role of ventral medial wall motor areas in bimanual co-ordination. A combined lesion and activation study. *Brain*, *122*, 351.

Stroop, J. R. (1935). Studies of interference in serial verbal reactions. *Journal of Experimental Psychology*, *18*, 643–662.

Swayze, V. W. 2nd, Johnson, V. P., Hanson, J. W., Piven, J., Sato, Y., Giedd, J. N., et al. (1997). Magnetic resonance imaging of brain anomalies in fetal alcohol syndrome. *Pediatrics*, *99*(2), 232–240.

Talairach, J., & Tournoux, P. (1988). *Co-planar stereotaxic atlas of the human brain*. New York: Thieme Medical Publishers.

Talcott, J. B., Witton, C., McLean, M. F., Hansen, P. C., Rees, A., Green, G. G., & Stein, J. F. (2000). Dynamic sensory sensitivity and children's word decoding skills. *Proceedings of the National Academy of Sciences of the USA*, *97*(6), 2952–2957.

Thapar, A., Langley, K., Fowler, T., Rice, F., Turic, D., Whittinger, N., et al. (2005). Catechol O-methyltransferase gene variant and birth weight predict early-onset antisocial behavior in children with attention-deficit/hyperactivity disorder. *Archives of General Psychiatry*, *62*, 1275–1278.

Theokas, C., Almerigi, J. B., Lerner, R. M., Dowling, E. M., Benson, P. L., Scales, P. C., & von Eye, A. (2005). Conceptualizing and modeling individual and ecological asset components of thriving in early adolescence. *Journal of Early Adolescence*, *25*(1), 113–143.

The Stationery Office (2002). *Infant Feeding Survey 2000*. London: The Stationery Office.

Toschke, A. M., Montgomery, S. M., Pfeiffer, U., & von Kries, R. (2003). Early intrauterine exposure to tobacco-inhaled products and obesity. *American Journal of Epidemiology*, *158*, 1068–1074.

Vaillancourt, T., Brendgen, M., Boivin, M., & Tremblay, R. E. (2003). A longitudinal confirmatory factor analysis of indirect and physical aggression: Evidence of two factors over time? *Child Development*, *74*, 1628–1638.

Von Kries, R., Toschke, A. M., Koletzko, B., & Slikker, W. Jr. (2002). Maternal smoking during pregnancy and childhood obesity. *American Journal of Epidemiology*, *156*, 954–961.

Wakschlag, L. S., Lahey, B. B., Loeber, R., Green, S. M., Gordon, R. A., & Leventhal, B. L. (1997). Maternal smoking during pregnancy and the risk of conduct disorder in boys. *Archives of General Psychiatry*, *54*, 670–676.

Wang, S., & Zhao, H. (2003). Sample size needed to detect gene–gene interactions using associated design. *American Journal of Epidemiology*, *158*, 899–914.

Wang, X., Zuckerman, B., Pearson, C., Kaufman, G., Chen, C., Wang, G., et al.

(2002). Maternal cigarette smoking, metabolic gene polymorphism, and infant birth weight. *JAMA, 287,* 195–202.

Wideroe, M., Vik, T., Jacobsen, G., & Bakketeig, L. S. (2003). Does maternal cigarette smoking during pregnancy cause childhood overweight? *Paediatric and Perinatal Epidemiology, 17,* 171–179.

Weir, K., & Duveen, G. (1981). Further development and validation of the prosocial behaviour questionnaire for use by teachers. *Journal of Child Psychology and Psychiatry, 22,* 357–374.

Weiss, R., Dziura, J., Burgert, T., Tamborlane, W. V., Taksali, S. E., Yeckel, C. W., et al. (2004). Obesity and the metabolic syndrome in children and adolescents. *New England Journal of Medicine, 35,* 2362–2374.

Weissman, M. M., Wickramaratne, P. J., & Kandel, D. B. (2000). Maternal smoking during pregnancy and psychopathology in offspring followed to adulthood. *Journal of the American Academy of Child and Adolescent Psychiatry, 38,* 892–899.

Williams, S., & Poulton, R. (1999). Twins and maternal smoking: Ordeals for the fetal origins hypothesis? A cohort study. *British Medical Journal, 318,* 1–5.

Wolff, S. D., & Balaban, R. S. (1989). Magnetization transfer contrast (MTC) and tissue water proton relaxation in vivo. *Magnetic Resonance in Medicine, 10*(1), 135–44.

Zijdenbos, A. P., Forghani, R., & Evans, A. C. (2002). Automatic "pipeline" analysis of 3D MRI data for clinical trials: Application to multiple sclerosis. *IEEE Transactions on Medical Imaging, 21,* 1280–1291.

Zoccolillo, M., Price, R. K., Ji, T., & Hwu, H.-G. (1999). Antisocial personality disorder: Comparisons of prevalence, symptoms, and correlates in four countries. In P. Cohen, C. Slomkowski, & L. L. L. Robins (Eds.), *Historical and geographic effects on psychopathology* (pp. 249–277). Hillsdale, NJ: Lawrence Erlbaum Associates, Inc.

5 The development of chronic physical aggression[1]

Genes and environments matter from the beginning

Richard E. Tremblay

As medicine is now practised it contains little that is very useful; but without any desire to depreciate, I am sure that there is no one, even among professional men, who will not declare that all we know is very little as compared with that which remains to be known; and that we might escape an infinity of diseases of the mind, no less than of the body, and even perhaps from the weakness of old age, if we had sufficient knowledge of their causes, and all the remedies with which nature has provided.

(Descartes, 1637/1982)

Descartes obviously anticipated the important progress of medicine for physical health over the four centuries that followed. However, the progress for the "diseases of the mind", which some of us now call "diseases of the brain", has been much less important. The brain is clearly a more complex organ than the heart and the kidneys. Part of this complexity is the fact that it is the central regulator of Descartes' human machine. Diseases of the brain can affect physical health as well as social behaviour. The World Health Organization recently reminded us that physical violence is a social behaviour that has an impact on physical health and can be caused by mental health problems (Krug, Dahlberg, Mercy, Zwi, & Lozano, 2002).

The aim of this chapter is to summarize recent research on the development of physical aggression, on the causes of chronic physical aggression, and on its prevention. It is well-known by criminologists that the risk of committing a physically violent crime is highest from middle adolescence to early adulthood. This was first shown in the early 19th century by Adolphe Quetelet, a Belgian astronomer and mathematician, who was also a statistician, epidemiologist, and developmentalist (Figure 5.1). Because adult violence is generally linked to a history of youth violence (McCord, Widom, & Cromwell, 2001), and because all adults are former youth, one would expect that reducing youth violence would also reduce adult violence. Thus, the reduction of youth violence should in the long run have a very large impact on total violence in a given society.

114   *Tremblay*

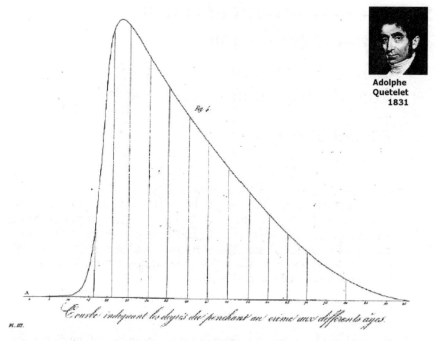

Figure 5.1 Quetelet's age–crime curve published in 1831.

Recently, the World Health Organization published a report on Violence and Health that concluded: "The majority of young people who become violent are adolescent-limited offenders who, in fact, show little or no evidence of high levels of aggression or other problem behaviours during their child-hood." (Krug et al., 2002, p. 31). This conclusion was following the footsteps of a Surgeon General (US) 2001 report, based almost exclusively on the analysis of physical violence during adolescence. Indeed, most criminological studies of youth violence have focused on 12- to 18-year-old youth. During this period they become stronger physically, their cognitive competence increases (e.g., they are better at hiding their intentions), they become sexually mature, they ask and obtain a greater freedom to use their time without adult supervision, and they have access to more resources such as money and transportation, which increases their capacity to satisfy their needs.

This rapid bio-psychosocial development might be sufficient to explain why adolescence is a period of life when there are more opportunities and motives for antisocial behaviour. Adolescents lack experience and feel pres-sured to choose a career, or to perform in school, within their peer groups, or with possible sexual partners. These factors, and many others, may explain why, compared to adults, proportionally more adolescents and young adults resort to violent behaviour.

Although a majority of adolescents will commit some delinquent acts, most of these are minor legal infractions. Population-based surveys have systematically shown that a small proportion of adolescents (approximately 6%) account for the majority of violent acts and arrests (McCord et al., 2001). The challenge is to explain why some adolescents and some adults frequently resort to physically aggressive behaviour while others do not. Although they are relatively small in number, they frighten a large part of the population, and they represent a heavy burden of suffering for their victims, their families, and themselves. Adolescents with behavioural problems are also much more likely to be unemployed, suffer poor physical health, or have mental health problems.

Physical aggression during middle childhood

Over the past 22 years I have been following the development of thousands of children from school entry to early adulthood to try to understand the early development of these serious behaviour problems. With my colleague from Carnegie-Mellon University in Pittsburg (Nagin & Tremblay, 1999) we described the developmental trajectories of teacher-rated physical aggression in a sample of boys from poor socio-economic areas in Montreal. Those boys were assessed regularly from kindergarten to high school (Figure 5.2): 17% of the boys appeared never to have been physically aggressive; 4% showed a high frequency of physical aggression from 6 to 15 years of age; 28% started with a high level of physical aggression at age 6 and became less and less physically aggressive with time; while the majority (52%) had a low level of physical aggression at age 6 and also became less and less aggressive with time.

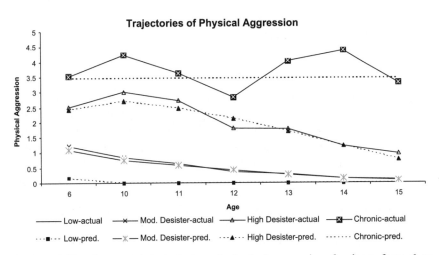

Figure 5.2 Developmental trajectories of physical aggression for boys from 6 to 15 years of age (Nagin & Tremblay, 1999).

In contrast to hypotheses concerning late onset of antisocial behaviour, we did not find any group of boys in which there appeared to be an "onset" and maintenance of high levels of physical aggression for a significant number of years after age 6. Self-report data during adolescence show that some individuals increase their frequency of physical aggression during adolescence. This can be seen especially with those who were already on a high trajectory of physical aggression during childhood. These boys are creating the famous peak in the age–crime curve (Farrington, 1987; Laub & Sampson, 2003; Quetelet, 1833/1984; Sampson & Laub, 2003), mainly because they are more likely to get arrested for physical aggressions as they grow taller and stronger. The same physical assault done by the same boy at 11 and 17 will be followed by a very different police reaction. There is a small group of boys who appear to start to use physical aggression during adolescence, but the frequency of use remains below the frequency of the worst cases before they reached adolescence. There are two other important observations from these studies. First, the boys on the high physical aggression trajectory during childhood are the most likely to be arrested and convicted of physical violence during adolescence and early adulthood (Broidy et al., 2003; Nagin & Tremblay, 1999). Second, the boys on the chronic physical aggression trajectory had the highest frequency of physical aggression during their kindergarten year (Nagin & Tremblay, 2001). They also observed that for every group of boys the peak level for frequency of physical aggression was during the first year of the study when they were in kindergarten.

These results clearly challenge the idea that the frequency of acts of physical aggression increases with age through social learning or because of hormonal changes during adolescence. They also challenge the notion that there is a significant group of children who show chronic physical aggression during late childhood or adolescence after having successfully inhibited physical aggression throughout childhood. However, they beg the question, when do children learn to aggress physically?

Early childhood physical aggression

There are surprisingly few longitudinal studies that have tried to chart the development of physical aggression during the preschool years. This lack of attention to physical aggression during the early years appears to be the result of a long-held belief that physical aggression appears during late childhood and early adolescence as a result of bad peer influences, television violence, and increased levels of male hormones. This view of antisocial development was very clearly described approximately 250 years ago by Jean-Jacques Rousseau. The first phrase of his book on child development and education, *Émile*, makes the point very clearly: "Everything is good as it leaves the hands of the author of things; everything degenerates in the hands of man." (Rousseau, 1762/1979). A few pages later he is still more explicit and appears to be writing the agenda for 20th-century research on the development of antisocial behaviour: "There is no original sin in the human heart, the how and why of the entrance of every vice can be traced." Rousseau's strong stance was in clear opposition to Hobbes, who, a century earlier, described infants as selfish machines striving for pleasure and power, and declared: "It is evident therefore that all men (since all men are born as infants) are born unfit for society; and very many (perhaps the majority) remain so throughout their lives, because of mental illness or lack of discipline . . . Therefore man is made fit for Society not by nature, but by training." (Hobbes, 1647/1998).

This debate has far-reaching consequences, not only for child development investigators and educators, but also for political scientists, philosophers, and policy makers. Because the underlying debate is clearly grounded in our views of human nature, it is not surprising that investigators are likely to prefer the "origin of aggressive behaviour" that best fits their view of human nature, and their political commitment. However, since most political philosophers appear to agree that society must be built on the natural tendencies of man, it is surprising that research on early childhood development has not been a priority for the social sciences.

Recent longitudinal studies starting around birth are showing that there is more to the weakling's aggressions than the disciples of Rousseau could imagine. Within a longitudinal study of a large sample of babies born in the Canadian province of Quebec in the mid-1990s, we asked mothers to rate the frequency of physical aggressions at ages 17 and 30 months and, at both times, to indicate at what age the child had started to show such behaviour. At age 17 months, close to 90% of the mothers reported that their child, at least sometimes, was physically aggressive toward others. One of the interesting results of that study is the fact that mothers who were reporting that their 17-month-old child had started to hit others in the previous months appeared to have forgotten this early onset, since they were reporting that at age 30 months their child had started to hit others after 17 months of age. This memory failure as children grow older, taller, and bigger could in part explain why parents of physically aggressive adolescents report that the aggression problems started only a year or two before (Loeber & Stouthamer-Loeber, 1998).

The long-term follow-up of this cohort, as well as two others from Canada and the United States, shows that most children substantially increase the frequency of physical aggressions from 9 to 48 months (Tremblay et al., 2004), and then decrease the frequency of use until adolescence (Côté, Vaillancourt, LeBlanc, Nagin, & Tremblay, 2006; NICHD-ECCR, 2004). Figure 5.3 shows the different developmental trajectories of physical aggression from 2 to 11 years of age for a random sample of Canadian children ($N = 10,658$) first assessed in 1994. We clearly see that the frequency of physical aggressions among children decreases substantially from the preschool years to pre-adolescence, except for a small group who use physical aggression most often throughout that period.

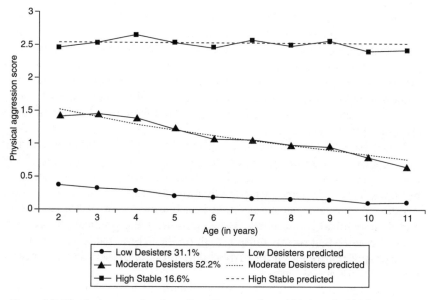

Figure 5.3 Physical aggression from 2 to 11 years of age (Côté et al., 2006).

Studies of antisocial behaviour during adolescence and pre-adolescence show that family characteristics and parental behaviour are good predictors of antisocial behaviour (McCord et al., 2001). Is this also true for preschool children on trajectories of chronic physical aggression? First, because one needs a target to physically aggress, the best predictor is having an older sibling. Parent separation before birth and low income, two of the classic family risks, also predict high physical aggression during early childhood. It will be no surprise that mothers' characteristics before birth are among the best predictors: frequent antisocial behaviour during adolescence, giving birth before 21 years of age, not having finished high school, and smoking during pregnancy. Smoking apparently affects the development of the brain (e.g., Huijbregts, Séguin, Zoccolillo, Boivin, & Tremblay, 2008; Wakschlag, Pickett, Cook, Benowitz, & Leventhal, 2002). Of course, males were more at risk than females of being on the high physical aggression trajectory, even when the assessment started at 17 months of age (see Chapter 7 of this book). After controlling for prenatal assessments, the assessments that were done 5 months after birth revealed two significant predictors: family dysfunction and coercive-hostile parenting by the mothers. Thus, the traditional predictors of adolescent antisocial behaviour are predicting chronic physical aggression during the preschool years. Interestingly, a twin study also shows that at 17 months of age more than half of the variation in frequency of physical aggression is explained by genetic factors (Dionne, Tremblay, Boivin, Laplante, & Pérusse, 2003).

Genetics and physical aggression development

Onset of physical aggression and individual differences

The longitudinal data on physical aggression from infancy onwards, summarized in the previous section, indicate that physical aggression is not a behaviour that children learn, like reading or writing, nor an illness that children "catch", like poliomyelitis or smallpox. It is rather a behaviour like crying, eating, grasping, throwing, and running, which young humans do when the physiological structure is in place. The young human learns to regulate these "natural" behaviours with age, experience, and brain maturation. The learning to control process implies regulating your needs to adjust to those of others, and this process is generally labelled "socialization".

It is not hard to imagine why the evolutionary process would have given humans a genetic programme coding for all the basic mechanisms in order to react to hunger and to threat. Young children's muscles are activated to run, push, kick, grab, hit, throw, and yell with extreme force when hungry, when angry, or when they are strongly attracted by something. However, stating that humans are genetically programmed to be able to physically aggress when needed is different from stating that the frequency of the physical aggressions they use is genetically programmed. Since all 18-month-olds who have developed normally can, and possibly do, physically aggress but not all do so at the same frequency and with the same vigour, to what extent are these individual differences due to the genetic programme they have inherited or to the environment in which they have been growing?

The trajectories shown in Figures 5.2 and 5.3 clearly indicate that these individual differences exist at any given point, starting in early childhood; but the most interesting phenotype is the development over time. There is obviously intra-individual change over time. Most children learn to reduce the frequency of the use of a behaviour that they apparently did not need to learn. However, relatively stable differences among individuals remain. What are the gene–environment mechanisms that explain the change and stability? They are possibly very similar to the mechanisms that explain the developmental trajectories of growth in height. Genes code for the growth mechanisms, but there are individual differences in these codings, as well as environmental, differences (e.g., access to food) that lead to stable individual differences. Thus the individual differences in the frequency of physical aggression at one point in time, and over time, can be due to a large number of "causes", e.g., to individual differences in the genetic coding for serotonin (Pihl & Benkelfat, 2005), testosterone (Van Goozen, 2005), language development (Dionne, 2005), or cognitive development (Séguin & Zelazo, 2005), or to environmental differences such as mother's tobacco use during pregnancy (Wakschlag et al., 2002), birth complications (Arseneault, Tremblay, Boulerice, & Saucier, 2002), parental care (Gatti & Tremblay, 2005; Raine, Brennan, & Mednick, 1997; Zoccolillo, Paquette, & Tremblay, 2005), and peer characteristics (Boivin, Vitaro, & Poulin, 2005). However, the individual differences that we observe are very likely to be due to interactions between many of these mechanisms, hence to epigenetic mechanisms (Francis, Diorio, Plotsky, & Meaney, 2002; Francis, Szegda, Campbell, Martin, & Insel, 2003; Weaver et al., 2004; Chapter 3 of this book).

Twin studies

Knowledge on gene–environment interactions that could explain the development of chronic physical aggression is perilously close to zero. The first reason is that gene–environment interaction studies are recent. The second reason is that there are very few longitudinal studies that have included repeated assessments of physical aggression from early childhood to adulthood (Rhee & Waldman, 2002). However, the most important problem is that molecular genetic studies and twin studies have concentrated on global antisocial behaviour phenotypes, generally assessed at one point in time. This is an old problem in the antisocial behaviour literature (e.g., Barker, et al., 2007; Blumstein, Cohen, & Farrington, 1988; Gottfredson & Hirschi, 1990; Tremblay, 2000a; Tremblay 2003; Tremblay, Loeber, Gagnon, Charlebois, Larivée, & LeBlanc, 1991). Genetic studies have simply followed the main trend, which tends to rely on measurement scales constructed by lumping items that are shown to correlate at one point in time.

A strong heritability of the aggression (i.e., disruptive or obnoxious) score of the Cognitive Behavior Checklist (CBCL) was shown with British, Swedish, and American pre-adolescent samples (Edelbrock, Rende, Plomin, & Thompson, 1995; Eley, Lichtenstein, & Stevenson, 1999). In fact the heritability for the aggressive behaviour scale was stronger than for the delinquency scale. Eley et al. (1999) went on to compare the pre-adolescent sample to an adolescent sample. They observed high heritability for both groups on the aggressive scale, and observed higher shared environmental effects for the delinquency scale, especially for the adolescent group. These results led them to conclude: (a) that aggressive antisocial behaviour (CBCL aggression scale) is highly heritable, and this confirms that life-course persistent antisocial behaviour is highly heritable (Moffitt, 1993); (b) that non-aggressive antisocial behaviour (CBCL delinquency measure: e.g., bad friends, truant, alcohol, drugs, run away, prefers older kids) is more influenced by the shared environment, confirming that adolescent-limited antisocial behaviour is caused by environmental factors (Moffitt, 1993). Note that these conclusions concerning a life-course developmental model were drawn from a cross-sectional study with an aggression scale that looks like an extraversion personality scale, and a delinquency scale that focuses on behaviour that tends to start when children have become adolescents (drugs, alcohol, truant, run away). The phenotypes that are being assessed are not the developmental trajectories hypothesized by the theory. They are assessments at one point in time.

We initiated a study that started at the earliest point during development to assess gene–environment effects on physical aggression and used a large sample of 18- to 19-month-old twins (Dionne et al., 2003). Results showed, with a large sample of female and male twins, that variance in mothers' reports of physical aggression were explained somewhat more by genetic factors (58%) than by environmental factors (42%), suggesting that there are strong genetic effects on physical aggression during early childhood. Based on the longitudinal studies described above, which show that physical aggression decreases with age, we would expect to observe increased environmental effects as they grow older, if the pressures on learning alternatives to physical aggression come from the environment. Unfortunately, studies with older samples of twins have used global scales of antisocial behaviour (Arseneault et al., 2003; Edelbrock et al., 1995; Eley et al., 1999). If their results are a true representation of genetic effects on physical aggression, we would have to conclude that learning to regulate physical aggression is largely determined by genetic factors (Arseneault et al., 2003). To settle this question we need genetically and environmentally informative longitudinal studies, such as twin studies, that will focus on the development of physical aggression from early childhood to adulthood, to understand the role of genetic and environmental factors throughout development. The Dionne et al. study (2003) shows that both the genetic and environmental causes of a very specific socially disruptive behaviour – physical aggressions – are in place by 19 months of age, long before the violent video games, the delinquent peers, and the effects of a Vietnam war.

Molecular genetic studies

Many molecular genetic studies have attempted to identify polymorphisms related to aggressive behaviour, mainly with animal and human adult samples (Pihl & Benkelfat, 2005). Caspi et al. (2002) used a longitudinal study to specifically address gene–environment interactions. They observed that the most maltreated males were at higher risk of being convicted of a violent crime before 27 years of age if they had the short version of the functional polymorphism in the gene coding for monoamine oxidase A (MAOA) activity. The MAOA enzyme metabolizes neurotransmitters linked in previous studies to behaviour problems (e.g., dopamine, norepinephrine, and serotonin), and the short version of the allele leads to low activity. Effects were similar for conduct disorder assessed between 10 and 18 years of age, antisocial personality symptoms, and disposition to violence measured at 26 years of age. Individuals with a history of chronic physical aggression may be the driving force in these associations, since they are the most likely to be found in each of the assessed categories. This study is a good illustration of gene–environment issues related to prevention that need to be addressed. First, although the study was a longitudinal study from birth to 26 years of age, the analyses did not provide information on the developmental impact of the gene–environment interaction. Was the effect of the gene–environment inter-action on physical aggression present in early childhood? Did it appear later during elementary school, adolescence, and even adulthood? These are important questions for preventive interventions. From the developmental data presented in the preceding section, one would expect that the effects were present early, and may have grown with time. A second question concerns the intervention strategies. Let us assume that the gene–environment interaction effects appear in early childhood and will increase with time if there are no early interventions. Which type of intervention should we use? For example, we could screen pregnant women soon after conception to identify those at risk of maltreating their child and offer a support programme to help prevent the family from abusing the child (Olds et al., 1998). An alternative strategy would be to give the child a chemical treatment that would correct or com-pensate for the low MAOA activity (Caspi et al., 2002; Weaver et al., 2004). Both strategies could also be used with some cases. Thus, much research is needed to understand the gene–environment impact on the development of physical aggression, but research is also needed on the use of that knowledge to prevent the *development* of chronic physical aggression.

Gene–environment interactions, epigenetics, and prevention experiments

To address causal issues and identify effective preventive interventions we need to be able to manipulate putative causal variables. Twin studies and molecular genetic studies can address the gene–environment interaction issue. However, concerning causal mechanisms leading to chronic physical aggression, they are still limited to a correlational analysis. Cross-fostering experiments like those done with rats, mice, and monkeys (e.g., Francis et al., 2003; Suomi, 2005; Weaver et al., 2004) would give better insights into causal mechanisms than studies that are limited to correlational analyses. Obviously, it is hard to conduct such studies with humans, except with adoption studies. However, prevention experiments aimed at helping high risk families and children can be used to understand the mechanisms that prevent children from chronic physical aggression.

Recent prevention experiments have shown that interventions with elemen-tary school children can also have relatively long-term positive impacts (e.g., Boisjoli, Vitaro, Lacourse, Barker, & Tremblay, 2007; Hawkins, Kosterman, Catalano, Hill, & Abbott, 2005; Kellam, Rebok, Ialongo, & Mayer, 1994; Lacourse, Côté, Nagin, Vitaro, Brendgen, & Tremblay, 2002; Vitaro, Brendgen, & Tremblay, 1999). However, from our present understand-ing of the development of physical aggression described above, we would expect that intensive preschool interventions would have more positive (or negative) long-term impact than intensive elementary school interventions (Côté et al., 2007).

For example, the Perry preschool experiment with 3- and 4-year-olds showed impressive long-term reduction of criminal behaviour among males (Schweinhart, Montie, Xiang, Barnett, Belfield, & Nores, 2005); unfortunately, there is apparently no information on the development of physical aggression in this study. Olds et al. (1998) experimented with an earlier intervention. They randomly allocated a nurse home visitation programme to young underprivileged pregnant women at high risk of child abuse and neglect. These children were obviously also at high risk of chronic physical aggression. The long-term follow-up of the children from the intervention group showed that they were less frequently abused and neglected, and were also less likely to exhibit delinquent behaviours during adolescence. One would expect that the intervention group learned more rapidly to regulate physical aggression and was less frequently involved in physical aggression during childhood and adolescence. Unfortunately, based on the published material, the development of physical aggression, or any other antisocial behaviour, appears not to have been included in the follow-up assessments. Regular assessments of physical aggression during childhood and adolescence in the two experiments would have helped us to understand whether an intervention starting 3 years after birth and targeting cognitive development has as much of an impact on developmental trajectories of physical aggression as an intervention that started during pregnancy and that could affect early brain development. These are important questions for assessing the cost and benefits of interventions during the developmental cycle, but they are also important questions for understanding the mechanisms that lead to or prevent chronic physical aggression. To what extent are the control mechanisms plastic, and over what period of time? The preventive study we did with disruptive children at school entry (Boisjoli et al., 2007; Lacourse et al., 2002) indicated that there is still some plasticity, but it is somewhat limited and costly to achieve.

Drug companies are developing a new research field that has been labelled "pharmacogenomics". Its aim is to create the knowledge that will enable the creation of pharmaceutical products specifically meant to match the genetic makeup of an individual. It is easy to imagine that we can do the same with psychosocial interventions: match the intervention to the genetic profile of the client. Weaver et al. (2004; Chapter 3 of this book) recently showed how an environmental event during early childhood (rat pups licked by their mothers) activated gene expression that influenced the development of the HPA axis and increased life expectancy. This phenomenon is a good illustration of the complex epigenetic mechanisms involved in gene–environment interactions. Genes need an environment to be turned on and off, and psychosocial interventions can offer programmes that will help to activate the right genes at the right time. This is more probable during pregnancy and early childhood than at later stages of development (Tremblay, 2008). Psychosocial interventions can also compensate for defective genes, as is often done with nutrition (e.g., Scriver & Kaufman, 2001).

The ultimate prevention experiment to test early interventions and gene–environment interactions is to use adoption studies. Instead of trying to change an individual's environment by attempting to modify the behaviour of his or her parents, adoption simply changes the parents. For example, Duyme, Dumaret, and Tomkiewicz (1999) showed that adoption into a family with a high social class compared to a lower social class had substantially increased the children's IQ by adolescence. An old study by Van Dusen, Mednick, Gabrielli, and Hutchings (1983) is another good example. Using Danish records over many years, they collected the criminal convictions of adopted females ($N = 6374$) and males ($N = 5649$) with reference to the biological and adoptive parents' socio-economic status (SES). Their results showed, as expected, that the level of criminal convictions for males was close to six times that of females. However, males with High SES biological parents were less likely to have a criminal conviction if they were adopted into a High SES family (9.3%) than if they were adopted into a Low SES family (13.8%). Similarly, males with Low SES biological parents were less likely to have a criminal record if they were adopted into a High SES family (12.98%) than if they were adopted into a family with the Low SES of their biological parents (18.04%). Note that the former (Low SES biological–High SES adoptive) were as likely to have a criminal record as the High SES biological–Low SES adoptive (12.98% vs. 13.8%). The largest differences between groups of males were between the High SES biological–High SES adoptive (9.3%) and the Low SES biological–Low SES adoptive (18.04%). The latter are close to twice as likely to have a criminal conviction. If we were successful in changing the behaviour of high risk, Low SES parents it would be surprising if we achieved better results than placing a High SES biological parent male into a High SES adoptive family. The data also indicated that the interventions with females may have proportionally more impact (0.64% vs. 3.02%), although the number – and probably the severity – of convictions is substantially lower for females.

Experiments using an adoption design could randomly allocate children available for adoption to parents who are offering to adopt children. These experiments can control for types of children (e.g., sex, age, families of origin, genetic characteristics) and types of adoptive families (e.g., parents' age, education, income, parenting skills, place of residence). By starting such adoption studies during pregnancy and by including regular assessments over time of environment, behaviour, physiology, and genetic expression we will be able to address genotype–environment interactions, including timing of the change in environment, from the perspective of epigenetic mechanisms with males and females.

The question is to what extent the environment during birth and after birth can modify the developmental trajectories that are expected from the genotype, and reduce the probability of criminal behaviour. An important subquestion is why are there such differences between females and males? To give a good answer to these questions we need well designed experiments starting as close as possible to conception.

Conclusion

Less than five centuries after the birth of Christ, St. Augustine of Thagaste may have written the most sensible page on the development of aggression. In the seventh chapter of his *Confessions* he describes the physical aggressions of infants and concludes:

> Thus it is not the infant's will that is harmless, but the weakness of infant limbs ... These things are easily put up with; not because they are of little or no account, but because they will disappear with increase in age. This you can prove from the fact that the same things cannot be borne with patience when detected in an older person.
>
> (St. Augustine, AD 397/1960)

More than a thousand years later Hobbes, in *De Cive* (Hobbes, 1647/1998), makes a similar statement when he refers to a wicked man as a robust child.

In his attempt to blame the arts, sciences, and civilization in general for inequalities among men, Rousseau invented a human child, born innocent, who had to be kept far away from society until early adolescence. Living alone with nature was the best way for a child to follow nature and avoid becoming corrupted by society (Cranston, 1991). Children had to be kept away from peers and from books. Whatever led Rousseau to this romantic perception of child development appears to be an extremely common experience. Many late 20th-century adults, including psychologists and psychiatrists, appear to be convinced that social behaviour is natural ("God-given" or "genetic") and antisocial behaviour is learned. For example, social learning has been one of the most influential theories in the area of aggression development in the last 30 years. In his 1973 book *Aggression*, Albert Bandura, one of the leading social learning theorists, starts his chapter "Origins of aggression" with the following phrase: "People are not born with preformed repertoires of aggressive behaviour; they must learn them in one way or another" (Bandura, 1973, p. 61).

For those who believe that Rousseau is the cause of this attitude toward child development, consider the fact that, 200 years before the publication of *Émile*, Erasmus in his *Declamation on the subject of early liberal education for children* criticized those "who maintained out of a false spirit of tenderness and compassion that children should be left alone until early adolescence" and argued that "one cannot emphasize too strongly the importance of those first years for the course that a child will follow throughout his entire life" (Erasmus of Rotterdam, 1529/1985).

Twentieth-century longitudinal studies of thousands of subjects from childhood to adulthood have confirmed the old philosopher's experience. Children who fail to learn alternatives to physical aggression during the pre-school years are at very high risk of a huge number of problems. They tend to be hyperactive, inattentive, anxious, and fail to help when others are in need;

they are rejected by the majority of their classmates, they get poor grades, and their behaviour disrupts school activities (Tremblay, Vitaro, Nagin, Pagani, & Séguin, 2003). They are thus swiftly taken out of their "natural" peer group and placed in special classes, schools, and institutions with other "deviants", the ideal situation to reinforce marginal behaviour (Dishion, McCord, & Poulin, 1999). They are among the most delinquent from pre-adolescence onward, are the first to initiate substance use, the first to initiate sexual intercourse, the most at risk of dropping out of school, having a serious accident, being gang members, being violent offenders, and being diagnosed as having a psychiatric disorder (Lacourse, Nagin, Vitaro, Côté, Arseneault, & Tremblay, 2006; Tremblay et al., 2003).

From this perspective, failure to learn alternatives to physical aggression in the early years appears to have the long-term negative consequences on the social adjustment of an individual that Hobbes described in his 1647 *De Cive*. The modern studies that have followed aggressive children into their adult years have indeed shown that there are extremely negative consequences not only for the aggressive individuals, but also for their mates, their children, and the communities in which they live (Tremblay, 2000b). The stage is set for early parenthood, unemployment, family violence, and a second generation of poor children brought up in a disorganized environment. We are learning from the epigenetic studies with animals that this intergenerational process may well be transmitted through genetic endowment but also through early parenting behaviour, which affects brain development and in turn affects the ability to become an adequate parent. From this perspective, the development of girls who become the next generation's mothers is especially important, as was suggested more than half a century ago by the Swiss psychiatrist Lucien Bovet (1951), in his brilliant synthesis of research on juvenile delinquency for the World Health Organization.

Note

1 This chapter was adapted from the inaugural lecture of the J. J. Groen Professor-ship at Utrecht University in June 2006 and with permission from the article: Tremblay, R. E. (2000b). The origins of youth violence (ISUMA). *Canadian Journal of Policy Research, 1*(2), 19–24.

References

Arseneault, L., Moffit, T. E., Caspi, A., Taylor, A., Rijsdijk, F. V., Jaffee, S. R., et al. (2003). Strong genetic effects on cross-situational antisocial behaviour among 5-year-old children according to mothers, teachers, examiner-observers, and twins' self-reports. *Journal of Child Psychology and Psychiatry, 44*(6), 832–848.

Arseneault L., Tremblay R. E., Boulerice B., & Saucier J.-F. (2002). Obstetrical complications and violent delinquency: Testing two developmental pathways. *Child Development, 73*(2), 496–508.

Barker, E. D., Séguin, J. R., White, H. R., Bates, M., Lacourse, E., Carbonneau, R., &

Tremblay, R. E. (2007). Development trajectories of physical violence and theft: relations to neuro-cognitive performance. *Archives of General Psychiatry, 64,* 592–599.

Bandura, A. (1973). *Aggression: A social learning analysis.* New York: Holt.

Blumstein, A., Cohen, J., & Farrington, D. P. (1988). Criminal career research: Its value for criminology. *Criminology, 26,* 11.

Boisjoli, R., Vitaro, F., Lacourse, E., Barker, E. D., & Tremblay, R. E. (2007). Impact and clinical significance of a preventive intervention for disruptive boys: 15 year follow-up. *British Journal of Psychiatry, 199,* 415–419.

Boivin, M., Vitaro, F., & Poulin, F. (2005). Peer relationships and the development of aggressive behavior in early childhood. In R. E. Tremblay, W. W. Hartup, & J. Archer (Eds.), *Developmental origins of aggression* (pp. 376–397). New York: Guilford.

Bovet, L. (1951). *Psychiatric aspects of juvenile delinquency.* Geneva: World Health Organization.

Broidy, L. M., Nagin, D. S., Tremblay, R. E., Bates, J. E., Brame, B., Dodge, K., et al. (2003). Developmental trajectories of childhood disruptive behaviors and adolescent delinquency: A six site, cross national study. *Developmental Psychology, 39*(2), 222–245.

Caspi, A., McClay, J., Moffitt, T., Mill, J., Martin, J., Craig, I. W., et al. (2002). Role of genotype in the cycle of violence in maltreated children. *Science, 297,* 851–854.

Côté, S. M., Boivin, M., Nagin, D. S., Japel, C., Xu, Q., Zoccolillo, M., et al. (2007). The role of maternal education and non-maternal care services in the prevention of children's physical aggression. *Archives of General Psychiatry, 64*(1), 1305–1312.

Côté, S. M., Vaillancourt, T., LeBlanc, J. C., Nagin, D. S., & Tremblay, R. E. (2006). The development of physical aggression from toddlerhood to pre-adolescence: A nation wide longitudinal study of Canadian children. *Journal of Abnormal Child Psychology, 34*(11), 71–85.

Cranston, M. W. (1991). *The noble savage: Jean-Jacques Rousseau, 1754–1762.* Chicago: University of Chicago Press.

Descartes, R. (1982). *Discours de la méthode.* Paris: Larousse. (Original work published in 1637)

Dionne, G. (2005). Language development and aggressive behavior. In R. E. Tremblay, W. W. Hartup, & J. Archer (Eds.), *Developmental origins of aggression* (pp. 330–352). New York: Guilford.

Dionne, G., Tremblay, R. E., Boivin, M., Laplante, D., & Pérusse, D. (2003). Physical aggression and expressive vocabulary in 19 month-old twins. *Developmental Psychology, 39*(2), 261–273.

Dishion, T. J., McCord, J., & Poulin, F. (1999). Iatrogenic effects in early adolescent interventions that aggregate peers. *American Psychologist, 54*(9), 755–764.

Duyme, M., Dumaret, A. C., & Tomkiewicz, S. (1999). How can we boost IQs of "dull children"? A late adoption study. *Proceedings of the National Academy of Sciences of the USA, 96,* 8790–8794.

Edelbrock, C., Rende, R., Plomin, R., & Thompson, L.A. (1995). A twin study of competence and problem behavior in childhood and early adolescence. *Journal of Child Psychology and Psychiatry, 36*(5), 775–785.

Eley, T. C., Lichtenstein, P., & Stevenson, J. (1999). Sex differences in the etiology of aggressive and nonaggressive antisocial behavior: Results from two twin studies. *Child Development, 70*(1), 155–168.

Erasmus of Rotterdam (1985). A declamation on the subject of early liberal education for children. In G. K. Sowards (Ed.), *Collected works of Erasmus, literary and educational writings* (pp. 297–346). Toronto: University of Toronto Press. (Original work published in 1529)

Farrington, D. P. (1987). Epidemiology. In H. C. Quay (Ed.), *Handbook of juvenile delinquency* (pp. 33–61). New York: John Wiley & Sons.

Francis, D. D., Diorio, J., Plotsky, P. M., & Meaney, M. J. (2002). Environmental enrichment reverses the effects of maternal separation on stress reactivity. *Journal of Neuroscience, 22*, 7840–7843.

Francis, D. D., Szegda, K., Campbell, G., Martin, W.D., & Insel, T. (2003). Epigenetic sources of behavioral differences in mice. *Nature Neuroscience, 6*, 445–446.

Gatti, U., & Tremblay, R. E. (2005). Social capital and physical violence. In R. E. Tremblay, W. W. Hartup, & J. Archer (Eds.), *Developmental origins of aggression* (pp. 398–424). New York: Guilford.

Gottfredson, M. R., & Hirschi, T. (1990). *A general theory of crime.* Stanford, CA: Stanford University Press.

Hawkins, J. D., Kosterman, R., Catalano, R. F., Hill, K. G., & Abbott, R. D. (2005). Promoting positive adult functioning through social development intervention in childhood: Long-term effects from the Seattle Social Development Project. *Archives of Pediatrics and Adolescent Medicine, 159*(1), 25–31.

Hobbes, T. (1998). *De Cive; on the citizen.* New York: Cambridge University Press. (Original work published in 1647)

Huijbregts, S. C. J., Séguin, J. R., Zoccolillo, M., Boivin, M., & Tremblay, R. E. (2008). Maternal prenatal smoking, parental antisocial behavior, and early childhood physical aggression. *Development and Psychopathology, 20*, 437–453.

Kellam, S. G., Rebok, G. W., Ialongo, N., & Mayer, L. S. (1994). The course and malleability of aggressive behavior from early first grade into middle school: Results of a developmental epidemiologically-based preventive trial. *Journal of Child Psychology and Psychiatry, 35*(2), 259–281.

Krug, E. G., Dahlberg, L. L., Mercy, J. A., Zwi, A. B., & Lozano, R. E. (2002). *World report on violence and health.* Geneva: World Health Organization.

Lacourse, E., Côté, S., Nagin, D. S., Vitaro, F., Brendgen, M., & Tremblay, R. E. (2002). A longitudinal-experimental approach to testing theories of antisocial behavior development. *Development and Psychopathology, 14*, 909–924.

Lacourse, E., Nagin, D. S., Vitaro, F., Côté, S., Arseneault, L., & Tremblay, R. E. (2006). Prediction of early onset deviant peer group affiliation: A 12 year longitudinal study. *Archives of General Psychiatry, 63*, 562–568.

Laub, J. H., & Sampson, R. J. (2003). *Shared beginnings, divergent lives: Delinquent boys to age 70.* Cambridge, MA: Harvard University Press.

Loeber, R., & Stouthamer-Loeber, M. (1998). Development of juvenile aggression and violence. Some common misconceptions and controversies. *American Psychologist, 53*(2), 242–259.

McCord, J., Widom, C. S., & Crowell, N. E. (2001). *Juvenile crime, juvenile justice.* Washington: National Academy Press.

Moffitt, T. E. (1993). Adolescence-limited and life-course persistent antisocial behavior: A developmental taxonomy. *Psychological Review, 100*(4), 674–701.

Nagin, D., & Tremblay, R. E. (1999). Trajectories of boys' physical aggression, opposition, and hyperactivity on the path to physically violent and non violent juvenile delinquency. *Child Development, 70*(5), 1181–1196.

Nagin, D., & Tremblay, R. E. (2001). Parental and early childhood predictors of persistent physical aggression in boys from kindergarten to high school. *Archives of General Psychiatry, 58*, 389–394.

NICHD-ECCRN (2004). Trajectories of physical aggression from toddlerhood to middle school. *Monographs of the Society for Research in Child Development, 69* (4, Serial No. 278).

Olds, D., Henderson, C. R., Cole, R., Eckenrode, J., Kitzman, H., Luckey, D., et al. (1998). Long-term effects of nurse home visitation on children's criminal and antisocial behavior: Fifteen-year follow-up of a randomized controlled trial. *JAMA, 280*(14), 1238–1244.

Pihl, R. O., & Benkelfat, C. (2005). Neuromodulators in the development and expression of inhibition and aggression. In R. E. Tremblay, W. W. Hartup, & J. Archer (Eds.), *Developmental origins of aggression* (pp. 261–280). New York: Guilford.

Quetelet, A. (1984). *Research on the propensity for crime at different ages.* Cincinnati, OH: Anderson. (Original work published in 1833)

Raine, A., Brennan, P., & Mednick, S.A. (1997). Interaction between birth complications and early maternal rejection in predisposing individuals to adult violence: Specificity to serious, early-onset violence. *American Journal of Psychiatry, 154*, 1265–1271.

Rhee, S. H., & Waldman, I.D. (2002). Genetic and environmental influences on antisocial behavior: A meta-analysis of twin and adoption studies. *Psychological Bulletin, 128*(3), 490–529.

Rousseau, J.-J. (1979). *Emile or on education.* New York: Basic Books. (Original work published in 1762)

Sampson, R. J., & Laub, J. H. (2003). Life-course desisters? Trajectories of crime among delinquent boys followed to age 70. *Criminology, 41*, 301–339.

Schweinhart, L., Montie, J., Xiang, Z., Barnett, W. S., Belfield, C. R., & Nores, M. (2005). *Lifetime effects: The High/Scope Perry preschool study through age 40.* Ypsilanti, MI: High/Scope Press.

Scriver, C. R., & Kaufman, S. (2001). Hyperphenylalaninemia: Phenylalanine hydroxylase deficiency. In C. R. Scriver, A. L. Beaudet, W. S. Sly, & D. Valle (Eds.), *The metabolic and molecular bases of inherited disease* (pp. 1667–1724). New York: McGraw-Hill.

Séguin, J. R., & Zelazo, P. (2005). Executive function in early physical aggression. In R. E. Tremblay, W. H. Hartup, & J. Archer (Eds.), *Developmental origins of aggression* (pp. 307–329). New York: Guilford.

St. Augustine (1960). *Confessions.* New York: Doubleday. (Original work published in AD 397)

Suomi, S. J. (2005). Genetic and environmental factors influencing the expression of impulsive aggression and serotonergic functioning in rhesus monkeys. In R. E. Tremblay, W. W. Hartup, & J. Archer (Eds.), *Developmental origins of aggression* (pp. 63–82). New York: Guilford.

Tremblay, R. E. (2000a). The development of aggressive behaviour during childhood: What have we learned in the past century? *International Journal of Behavioral Development, 24*(2), 129–141.

Tremblay, R. E. (2000b). The origins of youth violence (ISUMA). *Canadian Journal of Policy Research, 1*(2), 19–24.

Tremblay, R. E. (2003). Why socialization fails: The case of chronic physical aggression. In B. B. Lahey, T. E. Moffitt, & A. Caspi (Eds.), *Causes of conduct disorder and juvenile delinquency* (pp. 182–224). New York: Guilford.

Tremblay, R. E. (2008). Understanding development and prevention of chronic physical aggression: Towards experimental epigenetic studies. *Philosophical Transactions of the Royal Society of London, Series B: Biological Sciences, 363,* 2613–2622.

Tremblay, R. E., Loeber, R., Gagnon, C., Charlebois, P., Larivée, S., & LeBlanc, M. (1991). Disruptive boys with stable and unstable high fighting behavior patterns during junior elementary school. *Journal of Abnormal Child Psychology, 19,* 285–300.

Tremblay, R. E., Nagin, D. S., Séguin, J. R., Zoccolillo, M., Zelazo, P., Boivin, M., et al. (2004). Physical aggression during early childhood: Trajectories and predictors. *Pediatrics, 114*(1), e43–e50.

Tremblay, R. E., Vitaro, F., Nagin, D. S., Pagani, L., & Séguin, J. R. (2003). The Montreal longitudinal and experimental study: Rediscovering the power of descriptions. In T. Thornberry (Ed.), *Taking stock of delinquency: An overview of findings from contemporary longitudinal studies* (pp. 205–254). New York: Kluwer Academic/Plenum.

Van Dusen, K. T., Mednick, S. A., Gabrielli, W. F., & Hutchings, B. (1983). Social class and crime in an adoption cohort. *Journal of Criminal Law in Criminology, 74*(1), 249–269.

Van Goozen, S. H. M. (2005). Hormones and the developmental origin of aggression. In R. E. Tremblay, W. W. Hartup, & J. Archer (Eds.), *Developmental origins of aggression* (pp. 281–306). New York: Guilford.

Vitaro, F., Brendgen, M., & Tremblay, R. E. (1999). Prevention of school dropout through the reduction of disruptive behaviors and school failure in elementary school. *Journal of School Psychology, 37*(2), 205–226.

Wakschlag, L., Pickett, K. E., Cook, E., Benowitz, N. L., & Leventhal, B. (2002). Maternal smoking during pregnancy and severe antisocial behavior in offspring: A review. *American Journal of Public Health, 92*(6), 966–974.

Weaver, I. C. G., Cervoni, N., Champagne, F. A., D'Alessio, A. C., Sharma, S., Seckl, J. R., et al. (2004). Epigenetic programming by maternal behavior. *Nature Neuroscience, 7*(8), 847–854.

Zoccolillo, M., Paquette, D., & Tremblay, R. E. (2005). Maternal conduct disorder and the risk for the next generation. In D. Pepler, K. Masden, C. Webster, & K. Levene (Eds.), *Development and treatment of girlhood aggression* (pp. 225–252). Mahwah, NJ: Lawrence Erlbaum Associates, Inc.

6 Personality in children and adolescents[1]

Development and consequences

Marcel A. G. van Aken

This chapter focuses on individual differences between children, as indicated by the concepts of temperament and personality. It describes how children's personalities are clearly observable from an early age and show moderate stability. It points out how personality and environmental factors determine a child's functioning through person–environment correlations as well as person–environment interactions. Furthermore, several possible connections between personality and psychopathology in children are illustrated. To conclude, the implications of the above for interventions with children are discussed.

People have different personalities. Some live their lives in a very positive manner; they deal with life's demands and possibilities with enthusiasm and focus, and are not easily taken aback when they meet with adversity. Others are more withdrawn or more irritable, find it hard to conform to society's expectations and to meet its demands, or are easily upset.

These differences can also be found in children and adolescents. Some babies are contented, whereas others get easily upset when their normal daily routines, such as feeding and sleeping patterns, are disturbed. Some adolescents are resilient and capable of dealing with the challenges of this phase in their lives, while others are inclined to confront the same challenges by exhibiting rebellious or introverted behaviour.

These individual differences, both in adults and children, mostly fall within a more or less normal and acceptable range. However, sometimes they can be categorized as near-pathological behaviour, or even as real psychopathology. These individual differences, which encompass "personality", constitute the subject of this chapter.

From temperament to personality

As mentioned above, differences in behavioural styles between children, the way they cope with life, can be observed from a very young age. At that age these differences are usually described in terms of temperament. Temperament research goes back to the ancient Greek philosophers who developed the theory of humours, which was based on the belief that temperament is determined by the "four body fluids": blood, phlegm, yellow bile and black bile. Modern temperament research, however, is mostly assumed to have started with studies by Thomas and Chess (1984) in the second half of the last century. They were the first to study children's personalities empirically and to develop a taxonomy of individual differences.

By now, a consensus appears to have been established among temperament researchers on the existence of two main dimensions for classifying differences between children (Rothbart & Bates, 2006). The first dimension is formed by *reactivity*, the two poles of which are sometimes considered independent dimensions: negative emotionality and positive emotionality. The second dimension is constituted by *self-regulation*, which is defined as the processes that are necessary for controlling reactivity, in other words for expressing or suppressing negative or positive emotionality, depending on the circumstances.

This chapter will not deal with the temperament of very young children, but with differences in behavioural styles between older children, from the age of about 3 years. In children of that age it is justifiable to speak of personality differences instead of temperament differences (Shiner & Caspi, 2003).

As has been indicated above, the main differences between young children can apparently be traced back to differences in their reactivity and in their regulation of reactivity. Consequently, it seems logical to think about children's personalities along the same lines. That is exactly what the personality theory of *ego-resilience* and *ego-control* does, described by Jack and Jeanne Block (Block & Block, 2006). Block and Block define ego-control as the threshold between either containing or expressing emotions, feelings, impulses, etc., while ego-resilience is the capacity to adjust this threshold, as circumstances require. Children high on ego-resilience can be spontaneous and impulsive at birthday parties, but also task-oriented in lesson time. Children low on ego-resilience are less capable of modulating these traits and are always either task-oriented and quiet, also at birthday parties, or impulsive and easily distracted, also in lesson time.

Various studies have been conducted on the basis of the theoretical work by Block and Block, which have established three types of children: "resilients", "over-controllers" and "under-controllers". Through our own studies, we also demonstrated the existence of these types and, moreover, we discovered that children of these particular types display differences in functioning and even in the course their lives take. The LOGIC study, on which I worked in collaboration with my German colleague Jens Asendorpf, and recently also with Jaap Denissen, has shown that personality types at the age of 5 years can predict developmental patterns of aggression and shyness in children until the age of 22 years (Denissen, Asendorpf, & van Aken, 2008a).

So far, so good, one could say. However, at this point we are confronted with a problem in the history of research on individual differences: there is a gap between research into individual differences between children, particularly consisting of temperament research, and research into individual differences between adults, consisting of more or less traditional personality research.

Research into personalities of adults is based on another gold standard, the so-called *Big Five Model* (John & Srivastava, 1999). It has been shown that differences between adults can very well and exhaustively be described in terms of five personality dimensions: *Extraversion*, which relates to energy or dominance differences; *Agreeableness*, which relates to differences in social skills and compassion; *Conscientiousness*, which describes differences in task-orientedness, orderliness and reliability; *Emotional Stability*, which distinguishes between stress resistance and neuroticism or self-doubt; and *Openness* (also called Intellect or Creativity), which describes differences in the way people are open to or handle new experiences or intellectual challenges.

The conceptual connection between the above-mentioned temperament dimensions and the Big Five can be fairly easily established. It can be assumed that positive emotionality mainly has to do with Extraversion, while negative emotionality to a large degree corresponds with Emotional Stability (or rather its opposite – Neuroticism). The dimension of self-regulation could in this perception be linked to Conscientiousness if it concerns controlling non-social tasks and to Agreeableness if it concerns controlling social tasks. Openness, or Intellect, would then be a dimension that only surfaces when children have reached a certain age, when cultural or intellectual issues become relevant.

Research into the connections between temperament and personality is mostly lacking, but studies have, however, been carried out into the presence of the Big Five in children. Various researchers have found that differences between children can be described using the Big Five dimensions (Halverson, Kohnstamm, & Martin, 1994) and can also be linked to differences in children's functioning in other domains. In the above-mentioned LOGIC study, for example, we (Asendorpf & van Aken, 2003) demonstrated that the five personality dimensions are fairly stable in children between 4 and 12 years of age. In other words, children scoring high regarding a certain dimension at the age of 4 years still scored high at the age of 12 years. Moreover, we discovered that the five personality dimensions are interrelated with other variables, also when measured using other methods. For instance, Conscientiousness is related to a child's school performance, (low) Extraversion to observations of inhibition, Agreeableness to low levels of aggression, etc. Apparently, the Big Five can also be found in children and refer to meaningful differences between them.

The importance of research into the personality of children and adolescents lies not so much in describing the development of individual differences, but in the fact that personality differences influence children's functioning and their social interactions with, for instance, parents or peers, as various studies have proved.

Correlations and interactions between environment and personality

The way in which personality and environment are interrelated and the way in which they shape children's development will now be discussed and in so doing we enter the field of person–environment correlations and person–environment interactions (comparable to the gene–environment interplay; see Rutter, Moffitt, & Caspi, 2006).

Person–environment *correlations* refer to the fact that a child's personality and its environment can be interrelated through a number of mechanisms. These mechanisms can be reactive, which means that people interpret environmental aspects in such a way that the environment fits their personality. They can be active, which means that people consciously select or shape an environment to suit their personality, and they can be evocative, which means that a type of personality can evoke a type of environment. Person–environment correlations are important because they lead to an improved rapport between people and their environment. Although this can have both positive and negative consequences, it can make personalities more stable.

Person–environment *interactions* refer to the fact that personality traits may have a certain effect on a child's functioning only in combination with certain environmental characteristics. Contrastingly, it can also happen that certain environmental aspects under some circumstances must be considered a risk whereas they do not constitute a risk in other circumstances, depending upon the type of person involved.

Studies by Caspi and others using the Dunedin study data have become famous across the world. Caspi and others have demonstrated three important gene–environment interactions. In a first study (Caspi et al., 2002), they showed that the effect of child abuse may depend on a gene encoding for monoamine oxidase A, which is a neurotransmitter (the MAOA gene). In persons with low MAOA activity, child abuse will more likely cause problem behaviour later in life. In a second study (Caspi et al., 2003), they showed that the effects of stressful life events depend upon a gene encoding for a serotonin transporter (the 5-HTT gene). Persons with a short version of this gene more often suffer from depression and suicidality as a result of serious life events compared to persons who have a long version of the same gene. Finally, they showed (Caspi et al., 2005) that the effect of cannabis use may be genetically determined. The so-called COMT gene (a catechol O-methyltransferase gene) seems to determine if excessive cannabis use during adolescence will lead to psychoses in adulthood.

This has nothing to do with personality, has it? Strictly speaking it has not, but for the above-mentioned genes it has already been demonstrated that they are also related to personality dimensions. Moreover, apart from these actual "gene"–environment interactions, various person–environment interactions have been found, which can often be more readily proven by developmental psychologists. I will provide some examples from our own research group.

Recently, we have found in a study by Cathelijne Buschgens (Buschgens, van Aken, Swinkels, Ormel, Verhulst, & Buitelaar, 2008), who used an extensive database from the north of The Netherlands, the TRAILS data, that the effects of parental rejection are linked to a certain degree of genetic-behavioural vulnerability in children. Children with a high genetic vulnerability (as measured on the basis of problem behaviour in the parents, assuming that this behaviour is hereditary to some extent) appeared to display a higher degree of problem behaviour as a consequence of parental rejection, whereas children with a low genetic vulnerability did not.

Research by Chantal van Aken (van Aken, Junger, Verhoeven, van Aken, & Deković, 2007) has demonstrated that the effects of a lack of sensitivity in the mother depend upon the temperament of the child. For children with an easy temperament, in this study operationalized as a high degree of self-regulation, a lack of sensitivity does not have much impact on their problem behaviour. For children with a difficult temperament, or a low degree of self-regulation, a lack of sensitivity leads to more serious problem behaviour.

Finally, in research by Annemiek Karreman (Karreman, van Tuijl, van Aken, & Deković, in press) we found again that for various parenting and co-parenting styles the effects are determined by the child's temperament. Problem behaviour of children with an easy temperament is less affected by inadequate parenting and co-parenting than that of children with a difficult temperament.

Apart from temperament–parenting interactions, we have found other person–environment interactions as well. Earlier, we established (van Aken, van Lieshout, Scholte, & Haselager, 2002) that for the three above-mentioned personality types it was important whether children had good relationships with peers. The "over-controllers" had a higher risk of internalizing problems, such as depression and loneliness, but only if they had not established good peer relationships. The "under-controllers" had a higher risk of externalizing problems, such as antisocial and risky behaviour, but again only if they had not established good peer relationships.

It should, however, be realized that these types of person–environment interactions can be explained either in favour of the person or in favour of the environment. More specifically, in the examples above it could be said that the personality determines the impact of the environment (after all, a negative environment only influences a certain type of personality) and, vice versa, that the environment determines the implications of the personality (after all, the personality only causes problems in a certain type of environment). It goes to show that with these so-called transactional models there is no point in thinking in terms of causes and consequences. These models are about mutually reinforcing (or inhibiting) factors, and in proper transactional models the origins are not relevant and often cannot be traced.

Personality and psychopathology

The importance of studying the personalities of children and adolescents is emphasized by recent developments in thinking about psychopathology. Personality and problem behaviour may be partly overlapping fields, not only when problem behaviour is defined in terms of ill-adjusted behaviour by otherwise normal persons, but also when it is defined in terms of real "psychopathology".

Recently, various articles have been published in which links have been established between more or less normal differences between children, in temperament or personality, and differences on the basis of which a distinction between children with a psychopathological disorder and those without such a disorder could be made (see Mervielde, De Clercq, De Fruyt, & van Leeuwen, 2005). The gist of these articles is that much can be learnt from the "normal" personality development in order to understand the causes of psychopathological disorders, both in children and in adults. Hardly any empirical articles have been written on this subject, but in two recent overview articles both Shiner and Caspi (Shiner & Caspi, 2003) and Clark (Clark, 2005) have already described various perspectives for considering the relationship between the "normal" personality and pathology, be it personality pathology or another type of pathology. Firstly, they have formulated the "spectrum" hypothesis: Possibly psychopathology is nothing more and nothing less than an extreme score on one or more personality dimensions. Attention deficit hyperactivity disorder (ADHD), for example, may not be a separate category but reflect an extremely low score on self-regulation, in combination with an inclination towards impulsiveness. To give another example, anxiety disorders could represent an extremely low measure of self-regulation coupled with either a high level of negative emotionality or a high level of emotional instability.

Secondly, the relationship between personality and psychopathology may also be considered in terms of vulnerability or resilience. Perhaps some personality dimensions make children more vulnerable to developing a psychopathological disorder. As we have seen above, for example, children with a low degree of self-regulation may be more likely to be affected by external factors (such as inadequate parenting) and as a result be more vulnerable to the negative effects of these factors. This approach differs from the spectrum hypothesis in the sense that a child's vulnerability is accompanied by more or less external events (for instance a life event or a type of social environment) that may evoke the psychopathological disorder. Or it may be that some personality dimensions protect children against negative external influences instead of making them more vulnerable. Research has demonstrated that resilient children cope better with a number of risk factors, such as perinatal stress, poverty or serious family problems, which can lead to psychopathological disorders in less resilient children (Masten, 2001).

Thirdly, the relationship between personality and psychopathology may be said to have shaping effects. In this approach, personality may affect the course of psychopathology. Research testing this hypothesis aims at comorbidity, among other things. Attention disorders coupled with a high level of impulsiveness, for instance, appear to follow quite another course than attention disorders that are not coupled with impulsiveness (Nigg, 2006).

All three hypotheses are based on the assumption that psychopathology is developed as a consequence or under the influence of a normal personality. However, the opposite may also occur: serious psychopathology may cause temporary or permanent personality changes. This is called the "scar" hypothesis and leads us to another important aspect of the personality of children and adolescents, namely the degree of stability or changeability of the personality.

Stability and change in personality

Recently, some meta-analyses of stability and change in personality during the course of life have been published. A distinction should be made between the stability of mean levels and the stability of individual differences. The stability of mean levels refers to the question of whether people in general become more extravert, more task-oriented or more emotionally stable during the course of their lives, in other words whether they go through a sort of normative development. The stability of individual differences relates to the question of whether persons who at some point score high or low on a certain personality dimension will also do so later in life (the question of individual developmental pathways).

A meta-analysis of the normative development of the personality (in other words, the stability of mean levels; Roberts, Walton, & Viechtbauer, 2006) showed an increase of each of the Big Five dimensions. During the course of their lives, people become more extraverted, somewhat more agreeable, more conscientious and more emotionally stable. A curvilinear effect was found for openness to new experiences: an increase is followed by stability, and later in life by a decrease. For the periods of 0–10 years and 10–20 years, similar increases were found. Strikingly, the increases primarily occurred at the end of adolescence, what we nowadays would call "emerging adulthood" (see also Denissen, Geenen, van Aken, Gosling, & Potter, 2008b). Late adolescents particularly experience an increase in Openness during this period, be it that this is more specifically so in the student population rather than the working population (Barends, 2005).

A meta-analysis of the stability (or development) of individual personality differences (Roberts & DelVecchio, 2000) showed that although these differences become more stable, change can still be substantial until beyond the age of 50 years. A much lower stability was found for the periods of 0–10 years and 10–20 years. Apparently, differences between children of these ages have not become fixed, as will be discussed later within the context of the influenceability of the personality.

What are the origins of stability and change? What causes personality changes in people during the course of their lives, both absolute and in relation to each other? According to the *Social Investment Model* of Roberts and others (Roberts, Wood, & Smith, 2005) personality changes, both normative and as regards individual differences, can be activated by certain social roles that people take on at some point in their lives. It is thought that people develop their identity in reaction to the roles they assume, because these roles are associated with rewards for changes in personality dimensions. By assuming adult roles, people are guided towards a higher degree of social dominance, as well as higher degrees of agreeableness, conscientiousness and emotional stability. At the same time individual differences in the degree to which people succeed in assuming such roles also explain individual differences in personality development.

Recent studies have confirmed this model. For example, a study into personality changes in parents of adolescent children (van Aken, Denissen, Branje, Dubas, & Goossens, 2006) has demonstrated that changes are linked to a kind of general satisfaction with life, and also to satisfaction with specific roles during this particular period of their lives, such as the roles of spouse, employee and parent. The above-mentioned study by Denissen et al. (2008a) of adolescents during their so-called "emerging adulthood" also proved that assuming adult roles (for instance, a first job, a first house) was a significant factor in predicting aggression and shyness on the basis of their personality at a very young age.

This Social Investment Model seems to be important for understanding personality stability and change as well as the consequences of personality dispositions. Until now, this model has only been formulated in terms of adult roles and transitions. Developmental psychology is in need of a taxonomy of such transitions in the development of children and adolescents. A suitable theoretical model could be the model of development tasks, as initially formulated by Havighurst and later by Baltes and others (see van Aken, 1994). Just like specific adult roles, these development tasks could function as a window of opportunity for studying the development of personality in children and adolescents.

Influenceability of personality?

Obviously, the perception of a window of opportunity has another connotation as well. Apart from constituting an opportunity to study personality development, such a development task approach could serve as an opportunity for influencing personality. Possibly, when children or adolescents take up a development task, this not only represents a normative development of their personality but also an occasion at which interventions for changing the personality could be effective.

Some reservations, however, are in order. Firstly, the effect sizes of personality changes in studies by Roberts and others, and also by ourselves, are relatively small. That is to say, these studies have demonstrated that the personality is fairly stable and that changes, although significant and consequently reliable, are often small and mostly have an explained variance of no more than a few per cent. Secondly, the causal direction cannot be readily assessed, despite the fact that personality changes appear to be linked to roles, events or social relationships. In other words, personality does seem to change and sometimes does so at the same time or in the same way as, for instance, social relationships change, but until now few factors have been established that contribute to or even cause personality changes.

In a fine model article, Fraley and Roberts (2005) discuss the mechanisms underlying personality change. They have formulated three mechanisms that might lead to personality stabilization. The first mechanism, which we use most in our theoretical models, is the transactional model. This mechanism is based on the assumption that personality traits influence the environment, which again influences the person, who again influences the environment, and so on. The second mechanism mentioned by Fraley and Roberts is that of the so-called development constants. This mechanism is based on the idea that people have inborn and constant factors (for instance, the genetic "make-up"), that influence their personality throughout their lives. The third mechanism Fraley and Roberts have formulated is that of the stochastic or contextual influences. This mechanism takes account of the large influence of accidental factors on personality development, such as life events or major incidental changes to the environment.

Strikingly, a demonstration of this model by Fraley and Roberts showed that all three mechanisms play a role in explaining the development of Neuroticism (one of the Big Five dimensions, the opposite of Emotional Stability). Transactional mechanisms played the smallest role, followed by the mechanism of the development constants, with the largest influence being exerted by stochastic processes, or coincidence. This is pretty much in line with research literature in this field, showing that the personality is not absolutely stable and can change, although it does not become clear which factors cause personality change.

Our own studies (see Branje, van Lieshout, & van Aken, 2004) also demonstrate a certain degree of personality instability as well as correlations between personality and social relationships. We have even found that if the personality changes, the social relationships often change with it, although it cannot be said that the personality changes as a result of social relationships. This phenomenon has not been studied extensively enough. For instance, we have not yet sufficiently examined the effects of serious life events or of psychopathology (e.g., the "scar" hypothesis referred to above). Nevertheless, it does not seem unlikely that we will finally arrive at the conclusion that the personality does indeed undergo minor changes, but that we cannot ascertain the origins of these changes or, more importantly, if these changes can be influenced.

Consequences for interventions

This last conclusion also has implications for our thinking on prevention and intervention, particularly for our ideas on what we can and cannot expect from these. In his provocative book *Altering Fate: Why the Past Does Not Predict the Future*, Lewis (1997) describes that a too strong focus on early characteristics as predictors of later functioning leads to too much emphasis on "cure": the idea that once these early characteristics have been taken care of the child will develop without problems. Lewis advocates more thinking in terms of "care": the idea that a social context should take care of a child at every moment in development. Interventions should perhaps be more embedded in a "culture of care", and more aimed at learning to live with problems rather than at curing them.

The implications for interventions in the development of children and adolescents are that we should not think too much in terms of launching them into desirable development paths, but more in terms of supplying tools for dealing with their temperament or personality, both by themselves and by their environment. Lewis makes the comparison with providing glasses to a person: not an intervention with a curative long-term effect, but at the same time a most effective intervention aimed at learning to live with a problematic visual condition. Similar ideas could be helpful in the domain of temperament and personality, where the child itself and its environment could be assisted in dealing with a sometimes very difficult way of dealing with impulses and environmental demands.

Summarizing the studies referred to above, it appears that the personality of children, as preceded by their temperament, is a major factor in their development. It has been demonstrated that children's personality is fairly stable, that it is connected to their functioning and can be linked to the development of psychopathology. A child's social environment (parents, peers) plays an important role in the sense that problem behaviour seems to be the result of a combination of a difficult personality and an ill-functioning environment.

We have acquired some knowledge about children's personality. However, much needs to be examined, particularly relating to personality stability and change, and to the role of the environment, in this case social relationships. As has been described in this chapter, these are the most important areas for further exploration and study.

Note

1 This chapter is a translation of the inaugural lecture presented, with the acceptance of a chair in Development Psychology, at Utrecht University on 9 June 2006.

References

Asendorpf, J. B., & van Aken, M. A. G. (2003). Validity of Big Five personality judgments in childhood: A 9 year longitudinal study. *European Journal of Personality, 17*, 1–17.

Barends, C. (2005). *De invloed van leeftijd op de Big Five persoonlijkheidstrekken: Een studie naar de periode van de emerging adulthood.* [The influence of age on the Big Five: A study in emerging adulthood]. Utrecht: Utrecht University.

Block, J., & Block, J. H. (2006). Venturing a 30-year longitudinal study. *American Psychologist, 61*, 315–327.

Branje, S. J. T., van Lieshout, C. F. M., & van Aken, M. A. G. (2004). Relations between Big Five personality characteristics and perceived support in adolescents' families. *Journal of Personality and Social Psychology, 86*, 615–628.

Buschgens, C. J. M., van Aken, M. A. G., Swinkels, S. H. N., Ormel, J., Verhulst, F. C., & Buitelaar, J. K. (2008). Externalizing behavior in pre-adolescents: Family-genetic vulnerability and perceived parenting styles. *European Child and Adolescent Psychiatry*. Retrieved June 28, 2008, from http://www.springerlink.com/content/j207p84333×3h2582/?p=0530b0b7d1f04cfeab5f44f28901efba&pi=0

Caspi, A., McClay, J., Moffitt, T. E., Mill, J., Martin, J., Craig, I. W., et al. (2002). Role of genotype in the cycle of violence in maltreated children. *Science, 297*, 851–854.

Caspi, A., Moffitt, T. E., Cannon, M., McClay, J., Murray, R., Harrington, H., et al. (2005). Moderation of the effect of adolescent-onset cannabis use on adult psychosis by a functional polymorphism in the catechol-O-methyltransferase gene: Longitudinal evidence of a gene × environment interaction. *Biological Psychiatry, 57*, 1117–1127.

Caspi, A., Sugden, K., Moffitt, T. E., Taylor, A., Craig, I. W., Harrington, H., et al. (2003). Influence of life stress on depression: Moderation by a polymorphism in the 5-HTT gene. *Science, 301*, 386–389.

Clark, L. A. (2005). Temperament as a unifying basis for personality and psychopathology. *Journal of Abnormal Psychology, 114*, 505–521.

Denissen, J. J. A., Asendorpf, J. B., & van Aken, M. A. G. (2008a). Childhood personality predicts long-term trajectories of shyness and aggressiveness in the context of demographic transitions in emerging adulthood. *Journal of Personality, 76*, 67–99.

Denissen, J. J. A., Geenen, R., van Aken, M. A. G., Gosling, S., & Potter, J. (2008b). Development and validation of a Dutch translation of the Big Five Inventory. *Journal of Personality Assessment, 90*, 152–157.

Fraley, R. C., & Roberts, B. W. (2005). Patterns of continuity: A dynamic model for conceptualizing the stability of individual differences in psychological constructs across the life course. *Psychological Review, 112*, 60–74.

Halverson, C. F., Kohnstamm, G. A., & Martin, R. P. (1994). *The developing structure of temperament and personality from infancy to adulthood.* Hillsdale, NJ: Lawrence Erlbaum Associates, Inc.

John, O. P., & Srivastava, S. (1999). The Big Five trait taxonomy: History, measurement and theoretical perspectives. In L. A. Pervin & O. P. John (Eds.), *Handbook of personality: Theory and Research* (pp. 102–138). New York: Guilford Press.

Karreman, A., van Tuijl, C., van Aken, M. A. G., & Deković, M. (in press). Predicting young children's externalizing problems: Interactions between child sex, effortful control, and parenting and coparenting behavior. *Merrill Palmer Quarterly*.

Lewis, M. (1997). *Altering fate: Why the past does not predict the future.* New York: Guilford Press.

Masten, A. S. (2001). Ordinary magic: Resilience processes in development. *American Psychologist, 56*, 227–238.

Mervielde, I., De Clercq, B., De Fruyt, F., & van Leeuwen, K. (2005). Temperament, personality, and developmental psychopathology as childhood antecedents of personality disorders. *Journal of Personality Disorders 19*, 171–201.

Nigg, J. T. (2006). Temperament and developmental psychopathology. *Journal of Child Psychology and Psychiatry and Allied Disciplines, 47*, 395.

Roberts, B. W., & DelVecchio, W. F. (2000). The rank-order consistency of personality traits from childhood to old age: A quantitative review of longitudinal studies. *Psychological Bulletin, 126*, 3–25.

Roberts, B. W., Walton, K. E., & Viechtbauer, W. (2006). Patterns of mean-level change in personality traits across the life course: A meta-analysis of longitudinal studies. *Psychological Bulletin, 132*, 1–25.

Roberts, B. W., Wood, D., & Smith, J. L. (2005). Evaluating Five Factor theory and social investment perspectives on personality trait development. *Journal of Research in Personality, 39*, 166–184.

Rothbart, M. K., & Bates, J. E. (2006). Temperament. In N. Eisenberg & W. Damon (Eds.), *Handbook of child psychology: Vol. 3. Social, emotional and personality development* (pp. 99–166). New York: Wiley.

Rutter, M., Moffitt, T. E., & Caspi, A. (2006). Gene-environment interplay and psychopathology: multiple varieties but real effects. *Journal of Child Psychology and Psychiatry, 47*, 226–261.

Shiner, R., & Caspi, A. (2003). Personality differences in childhood and adolescence: Measurement, development, and consequences. *Journal of Child Psychology and Psychiatry and Allied Disciplines, 44*, 2.

Thomas, A., & Chess, S. (1984). Genesis and evolution of behavioral disorders: From infancy to early adult life. *American Journal of Psychiatry, 141*, 1–9.

Van Aken, C., Junger, M., Verhoeven, M., van Aken, M. A. G., & Deković, M. (2007). The interactive effects of temperament and maternal parenting on toddlers' externalizing behaviors. *Infant and Child Development, 16*, 553–572.

Van Aken, M. A. G. (1994). The transactional relations between social support and children's competence. In F. Nestmann & K. Hurrelmann (Eds.), *Social networks and social support in childhood and adolescence* (pp. 131–148). New York: De Gruyter.

Van Aken, M. A. G., Denissen, J. J. A., Branje, S. J. T., Dubas, J. S., & Goossens, L. (2006). Associations of midlife concerns with short-term personality change in middle adulthood. *European Journal of Personality, 20*, 497–513.

Van Aken, M. A. G., van Lieshout, C. F. M., Scholte, R. H. J., & Haselager, G. J. T. (2002). Personality types in childhood and adolescence: Main effects and person–relationship transactions. In L. Pulkkinen, & A. Caspi (Eds.), *Pathways to successful development: Personality over the life course* (pp. 129–156). Cambridge: Cambridge University Press.

7 A developmental perspective on sex differences in aggressive behaviours*

Sylvana M. Côté

Introduction

Belle van Zuylen was a talented writer and music composer of the 18th century. She made an important contribution to women's emancipation with her avant-garde ideas about women's role in society. She was acutely conscious of the importance of women's education. She herself profited from high quality education and contributed, particularly through her writings, to the education of women.

Belle van Zuylen was a free spirit, and there are several examples of this in the way she led her life. Her marriage decision is a particularly good example. After Belle refused close to a dozen marriage proposals, she – at the age of 31 years – asked Charles-Emmanuel de Charrière, a Swiss man, to be her husband. He accepted, and she became Isabelle de Charrière and went to live in Switzerland. Monsieur de Charrière was a great supporter of her work and this union certainly encouraged her productivity.

Given Belle's open-mindedness and wide interests, it seems that she would have been very pleased to see her work interpreted through the lenses of different approaches – philosophy, literature, feminism and, with the present chair, life-span developmental psychopathology. She would be pleased to know that women from various countries and continents are associated with her work.

In this chapter, I review research findings on the evolution of the magnitude of sex differences in aggression and antisocial behaviours, and I distinguish between different types of aggressive behaviours while doing so. I then present an overview of two sets of explanations for sex differences in aggression: biological factors and social learning. Finally, I discuss the implications of this work for the intergenerational transmission of risk for maladjustment, and I illustrate how future violence could be prevented by improving women's education.

* This chapter is an account of the inaugural lecture given on 7 June 2007 at Utrecht University.

Sex differences in aggression

Sexual dimorphism is one of the most robust findings in studies on aggression. Men generally use aggression more than females when direct forms of aggression (e.g., physical or verbal) are considered. Conversely, females tend to use aggression more often than males when indirect forms of aggression are considered (e.g., relational, social) (Archer, 2000). However, both sexes use both direct and indirect forms of aggression, and the magnitude of sex differences varies over the course of development. What, then, are we referring to when we discuss "sex differences in aggression"? In their broadest expression, sex differences range from being nearly absolute to being simply statistical. Absolute or sex-dichotomous differences refer to aspects of development that are distinctly characteristic of one sex. Differences may be readily identifiable at a physiological level, the most obvious examples being sex-specific genital organs (e.g., the uterus or penis). Height and muscle mass differences constitute statistical differences: on average, males are taller and have greater muscle mass.

Sex differences in acts of aggression are often a matter of degree, but for some specific types of aggression sex differences are dramatic. For instance, infanticide is a type of homicide almost exclusively committed by human females (Hrdy, 1999). It may also be said that important sex differences exist in the contexts and motives associated with acts of aggression. For instance, women are as likely as men to use physical aggression in the context of intimate relationships (Archer, 2000; Moffitt, Caspi, Rutter, & Silva, 2001). Males, however, are much more likely than women to use physical aggression with strangers (Archer, 2000). Nonetheless, there is a great deal of overlap between the sexes in the distribution of aggressive behaviours.

The term physical aggression (PA) is used in this chapter to refer to physical acts that are directed at another person and that may cause bodily harm (e.g., kicking, pushing, hitting; e.g., Cairns, Cairns, Neckerman, Ferguson, & Gariépy, 1989; Straus & Gelles, 1990; Tremblay 2000). We use the term indirect aggression (IA) to refer to social manipulations (such as spreading rumours, excluding peers, betraying trust or divulging secrets) that are circuitous in nature and that can be socially harmful (Crick, 1995; Crick & Grotpeter, 1995; Lagerspetz, Björkqvist, & Peltonen, 1988). It may be noted that our use of the term IA (e.g., Björkqvist, Lagerspetz, & Kaukiainen, 1992a) is synonymous with both the term social aggression (e.g., Cairns et al., 1989; Galen & Underwood, 1997) and the term relational aggression (Crick & Grotpeter, 1995).

Sex difference in the development of physical aggression

Owing to a paucity of relevant longitudinal studies, information on the comparative development of human and non-human male and female physical aggression is limited. Longitudinal studies with data on PA during the first years of life – the period at which PA is most prevalent – are all the more scarce. However, over the past decade, data from longitudinal studies initiated during preschool years and comprising assessments of PA have started to become available.

Several studies have demonstrated that boys and men use PA more frequently than do girls and women after school entry (Broidy et al., 2003; Cairns et al., 1989; Tremblay et al., 1996). It has been less clear, however, whether boys are more physically aggressive in their preschool years. In their often-cited review of the literature, Keenan and Shaw (1997) posited that girls and boys exhibit similar levels of aggression during toddlerhood and that the rate of externalizing behaviours starts to diverge around 4–5 years of age (Keenan & Shaw, 1997). Indeed, some studies reported no sex differences in externalizing behaviours (Hay, Castle, & Davies, 2000) or in conduct problems (Keenan & Wakschlag, 2000) among preschoolers. By middle childhood, evidence of higher levels of physical aggression and conduct problems among males has been well established (American Psychiatric Association, 1994; Maccoby, 1998). But recent studies also provide evidence that boys are already more physically aggressive than girls during their preschool years (Baillargeon et al., 2007; Côté, Vaillancourt, LeBlanc, Nagin, & Tremblay, 2006; Côté, Vaillancourt, Barker, Nagin, & Tremblay, 2007b; NICHD-ECCRN, 2004; Tremblay et al., 1996, 2004).

For instance, Baillargeon et al. (2007) noted that sex differences had already emerged by 17 months, according to reports from mothers regarding specific acts of PA. In their study, boys were found to be twice as likely as girls to hit another child frequently. Alink et al. (2006) found boys to be slightly more physically aggressive than girls at the age of 12 months, although the effect size was small and the sex difference was not significant ($d = .18$). However, significant sex differences were observed among older infants. More specifically, the effect size of the sex differences among infant groups between 24 and 36 months of age ranged between .30 and .37. This study suggests a gradual increase in the magnitude of the sex differences in PA over the course of early childhood. Observational studies also showed substantial sex differences by 3 years of age (Hay et al., 2000; McGrew, 1972; Sears, Rau, & Alpert, 1965). Thus, these studies suggest that, as previously proposed by Keenan and Shaw (1997), there appears to be a gradual emergence of sex differences in PA during preschool years. However, sex differentiation appears to begin earlier than what was originally proposed: i.e., during infancy (12 months) as opposed to near the end of preschool years (around 4–5 years of age).

Is the next developmental period, from school entry to pre-adolescence, also characterized by a continued increase in the divergence of male–female PA levels? The results from Archer's meta-analysis (2000) suggest that this is the case, at least when self-report data are considered. According to a summary of cross-sectional studies of self-reported PA, the mean effect size of the sex differences increased from $d = .26$ (95% CI = .20–.31) during middle childhood (6–11 years) to $d = .35$ (95% CI = .28–.41) at 11–13 years.

In sum, the evidence reviewed suggests that the PA sex gap gradually widens during childhood. But, this hypothesis does not provide any insight into the direction of changes. For instance, is the increasing sex gap attributable to a faster increase in PA among boys? Or is it related to a faster decrease in PA among girls? For a more precise evaluation of these possibilities, let us turn our attention to longitudinal studies that offer repeated assessments of PA and data on both sexes.

Recently, two longitudinal studies provided information on the developmental patterns of PA and the magnitude of sex differences from toddlerhood to middle-childhood (NICHD-ECCRN, 2004) or pre-adolescence (Côté et al., 2006). These studies provided information on the changes in the magnitude of the PA sex gap, but they also distinguished between atypically elevated PA and normative levels of PA by modelling the development of PA with group-based developmental trajectories.

First, in our work with the National Longitudinal Survey of Children and Youth (NLSCY), we modelled the development of PA among a large ($n = 10,658$) nationally representative sample (in Canada), using data on males and females, from ages 2 to 11 (Côté et al., 2006). Using a group-based trajectory methodology, we found that at the earliest assessment, in toddlerhood (age 2), PA was already part of most children's behavioural repertoire. Typical developmental trajectories then declined in the frequency of PA (Figure 7.1). More specifically, the moderate-desister group represented

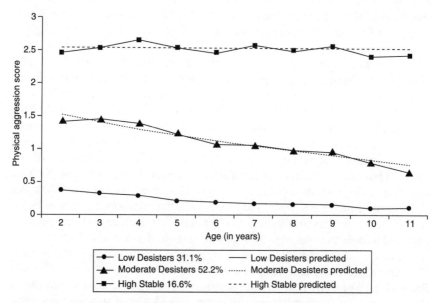

Figure 7.1 Developmental trajectories of physical aggression.

Source: Côté, S. M., Vaillancourt, T., LeBlanc, J. C., Nagin, D. S., & Tremblay, R. E. (2006). The development of physical aggression from toddlerhood to pre-adolescence: A nation wide longitudinal study of Canadian children. *Journal of Abnormal Child Psychology, 34* (1), 71–85.

52.2% of the sample group children, who used PA occasionally in toddler-hood and desisted to infrequent use by age 11. The low-level desister group represented 31.1% of the sample, who used PA infrequently in toddlerhood and virtually not at all by age 11. A third group of children, representing 16.6% of the sample, was also identified, showing high, stable levels of PA when compared with their peers. This particular developmental pattern was atypical in the sense that it was distinct from the general declining and lower levels of PA exhibited by the rest of the sample.

The overall pattern of the results from this Canadian study was similar to that found in the US-based National Institute for Child Health Development and Early Childhood Care Research Network study (NICHD-ECCRN, 2004), in which most children were also found to exhibit low-to-moderate levels of PA, with declining trajectories between toddlerhood and middle childhood. Similarly, the NICHD-ECCRN study results showed that a pro-portion of children exhibiting higher levels of PA during toddlerhood main-tained relatively high trajectories throughout childhood. These two studies replicate earlier analyses of PA trajectories during the elementary school years and high school in Canada, New Zealand and the USA (Brame, Nagin, & Tremblay, 2001; Broidy et al., 2003; Nagin & Tremblay, 1999), but show that the same phenomenon is found in preschool years.

In the NLSCY, comparisons between boys and girls indicated that boys were 1.67 times more likely to follow a high and stable PA trajectory. Thus, between 2 and 11 years of age boys tended to be more physically aggressive than girls. Similar sex differences were found among the participants in the NICHD-ECCRN study. More specifically, boys were more likely to follow a moderate (the second-highest odds ratio (OR): 1.68) or a high (OR: 2.89) PA trajectory when compared with the (two) lowest trajectories. Together, these results suggest that the PA sex gap is already substantial in toddlerhood, since girls are more likely to follow low, desisting PA trajectories and boys are more likely to follow high, stable PA trajectories. Overall, the male–female dichot-omy found in this study was consistent with previous studies on sex difference in various forms of social behaviour (Archer & Côté, 2005; Kochanska, Murray, & Harlan, 2000; Maccoby, 1998; Tremblay et al., 2004), and with other studies showing that a much larger proportion of males than females follow a chronic trajectory of PA or a persistent life course trajectory of antisocial behaviours from an early age (Moffitt et al., 2001). In fact, the sex gap grows wider as more extreme antisocial behaviours (measured for frequency and severity) are considered.

The results of these trajectory analyses illustrate the usefulness of examin-ing the magnitude of sex differences while accounting for the heterogeneity in the population – i.e., the existence of distinct groups. Indeed, these studies suggest that the widening of the PA sex gap over the course of childhood may be attributed to the relatively large proportion of boys who follow a high-level PA trajectory from their early infancy. Because most children cease to use PA, the fact that more boys than girls follow a high, stable trajectory instead of a low, declining trajectory appears to account, in large part, for the widening PA sex gap during childhood. This said, patterns of change in the growing gap between the sexes may also be masked when the heterogeneity in the population is not accounted for, or when cross-sectional data are used.

What about the sex differences in PA after childhood? Archer's meta-analysis (2000) indicates that the sex gap continues to widen at puberty, increasing from .26 (95% CI: .20–.31) during middle childhood to .35 (95% CI: .28–.41) at 11–13 years and .37 (95% CI: .35–.38) at 14–17 years (Archer, 2000). The widest gap during the life course is observed in adulthood, between the ages of 18 and 30 years (d = .66; 95% CI = .62–.69 between ages 18 and 21 and .60 between ages 22 and 30). These ages correspond to peak years for the development of several characteristics that enable young men to successfully compete with other males (Archer & Côté, 2005), and also to peak years for violent crime and of homicides (Courtwright, 1996; Daly & Wilson, 1990; Quetelet, 1833/1984). After this period, the sex gap decreases to .25 (95% CI: .2.0–.3.0) between 30 and 55 years of age (Archer, 2000).

Therefore, existing evidence suggests that boys and girls differ little in their use of PA during infancy, although boys exhibit slightly more PA than do girls as early as the first year of life (Alink et al., 2006). The PA sex gap widens over the life-course, reaching a peak in adulthood between ages 18 and 30, when males use PA more frequently than do females. This increasing gap between males and females is a reflection of females' greater capacities to regulate and inhibit their physically aggressive behaviour.

Sex differences in the development of indirect aggression

Over the past three decades, there has been a growing interest in the empirical study of forms of more covert, indirect aggression (IA). As mentioned earlier, IA refers to socially manipulative and circuitous forms of aggression (Lagerspetz et al., 1988). IA may be physically manifested in acts such as destroying another person's property. Verbal manifestations of IA may include deliberately attacking a person's social standing, partaking in malicious gossip or practising social ostracism (Archer, 2000). IA does not usually involve direct confrontation, and due to its covert nature it is more difficult to measure than PA. In this chapter, we focus on the interpersonal use of IA, manifested in behaviours such as betraying trust, divulging secrets, encouraging others to dislike another person, befriending a person as a form of revenge, making derogatory remarks about a person behind his or her back and telling others to avoid a person (Lagerspetz et al., 1988; Underwood, Galen, & Paquette, 2001).[1] Lagerspetz et al. (1988) were the first to carry out a systematic study of indirect aggression using peer ratings, a particularly well suited method for measuring covert forms of aggression. They documented considerable sex differences in IA during adolescence, which were corroborated in later studies (Björkqvist et al., 1992a, Björkqvist, Oesterman, &

Kaukiainen, 1992b). The magnitude of the sex differences in IA, and even the direction of the sex differences (i.e., males or females using more IA), appears to depend on the source of information (e.g., self-report, vs. peer report vs. parent report), the type of sample (e.g., school, college student, community) and the developmental period at which IA is measured (Archer, 2000). In this chapter, our primary focus lies in the latter of these three factors.

Several cross-sectional studies have shown that females are already more indirectly aggressive than males during their preschool years (Crick, Ostrov, Appleyard, Jansen, & Casas, 2004; Ostrov & Keating, 2004; Tremblay et al., 1996). There is evidence that the IA sex gap gradually widens over the course of childhood and adolescence (Archer, 2000; Björkqvist, 1994; Björkqvist et al., 1992a, 1992b). This finding is borne out when IA is reported by peers. Archer (2000) reports no sex differences in children under age 11 years, but reports subsequent negative effect sizes, indicating a more frequent use of IA by females. More specifically, the effect size was −.13 (95% CI: −.19,−.06) for studies including children from ages 12–13 years and −.35 (95% CI: −.46,−.24) for studies including ages 14–17 years (Archer, 2000). Interestingly, there is evidence that the IA sex gap narrows substantially during adulthood, to the point where males and females do not significantly differ in their use of IA by age 22 years (Archer, 2000).

Recent studies explain the widening gap between the sexes by the fact that girls are more likely to follow rising IA trajectories during middle childhood than boys (Côté et al., 2007b; Vaillancourt, Miller, Fagbemi, Côté, & Tremblay, 2007). Whereas girls' use of PA gradually declines over the course of childhood, the use of IA appears to increase in frequency with age. In fact, while the peak frequency of PA appears to occur in toddlerhood, the peak frequency in IA is likely to occur in adolescence. Vaillancourt et al. (2007) modelled the development of IA in children from ages 4 to 10 years and identified two groups of children who followed distinct IA trajectories. More specifically, most children (65%) rarely used IA from ages 4 to 10 years, while others (35%) used IA with increasing frequency during this period of development. The latter group is mostly comprised of girls (57.5%). Figure 7.2 presents the trajectories of IA.

Sex differences in the joint development of PA and IA

Björkqvist et al. (1992a, 1992b) modelled the development of PA and IA during childhood and adolescence. These authors hypothesized that children's use of aggression is normative, and that the different types of aggression used are determined by specific developmental stages. For instance, children's first expressions of aggression are typically manifested through PA. Hence, this hypothesis predicted that toddlers would use PA to fulfil their needs, since they are limited in their capacity to express themselves verbally. As children mature cognitively, they are expected to reduce their use of direct (physical or verbal) forms of aggression and to increase their use of indirect forms of

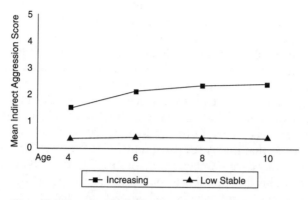

Figure 7.2 Developmental trajectories of indirect aggression.

Source: Vaillancourt, T., Miller, J., Fagbemi, J., Côté, S.M., & Tremblay, R. E. (2007). Trajectories and predictors of indirect aggression: Results from a nationally representative longitudinal study of Canadian children aged 2 to 8. *Aggressive Behavior, 33*, 1–13.

aggression. It was further hypothesized that IA represents a more sophisticated form of aggression, one that would be used more often by older rather than younger children (Björkqvist, 1994; Björkqvist et al., 1992a, 1992b; Lagerspetz et al., 1988). Thus, this model predicted that direct, physical forms of aggression would become less prevalent as childhood progresses, while indirect, relational forms of aggression would become increasingly more common during middle childhood. In other words, children are expected to switch from using PA to using IA. In order to test Björkqvist et al.'s (1992a, 1992b) developmental hypothesis, PA and IA development need to be examined jointly. While most studies have examined the exclusive use of PA and IA, recent empirical evidence on the joint development of PA and IA provides some support for Björkqvist et al.'s hypothesis. Using the person-oriented approach of the NLSCY, Côté et al. (2007b) studied children's exclusive and joint use of PA and IA during their preschool and elementary school years. The 1183 study participants were 2 years of age when the initial assessment took place and were followed over 6 years. Children followed either low or declining PA trajectories, but 14.6% followed high, stable trajectories. Approximately two-thirds of participants followed low IA trajectories (67.9%) and one-third (32.1%) followed high, rising IA trajectories. If we combine both PA and IA groups, most children (62.1%) exhibited desisting levels of PA and low levels of IA. A significant proportion of participants shared moderately desisting PA trajectories and rising IA (14.2%) trajectories. Among 13.5% of the participants there were high-level trajectories in both forms of aggression. Virtually no children scored high in one form of aggression and low in the other. Significant sex differences were found: Girls were 2.66 times more likely than boys to follow a trajectory of desisting PA and rising IA. These results suggest that PA and IA sex differences between boys and girls diverge increasingly as childhood progresses, with PA in boys being more likely to remain on a high-level trajectory and PA in girls being more likely to decrease as their use of IA increases. However, when adulthood is reached, important sex differences in PA aggression remain but sex differences in social aggression have practically disappeared. This suggests that, when considering both forms of aggression, males are more aggressive than females.

Summary of sex differences in PA and IA

Existing empirical evidence indicates that most children cease to use PA over the course of childhood but that a minority fails to do so. This group is mostly comprised of male children with high, stable PA levels. Overall, most children of both sexes use low levels of IA, but one group of children uses this type of aggression with increasing frequency. This group is mostly female. Importantly, the gap between the sexes does not remain stable over time, but rather widens considerably during childhood and pre-adolescence. In the following section, we will review two hypotheses based, respectively, on the fields of biology and social learning to provide critical insight into the origins and development of sex differences in aggression.

Hypotheses on the development of sex differences in aggression

Why are boys generally more likely to exhibit PA and girls generally more likely to exhibit IA? And why does the magnitude of the differences between the two sexes vary over the life-course? Broadly, two classes of factors should be considered: First, individual biology inevitably plays a part (e.g., genetics, hormones and anatomy). Second, social learning factors (e.g., socialization or societal norms) may also constitute crucial factors. Most sex differences, including differences in complex phenomena such as aggression, appear to be influenced by the two classes of factors.

Hypotheses on the causes of sex differences in aggression should account for variations in the IA–PA sex gap in the course of development and sex differences in the most prevalent types of aggression. In the next section, we will consider the relative value of the biological and social learning hypotheses in explaining the development of sex differences in aggression.

The biological hypothesis

Sexual differentiation takes place during the development of male or female physical traits in an undifferentiated zygote (fertilized egg). As male and female zygotes develop into foetuses, infants, children, adolescents and then into adults, sex differences appear at all levels: genes, chromosomes, gonads, hormones, anatomy and social behaviour. At the most basic level, male and female genes encode dichotomous development paths, determining a host of biological configurations. These factors include obvious differences in physical size and strength, reproductive functions and (prenatal and postnatal) hormone levels. All of these factors are important considerations in measuring aggression.

Sex differences in the gametes (i.e., sperms and ova in humans) are determined by the presence or absence of the Y chromosome. The Y chromosome triggers prenatal chemical reactions that result in marked sex differences in the production and sensitivity to the key masculinizing hormone, testosterone. In the first weeks of life, a foetus has no anatomic or hormonal gender, and only sex chromosomes differentiate females (XX) from males (XY). Early in foetal life, specific genes induce gonadal differences, thereby producing hormonal differences that lead to anatomic differences. Since the testosterone is mostly responsible for the process of masculinization, the prenatal influence of testosterone on the developing brain is probably the most important source of sexual differentiation. During puberty, hormones (testosterone in males and oestrogen in females) have a different function, triggering the onset of reproductive functions. Thus, dramatic differences between the sexes are established at birth, differences that form the basis of further sexual differentiation as psychological and behavioural differences develop.

Genetic and hormonal sex differences also lead to important brain differences. In fact, the brains of males and females differ both in their structure and function (Cahill, 2005). With technologic advances in brain imaging, researchers have now increased their capacity to detect sex differences in brain morphology and functioning. These new-found differences will greatly help in understanding sex differences in behaviour and aggression.

At a structural level, major sex differences have been discovered in the brain lobes and the regions involved in cognitive functions and emotion processing, such as the hippocampus, amygdala and neocortex (Goldstein et al., 2001). The hippocampus, a region associated with learning and memory, is sexually dimorphic in its structure and function (Cahill, 2005). Sex differences in the amygdala are also substantial. The amygdala plays a vital role in memory functions, especially in memories of emotional events. The sex-related lateralization of the amygdala has been documented in humans. Studies indicate a preferential involvement of the left amygdala in emotional memory for women, but a preferential involvement of the right amygdala for males (Cahill, 2005). In addition, differences in the size of the amygdala have been documented, with male amygdala being larger than that of females (relative to the size of the cerebellum).

Most sex differences are functional differences, and some have considerable implications in determining normative levels of aggression between the sexes. For instance, important sex differences were found with respect to serotonin synthesis following tryptophan depletion. Specifically, Nishizawa et al. (1997) found the mean rate of serotonin synthesis to be 52% higher in males than in females. Higher serotonin synthesis leads to low levels of serotonin in the cerebrospinal fluid, and low serotonin is a strong correlate of impulsive aggression (e.g., Haberstick, Smolen, & Hewitt, 2006; Halperin, Kalmar, Schulz, Marks, Sharma, & Newcorn, 2006).

In humans, X-linked genotypes representing risk for antisocial behaviours are related to sex differences in aggression. For instance, genetic deficiencies in monoamine oxidase A (MAOA) activity have been linked with aggression in mice and humans, and the MAOA gene is located on the X chromosome. Males, having a single X chromosome, yield two MAOA genotypes: high activity and low activity. Females, however, having two copies of the X chromosome, fall into four groups, one of which is the rare combination of the low–low MAOA genotype. Thus, the proportion of females with this risk for aggression is much smaller (Caspi et al., 2002).

With regard to sex differences in pathological aggression, sex differences in the prevalence of dysregulated neurochemical functioning may have significant implications for impulsive behaviour, and especially a predisposition to impulsive violence has been correlated with a low brain serotonin turnover rate, as indicated by a low concentration of 5-hydroxyindoleacetic acid (5-HIAA) in the cerebrospinal fluid (CSF) (Virkkunen, Goldman, Nielsen, & Linnoila, 1995). Such types of central serotonin metabolism deficits have been found in both humans and other primate species (Higley, Mehlman, Taub, Higley, Suomi, & Linnoila, 1996; Suomi, 2003). Among rhesus monkeys, low 5-HIAA appears to be related to aggressive and impulsive behaviour among both males and females.

Two important points should be noted regarding violence and low 5-HIAA concentrations in the rhesus monkey studies (Higley et al., 1996; Suomi, 2003). First, in primates, there are many more males than females with low CSF 5-HIAA concentrations. Second, compared with members of their own sex, aggressive males and females with low 5-HIAA concentrations engaged in a disproportionate number of aggressive interactions. This said, low CSF 5-HIAA females typically engaged in fewer overt acts of PA than did the males (Higley et al., 1996). Therefore, while low CSF 5-HIAA concentrations are associated with aggressive behaviour among both sexes, there are more males with low CSF 5-HIAA levels and more manifestations of aggression among low-level CSF 5-HIAA males than females. The example of low CSF 5-HIAA as a risk factor for aggression illustrates how a risk factor common to both sexes can produce significant sex differences with regard to the proportion and severity of aggression.

Biological hypotheses on sex differences do not necessarily explain changes in the magnitude of these differences over the course of development. However, there is evidence indicating that at least some changes in sex differences could result from differential rates of maturation between males and females. For instance, girls experience faster cognitive development during the preschool years. This accelerated maturation may lead to a faster rate of inhibition and regulation of PA in girls, and may produce sex differences in the development of IA. Faster language development in girls is of particular interest, since verbal requests may facilitate the regulation of physical aggression. Thus, males may have a higher prevalence of risk factors that interfere with the regulation of aggression.

In sum, there are numerous major biological differences between males and females that are likely to explain most, if not all, of the differences in anti-social behaviours. Biological research that systematically tests the extent to which a given biological mechanism applies to both sexes is needed. As illustrated in this section, the studies that tested for potential sex differences have begun to uncover the breadth and importance of the differences. Humans are not, however, developing in a vacuum and several lines of research point to the importance of socialization and contextual influences in the emergence of sex difference in aggressive behaviours.

The social learning hypothesis

The social learning hypothesis has provided an influential account of the development of prosocial and aggressive behaviours (Bandura, 1973; Loeber & Stouthamer-Loeber, 1998; Reiss & Roth, 1993). According to this hypothesis, aggressive and violent behaviours are learned during childhood and adolescence through exposure to social influences such as violent television programmes, aggressive role models or deviant peers (Johnson, Cohen, Smailes, Kasen, & Brook, 2002; Patterson, Dishion, & Bank, 1984; Thornberry, 1998). Based solely on this hypothesis, children would logically become more aggressive and violent as they grow older.

As summarized in the first section of this chapter, recent longitudinal studies indicate that children become less, not more, physically aggressive and violent over time (Broidy et al., 2003; Cairns et al., 1989; Côté et al., 2006; Nagin & Tremblay, 1999; Tremblay et al., 1999). In fact, developmental trajectory studies have found that most children followed declining trajectories of PA between kindergarten and grade 6. If the development of aggression were solely based on the cumulative effects of social influences that purportedly promote aggressive behaviour, we would expect a significant group of children to begin their use of PA during their elementary school years. Such a group has not been identified (Broidy et al., 2003; Côté et al., 2006; Nagin & Tremblay, 1999; NICHD-ECCRN, 2004).

Furthermore, the evidence reviewed in the first section of this chapter clearly indicates that PA appears during the first 12 months after birth and seems to be a normal part of early social interaction. Rather than learning to aggress over time, children apparently learn not to aggress. This learning curve appears to be supported by brain maturation but is also most likely the result of social learning, which involves learning the rules that guide appropriate social behaviours.

In its explanation of the developmental progression of aggression, social learning theory places a heavy emphasis on how specific forms of aggressive behaviour are learned. But, while it is true that specific aggressive actions may be learned from peers, parents and the media, they do not account for broad changes in the frequency of aggression manifested at different ages (Archer & Côté, 2005). In reality, it is more plausible that social factors such as coercive parenting, violent models or violent media account for the failure, for a minority of children, to fail to learn how to regulate and inhibit their aggressive behaviour.

Social learning theory may produce sex differences in aggression through four mechanisms. First, social factors may have a stronger impact on girls than on boys in learning alternatives to PA. For instance, parents proposing an alternative strategy to aggression (e.g., asking for a toy instead of grabbing the toy) may be more successful with girls than boys in modifying the behaviour, as girls are less inclined to aggression and have generally better verbal abilities in early childhood. Second, compared with boys, girls may be exposed to more social influences conducive to learning alternatives to PA and greater consciousness. For example, given the segregation of the sexes during middle childhood, girls are exposed to many more friendships that involve verbal negotiation instead of PA. Third, social factors against aggression may have a stronger disinhibitory impact on boys than on girls. For instance, boys exposed to a violent television programme may be more likely to act out aggression than are girls. Fourth, compared with girls, boys may be exposed to a larger number of social influences that encourage the dishinhibition of aggression. For instance, socializing agents (such as peers and parents) may be more likely to encourage, rather than discourage, the use of aggression among boys, compared with girls. In fact, socializing agents may contribute to making aggression part of boys' conscientious reaction to an attack.

While few studies have formally tested these hypotheses, there is evidence that socializing agents (such as parents) selectively encourage traditional sex-typed behaviours (e.g., shyness, fearfulness and withdrawal in girls) and/or discourage non-sex-typed behaviours (e.g., aggressive behaviour in girls; Maccoby, 1998). There is also evidence supporting the importance of same-sex peer group influence during childhood, and the values of these groups, in explaining sex differences in PA. For instance, boys' play is more active, physical, group-oriented and competitive than is girls' play, thus creating more opportunities for physical contact and likely facilitating the expression of PA (Maccoby, 1998). Conversely, play among girls is typically more nurturing, caring, occurs in smaller groups (e.g., dyads or triads) and is oriented towards intimacy and social inclusion. Consequently, the structure of female friendships, which tends to be based on closeness and cohesiveness, is the basis for a more efficient use of indirect and relational forms of aggression among girls (Crick & Grotpeter, 1995; Green, Richardson, & Lago, 1996; Maccoby, 1998).

As peers play a significant role in reinforcing preferred modes of aggression, social interaction with a peer group is likely to account for some of the observed changes in the magnitude of sex differences during childhood. For instance, Fagot and Hagan (1985) showed that, as early as toddlerhood, aggressive actions (grabbing or taking objects, and hitting or verbally assault-ing others) are more prevalent in boys than in girls and that when girls do act aggressively their actions are ignored significantly more than are those initiated by boys. Boys have been shown to respond more to the actions of other boys than to the actions of girls, while girls respond more equally to the actions of boys and girls. It is suggested that responses to aggressive actions are seen as information sources for the child. The higher response rate to a boy's actions informs the child that this kind of behaviour will produce an effect on his world, while the lack of response to a girl's actions suggests the opposite. Over the course of development, if the sexes experience spe-cific types of reinforcements for their aggressive behaviours and conscious behaviours, the inhibition or the production of these behaviours will be modified accordingly.

Implications for intervention: Starting with mothers

Although males are responsible for the most severe and negative social consequences of violence and aggression, the solution to reduction of patho-logical aggression is likely to be in intervening with females, and specifically with mothers. Females are largely responsible for providing care to the next generation and experimental studies on animal and human subjects have repeatedly shown that adequate maternal care early in life is fundamental to the healthy development of offspring (Meaney, 2001; Repetti, Taylor, & Seeman, 2002; Weaver et al., 2004). The central role of females in the inter-generational transmission of aggression is vividly illustrated by Suomi's research in rhesus monkeys. Suomi (2005) suggested that a major biological vulnerability for impulsive and violent behaviours (low 5-HIAA concentra-tions) is passed on to the next generation of rhesus monkeys, primarily through the female genome. He showed that young female rhesus monkeys with low 5-HIAA concentrations are, like low 5-HIAA males, impulsive, aggressive and generally maladapted socially (Westergaard et al, 2003). Aggressive males, however, are rapidly expelled from their native troop and have a high risk of mortality prior to puberty, while aggressive females remain in their respective families for the rest of their lives. Moreover, unlike low 5-HIAA males, low 5-HIAA females engage in relatively normal repro-ductive behaviour. The offspring of mothers with low CSF 5-HIAA have a double dose of risks for pathological aggression. First, they have the genetic risks associated with being born to a mother with low CSF 5-HIAA. Second, they have the environmental risks associated with living with a mother who may exhibit significant abnormalities in maternal behaviour, behaviour that often results in insecure and/or disorganized bonding patterns in parent–child relationships. Thus, the intergenerational transmission of risks for aggression is likely to occur via genetic transmission through the female genome, inadequate maternal care or both (Suomi & Levine, 1998).

Studies with primates and rodents showed that the effects of poor maternal care and genetic vulnerabilities could be reversed by transferring the offspring to a mother who would provide better care (Kippin, Cain, Masum, & Ralph, 2004; Meaney, 2001; Suomi, 2003; Weaver et al., 2004). In humans, exposure to a high-risk family environment is reduced when children receive child care services (CCS). Results from experimental studies offering high-quality CCS to at-risk children provide robust evidence for the protective role of high-quality CCS. For instance, children of mothers with low levels of education and low SES (socio-economic status) benefited from receiving intensive, high-quality CCS during their preschool years. More specifically, CCS services in the form of preschool education were shown to have a long-term positive impact on violence and unemployment in adulthood (Campbell, Ramey, Pungello, Sparling, & Miller-Johnson, 2002; Schweinhart, Barnes, & Weikart, 1993).

Correlational studies show similar result patterns. Recent longitudinal studies have shown that young Canadian children born to high-risk mothers (i.e., mothers with low levels of education or low SES) benefited from receiving CCS early in life (Borge, Rutter, Côté, & Tremblay, 2004; Côté et al., 2007a; Côté, Borge, Rutter, Geoffroy, & Tremblay, 2008). More specifically, toddlers exposed to high levels of family risk were less likely to exhibit high levels of PA if they were in CCS than if they remained in maternal care (Borge et al., 2004). Furthermore, Geoffroy, Côté, Borge, Larouche, Séguin, and Rutter (2007) showed that children from low-SES families receiving regular CCS in infancy had better cognitive performance prior to school entry as compared with low-SES children who remained in maternal care. Other studies stress the importance of providing high quality care (e.g., Geoffroy, Côté, Parent, & Séguin, 2006; NICHD, 2005a, 2005b; Peisner-Feinberg et al., 2001). These studies suggest that early and high-quality CCS constitute an effective means of intervention that could significantly contribute to preventing the intergenerational transmission of risks for high aggression.

Social support to high-risk mothers (isolated and living in poverty) may also reduce the risk of intergenerational transmission. For instance, Olds and colleagues (Olds et al., 1998; Olds, Henderson, Kitzman, Eckenrode, Cole, & Tatelbaum, 1999; Olds et al., 2002) tested the impact of a programme aimed to improve parental behaviours and environmental conditions during pregnancy and early childhood. The programme was effective in improving parental care (as reflected in the lower numbers of injuries and accidental ingestion of foreign substances by infants) and in reducing the number of convictions, arrests, emergent substance abuse and promiscuous sexual activities among adolescents (15 years old) whose mothers were home-visited by nurses. Furthermore, this intervention led to a reduction in the mothers' subsequent number of pregnancies and their use of public assistance, and improved their work force participation. In sum, the reviewed evidence indicates that although a much greater proportion of males than females present severe aggression problems, intervention with mothers is the most promising

158   *Côté*

avenue for the prevention of intergenerational transmission of aggression problems.

Future studies should adopt experimental designs in order to formally test the timing hypothesis: i.e., that an intervention received earlier in life is more beneficial and cost-effective than intervention received later in life. Such an experiment would involve comparing the efficacy of an intervention during pregnancy (focused on maternal behaviour during pregnancy) versus in infancy (focused on high-quality CCS) versus later in childhood (focused on preschool education). Interventions involving these different timing and modalities have shown their efficacy. They have not, however, been compared within a single study. Such a comparison is necessary in order to gain a better understanding of the most efficient and cost-effective intervention for reducing aggression and violence.

Notes

1 There has been much discussion about the extent to which social (e.g., Crick & Grotpeter, 1995; Underwood, Galen, & Paquette, 2001) and indirect aggression (Björkqvist, 2001) are distinct constructs. In a recent meta-analysis, Archer and Coyne (2005) concluded that these two types of aggression are essentially part of the same construct. In this chapter, our use of the term indirect aggression is in line with that of Feshbach's pioneering work (1970).

References

Alink, L. R. A., van Zeijl, J., Stolk, M. N., Juffer, F., Koot, H. M., Bakersman-Kranenburg, M. J., et al. (2006). The early childhood aggression curve: Development of physical aggression in 10- to 50-months-old children. *Child Development*, 77(4), 954–966.

American Psychiatric Association (1994). *Diagnostic and statistical manual of mental disorders* (DSM-IV-TR) Washington, DC: APA.

Archer, J. (2000). Sex differences in aggression between heterosexual partners: A meta-analytic review. *Psychological Bulletin*, 126(5), 651–680.

Archer, J., & Côté, S. (2005). Sex differences in aggressive behavior: A developmental and evolutionary perspective. In R. E. Tremblay, W. H. Hartup, & J. Archer (Eds.), *Developmental origins of aggression* (pp. 425–446). New York: Guilford Press.

Archer, J., & Coyne, J. C. (2005). Why are girls more socially aggressive than boys? An integrated review of indirect, relational, and social aggression. *Personality and Social Psychology Review*, 9(3), 212–230.

Baillargeon, R. H., Zoccolillo, M., Keenan, K., Côté, S. M., Pérusse, D., Boivin, M., et al. (2007). Gender differences in the prevalence of physical aggression: A prospective population-based survey of children before and after two years of age. *Developmental Psychology*, 43 (1), 13–26.

Bandura, A. (1973). *Aggression: A social learning analysis*. New York: Holt.

Björkqvist, K. (1994). Sex differences in physical, verbal and indirect aggression: A review of recent research. *Sex Roles*, 30, 177–188.

Björkqvist, K. (2001). Different names, same issue. *Social Development*, 10, 272–275.

Björkqvist, K., Lagerspetz, K. M., & Kaukiainen, A. (1992a). Do girls manipulate and boys fight? Developmental trends in regard to direct and indirect aggression. *Aggressive Behavior, 18*(2), 117–127.

Björkqvist, K., Oesterman, K., & Kaukiainen, A. (1992b). The development of direct and indirect aggressive strategies in males and females. In K. Björkqvist & P. Niemelae (Eds.), *Of mice and women: Aspects of female aggression* (pp. 51–64). San Diego, CA: Academic Press.

Borge, A., Rutter, M., Côté, S., & Tremblay, R. E. (2004). Early childcare and physical aggression: Differentiating social selection and social causation. *Journal of Child Psychology and Psychiatry, 45*(2), 367–376.

Brame, B., Nagin, D. S., & Tremblay, R. E. (2001). Developmental trajectories of physical aggression from school entry to late adolescence. *Journal of Child Psychology and Psychiatry, 58*, 389–394.

Broidy, L. M., Nagin, D. S., Tremblay, R. E., Bates, J. E., Brame, B., Dodge, K., et al. (2003). Developmental trajectories of childhood disruptive behaviors and adolescent delinquency: A six site, cross national study. *Developmental Psychology, 39*(2), 222–245.

Cahill, L. (2005). His brain, her brain. *Scientific American, April*, 40–47.

Cairns, R. B., Cairns, B. D., Neckerman, H. J., Ferguson, L. L., & Gariépy, J. L. (1989). Growth and aggression: 1. Childhood to early adolescence. *Developmental Psychology, 25*(2), 320–330.

Campbell, F. A., Ramey, C. T., Pungello, E. P., Sparling, J., & Miller-Johnson, S. (2002). Early childhood education: Young adult outcomes from the Abecederian project. *Applied Developmental Science, 6*, 42–57.

Caspi, A., McClay, J., Moffitt, T., Mill, J., Martin, J., Craig, I. W., et al. (2002). Role of genotype in the cycle of violence in maltreated children. *Science, 297*, 851–854.

Côté, S. M., Boivin, M., Nagin, D. S., Japel, C., Xu, Q., Zoccolillo, M., et al. (2007a). The role of maternal education and non-maternal care services in the prevention of children's physical aggression. *Archives of General Psychiatry. 64*(11), 1305–1312.

Côté, S. M., Borge, A. I., Rutter, M., Geoffroy, M.-C., & Tremblay, R. E. (2008). Type of child care in infancy and emotional/behavioral difficulties at 4 years: Moderation by family risks and characteristics. *Developmental Psychology, 44*(1), 155–168.

Côté, S. M., Vaillancourt, T., LeBlanc, J. C., Nagin, D. S., & Tremblay, R. E. (2006). The development of physical aggression from toddlerhood to pre-adolescence: A nation wide longitudinal study of Canadian children. *Journal of Abnormal Child Psychology, 34*(11), 71–85.

Côté, S. M., Vaillancourt, T., Barker, E. D., Nagin, D. S., & Tremblay, R. E. (2007b). Predictors of continuity and change in the joint development of physical and indirect aggression. *Development and Psychopathology, 19*(1), 37–55.

Courtwright, D. T. (1996). *Violent land: Single men and social disorder from the frontier to the inner city*. Cambridge, MA: Harvard University Press.

Crick, N. R. (1995). Relational aggression: The role of intent attributions, feelings of distress, and provocation types. *Development and Psychopathology, 7*(2), 313–322.

Crick, N. R., & Grotpeter, J. K. (1995). Relational aggression, gender and social-psychological adjustment. *Child Development, 66*(3), 710–722.

Crick, N. R., Ostrov, J. M., Appleyard, K., Jansen, E. A., & Casas, J. F. (2004). Relational aggression in early childhood: "You can't come to my birthday party unless . . ." In M. Putallaz & K. L. Bierman (Eds.), *Aggression, antisocial behavior, and*

160   *Côté*

violence among girls: A developmental perspective (pp. 71–89). New York: Guilford Press.

Daly, M., & Wilson, M. (1990). Killing the competition: Female/female male/male homicide. *Human Nature, 1,* 81–107.

Fagot, B. I., & Hagan, R. (1985). Aggression in toddlers: Responses to the assertive acts of boys and girls. *Sex Roles, 12,* 341–351.

Feshbach, S. (1970). Aggression. In P. H. Mussen (Ed.), *Carmichael's manual of child psychology* (Vol. 2, 3rd edn, pp. 159–259). New York: John Wiley & Sons.

Galen, B. R., & Underwood, M. K. (1997). A developmental investigation of social aggression among children. *Developmental Psychology, 33*(4), 589–600.

Geoffroy, M.-C., Côté, S., Borge, A., Larouche, F., Séguin, J. R., & Rutter, M. (2007). Association between nonmaternal care in the first year of life and children's receptive language skills prior to school entry: The moderating role of the socioeconomic status. *Journal of Child Psychology and Psychiatry, 48*(5), 490–497.

Geoffroy, M.-C., Côté, S. M., Parent, S., & Séguin, J. R. (2006). Day-care attendance, stress and mental health. *Canadian Journal of Psychiatry, 51*(9), 607–615.

Goldstein, J. M., Seidman, L. J., Horton, N. J., Makris, N., Kennedy, D. N., Caviness, V. S., Jr., et al. (2001). Normal sexual dimorphism of the adult human brain assessed by in vivo magnetic resonance imaging. *Cerebral Cortex, 11*(6), 490–497.

Green, L. R., Richardson, D. R., & Lago, T. (1996). How do friendship, indirect, and direct aggression relate? *Aggressive Behavior, 22,* 81–86.

Haberstick, B. C., Smolen, A., Hewitt, J. K. (2006). Family-based association test of the 5HTTLPR and aggressive behavior in a general population sample of children. *Biological Psychiatry, 59,* 836–843.

Halperin, J. M., Kalmar, J. H., Schulz, K. P., Marks, D. J., Sharma, V., & Newcorn, J. H. (2006). Elevated childhood serotonergic function protects against adolescent aggression in disruptive boys. *Journal of the American Academy of Child and Adolescent Psychiatry. 45*(7), 833–840.

Hay, D. F., Castle, J., & Davies, L. (2000). Toddlers' use of force against familiar peers: A precursor of serious aggression? *Child Development, 71,* 457–467.

Higley, J. D., Mehlman, P. T., Taub, D. M., Higley, S. B., Suomi, S. J., & Linnoila, M. (1996). Stability of interindividual differences in serotonin function and its relationship to severe aggression and competent social behavior in rhesus Macaque females. *Neuropsychopharmacology, 7,* 67–76.

Hrdy, S. (1999). *Mother nature: A history of mothers, infants, and natural selection.* New York: Pantheon Books.

Johnson, J. G., Cohen, P., Smailes, E. M., Kasen, S., & Brook, J. S. (2002). Television viewing and aggressive behavior during adolescence and adulthood. *Science, 295,* 2468–2471.

Keenan, K., & Shaw, D. (1997). Developmental and social influences on young girls' early problem behaviors. *Psychological Bulletin, 121,* 95–113.

Keenan, K., & Wakschlag, L. S. (2000). More than the terrible twos: The nature and severity of behavior problems in clinic-referred preschool children. *Journal of Abnormal Child Psychology, 28*(1), 33–46.

Kippin, T. E., Cain, S. W., Masum, Z., & Ralph, M. R. (2004). Neural stem cells show bidirectional experience-dependent plasticity in the perinatal mammalian brain. *Journal of Neuroscience, 24,* 2832–2836.

Kochanska, G., Murray, K. T., & Harlan, E. T. (2000). Effortful control in early childhood: Continuity and change, antecedents, and implications for social development. *Developmental Psychology, 36*, 220–232.

Lagerspetz, K. M., Björkqvist, K., & Peltonen, T. (1988). Is indirect aggression typical of females: Gender differences in aggressiveness in 11- to 12-years-old children. *Aggressive Behavior, 14*, 403–414.

Loeber, R., & Stouthamer-Loeber, M. (1998). Development of juvenile aggression and violence. Some common misconceptions and controversies. *American Psychologist, 53*, 242–259.

Maccoby, E. (1998). *The two sexes.* Cambridge, MA: Harvard University Press.

McGrew, W. C. (1972). *An ethological study of children's behavior.* New York: Academic Press.

Meaney, M. J. (2001). Maternal care, gene expression, and the transmission of individual differences in stress reactivity across generations. *Annual Review of Neuroscience, 24*, 1161–1192.

Moffitt, T. E., Caspi, A., Rutter, M., & Silva, P. (2001). *Sex differences in antisocial behavior.* Cambridge, UK: Cambridge University Press.

Nagin, D., & Tremblay, R. E. (1999). Trajectories of boys' physical aggression, opposition, and hyperactivity on the path to physically violent and non violent juvenile delinquency. *Child Development, 70*(5), 1181–1196.

NICHD (2005a). Characteristics of infant child care: Factors contributing to positive caregiving. In NICHD Early Child Care Research Network (Ed.), *Child care and child development. Results from the NICHD study of early child care and youth development* (pp. 50–66). New York: Guilford Press.

NICHD (2005b). Early child care and children's development prior to school entry: results from the NICHD study of early child care. In NICHD Early Child Care Research Network (Ed.), *Child care and child development. Results from the NICHD study of early child care and youth development* (pp. 376–392). New York: Guilford Press.

NICHD-ECCRN (2004). Trajectories of physical aggression from toddlerhood to middle school. *Monographs of the Society for Research in Child Development, 69* (4, Serial No. 278).

Nishizawa, S., Benkelfat, C., Young, S. N., Leyton, M., Mzengeza, S., de Montigny, C., et al. (1997). Differences between males and females in rates of serotonin synthesis in human brain. *Proceedings of the National Academy of Sciences of the USA, 94*, 5308–5313.

Olds, D., Henderson, C. R., Cole, R., Eckenrode, J., Kitzman, H., Luckey, D., et al. (1998). Long-term effects of nurse home visitation on children's criminal and antisocial behavior: Fifteen-year follow-up of a randomized controlled trial. *Journal of the American Medical Association, 280*, 1238–1244.

Olds, D. L., Henderson, C. R., Jr., Kitzman, H., Eckenrode, J., Cole, R., & Tatelbaum, R. C. (1999). Prenatal and infancy home visitation by nurses: Recent findings. *The Future of Children, 9*, 44–65.

Olds, D. L., Robinson, J., O'Brien, R., Luckey, D. W., Pettitt, L. M., Henderson, C. R., et al. (2002). Home visiting by nurses and by paraprofessionals: A randomized controlled trial. *Pediatrics, 110*(3), 486–496.

Ostrov, J. M., & Keating, C. F. (2004). Gender differences in preschool aggression during free play and structured interactions: An observational study. *Social Development, 13*, 255–277.

162   *Côté*

Patterson, G. R., Dishion, T. J., & Bank, L. (1984). Family interaction: A process model of deviancy training. *Aggressive Behavior, 10*, 253–267.

Peisner-Feinberg, E. S., Burchinal, M., Clifford, R. M., Culkin, M., Howes, C., Kagan, S. L., et al. (2001). The relation of preschool child-care quality to children's cognitive and social development trajectories through second grade. *Child Development, 72*, 1534–1553.

Quetelet, A. (1984). *Research on the propensity for crime at different ages* (S. F. Sylvester, Trans.). Cincinnnati, OH: Anderson. (Original work published in 1833)

Reiss, A. J., & Roth, J. A. (1993). *Understanding and preventing violence.* Washington, DC: National Academy Press.

Repetti, R. L., Taylor, S. E., & Seeman, S. E. (2002). Risky family: Family social environments and the mental and physical health of offspring. *Psychological Bulletin, 128*, 330–366.

Schweinhart, L. L., Barnes, H. V., & Weikart, D. P. (1993). *Significant benefits. The High/Scope Perry School Study through age 27.* Ypsilanti, MI: High/Scope Press.

Sears, R. R., Rau, L., & Alpert, R. (1965). *Identification and childrearing.* Stanford, CA: Stanford University Press.

Straus, M. A., & Gelles, R. J. (1990). *Physical violence in American families: Risk factors and adaptations to violence in 8,145 families.* New Brunswick, NJ: Transaction Publishers.

Suomi, S. J. (2003). Social and biological mechanisms underlying impulsive aggressiveness in rhesus monkeys. In B. B. Lahey, T. E. Moffitt, & A. Caspi (Eds.), *Causes of conduct disorder and juvenile delinquency* (pp. 345–362). New York: Guilford Press.

Suomi, S. J. (2005). Genetic and environmental factors influencing the expression of impulsive aggression and serotonergic functioning in rhesus monkeys. In R. E. Tremblay, W. W. Hartup, & J. Archer (Eds.), *Developmental origins of aggression* (pp. 63–82). New York: Guilford Press.

Suomi, S. J., & Levine, S. (1998). Psychobiology of intergenerational effects of trauma: Evidence from animal studies. In Y. Danieli (Ed.), *Intergenerational handbook of multigeneration legacies* (pp. 623–637). New York: Plenum Press.

Thornberry, T. (1998). Membership in youth gangs and involvement in serious and violent offending. In R. Loeber & D. P. Farrington (Eds.), *Serious and violent juvenile offenders: Risk factors and successful interventions* (pp. 147–166). Thousand Oaks, CA: Sage Publications.

Tremblay, R. E. (2000). The development of aggressive behaviour during childhood: What have we learned in the past century? *International Journal of Behavioral development, 24*(2), 129–141.

Tremblay, R. E., Boulerice, B., Harden, P. W., McDuff, P., Pérusse, D., Pihl, R. O., et al. (1996). Do children in Canada become more aggressive as they approach adolescence? In Human Resources Development Canada and Statistics Canada (Eds.), *Growing up in Canada: National Longitudinal Survey of Children and Youth* (pp. 127–137). Ottawa: Statistics Canada.

Tremblay, R. E., Japel, C., Pérusse, D., McDuff, P., Boivin, M., Zoccolillo, M., et al. (1999). The search for the age of "onset" of physical aggression: Rousseau and Bandura revisited. *Criminal Behavior and Mental Health, 9*, 8–23.

Tremblay, R. E., Nagin, D. S., Séguin, J. R., Zoccolillo, M., Zelazo, P., Boivin, M., et al. (2004). Physical aggression during early childhood: Trajectories and predictors. *Pediatrics, 114*(1), e43–e50.

Underwood, M. K., Galen, B. R., & Paquette, J. A. (2001). Top ten challenges for understanding gender and aggression in children: Why can't we all just get along? *Social Development, 10*, 248–266.

Vaillancourt, T., Miller, J., Fagbemi, J., Côté, S.M., & Tremblay, R. E. (2007). Trajectories and predictors of indirect aggression: Results from a nationally representative longitudinal study of Canadian children aged 2 to 8. *Aggressive Behavior, 33*, 1–13.

Virkkunen, M., Goldman, D., Nielsen, D. A., & Linnoila, M. (1995). Low brain serotonin turnover rate (low CSF 5-HIAA) and impulsive violence. *Journal of Psychiatry and Neuroscience, 20*(4), 271–275.

Weaver, I. C. G., Cervoni, N., Champagne, F. A., D'Alessio, A. C., Sharma, S., Seckl, J. R., et al. (2004). Epigenetic programming by maternal behavior. *Nature Neuroscience, 7*(8), 847–854.

Westergaard, C. G., Suomi, S. J., Chavanne, T. J., Houser, L., Hurlye, A. C., Cleveland, A., et al. (2003). Physiological correlates of aggression and impulsivity in free-ranging female primates. *Neuropsychopharmacology, 28*, 1045–1055.

8 Intergenerational transmission of risk for antisocial behaviour

Sara Jaffee

Introduction

Antisocial behaviour carries a heavy cost to individuals and to society. As young adults, individuals who engage in antisocial behaviour are at risk for truncated educational attainment, persistent unemployment, incarceration, relationship conflict, physical health problems, and teen pregnancy and parenthood (e.g., Fergusson, Horwood, & Ridder, 2005; Jaffee, 2002; Maughan & Rutter, 2001; Moffitt, Caspi, Harrington, & Milne, 2002). Society members also pay for antisocial behaviour, both as victims and as taxpayers, in quantities that amount to billions of dollars per year (Welsh, 2003). Thus, antisocial behaviour is a significant public health concern. Even more concerning is the possibility that antisocial behaviour is transmitted across successive generations in a "cycle of violence" that clinicians and policy makers have found difficult to break. The goal of this chapter is to review the evidence on the familiality of antisocial behaviour, describe mechanisms by which risk for antisocial behaviour is transmitted from parents to children, and point to new directions for research that may inform efforts to prevent the emergence of antisocial behaviour.

Does antisocial behaviour run in families?

In a meta-analysis of risk factors for antisocial behaviour, parental criminal convictions emerged as one of the strongest predictors of an individual's own antisocial behaviour (Loeber & Stouthamer-Loeber, 1986) and studies of community samples in the United States and the United Kingdom have shown that a small number of families (approximately 10%) account for about half of all persons with arrest records (Farrington, Jolliffe, Loeber, Stouthamer-Loeber, & Kalb, 2001). Evidence for the familial aggregation of antisocial behaviour also comes from clinical samples. First degree relatives of children who have been diagnosed with conduct disorder or oppositional defiant disorder have elevated rates of antisocial personality disorder and other externalizing spectrum disorders (e.g., substance abuse disorders) compared with relatives of healthy controls or psychiatric controls (Faraone,

Biederman, Jetton, & Tsuang, 1997; Faraone, Biederman, & Monuteaux, 2000; Frick, Lahey, Christ, & Green, 1991; Lahey, Piacentini, McBurnett, Stone, Hartdagen, & Hynd, 1988; Stewart, deBlois, & Cummings, 1980; Wozniak, Biederman, Faraone, Blier, & Monuteaux, 2001). Children whose fathers have been diagnosed with antisocial personality disorder also have elevated rates of conduct disorder, oppositional defiant disorder, and attention deficit hyperactivity disorder (Moss, Baron, Hardie, & Vanyukov, 2001). Thus, evidence from clinic and community samples is consistent in demonstrating strong intergenerational continuities in antisocial behaviour.

Why does antisocial behaviour run in families?

The results of family studies demonstrate that antisocial behaviour runs in families, but less is known about *why* this is so. Researchers who have investigated this question can generally be divided into those who study psychosocial mechanisms of risk transmission versus those who study biological mechanisms (specifically, genetic mechanisms). In the past several years, investigators have begun to develop integrative models that estimate the joint and interactive effects of biological and psychosocial risk mechanisms. These models will be reviewed in turn.

Psychosocial models

Parents who have histories of antisocial behaviour tend to raise children in criminogenic environments and this effect is observed in studies that measure parent antisocial behaviour retrospectively (Loeber & Stouthamer-Loeber, 1986) as well as studies that follow young people prospectively across the transition to parenthood (Jaffee, Belsky, Harrington, Caspi, & Moffitt, 2006; Smith & Farrington, 2004). Indeed a recent study showed that parents who had been diagnosed with conduct disorder in adolescence provided even riskier care-giving environments for their children than parents who had been diagnosed with major depressive or anxiety disorders (Jaffee et al., 2006). These environments were characterized by relatively high rates of social disadvantage (e.g., unemployment, single parenthood, and low socio-economic status), adult partner violence, romantic relationship conflict, and suboptimal parenting practices.

Many researchers who study psychosocial mechanisms of risk transmission endorse a social learning perspective wherein children learn aggressive behaviour and aggressive parenting practices via their observations of their parents' behaviour and then carry these behaviours into the next generation (Conger, Neppl, Kim, & Scaramella, 2003; Patterson, 1998). Others note that social structural conditions (e.g., poverty, social disadvantage) remain stable across generations and propose that these may account for intergenerational continuities in suboptimal parenting as well as antisocial behaviour (Thornberry, Freeman-Gallant, Lizotte, Krohn, & Smith, 2003). Researchers interested in psychosocial risk mechanisms test whether child rearing practices (including authoritarian parenting style, harsh and inconsistent discipline, parental involvement, poor supervision and monitoring) or social structural conditions account for the association between parent and offspring antisocial behaviour.

A review of the literature provides mixed support for psychosocial models. Several studies have shown that continuity in antisocial behaviour across generations is accounted for by suboptimal parenting practices, such as low levels of monitoring and time spent together doing activities (Capaldi & Patterson, 1991), abuse (Verona & Sachs-Ericsson, 2005), marital tension and parental hostility (Caspi & Elder, 1988), and low parental warmth and disciplinary inconsistency (Thornberry et al., 2003). In contrast, other studies have either failed to detect intergenerational continuities in antisocial behaviour (Conger et al., 2003), failed to find that parenting practices explain intergenerational continuities in antisocial behaviour (Capaldi, Pears, Patterson, & Owen, 2003; Ehrensaft, Wasserman, Verdelli, Greenwald, Miller, & Davies, 2003; Verlaan & Schwartzman, 2002), or have found that these processes operate differently for mothers and fathers and across successive generations (Smith & Farrington, 2004). For example, Smith and Farrington (2004) tested whether authoritarian parenting style in mothers and fathers, paternal uninvolvement, poor parental supervision, inconsistent discipline, and partner conflict explained intergenerational continuities in antisocial behaviour. Although paternal and maternal antisocial behaviour in generation 1 were both predictive of offspring antisocial behaviour in generation 2, only the mother–offspring link was mediated by suboptimal parenting practices. Specifically, mothers who engaged in relatively high levels of antisocial behaviour provided inadequate supervision, which, in turn, explained high levels of antisocial behaviour in their children. In contrast, only maternal antisocial behaviour in generation 2 was predictive of offspring antisocial behaviour in generation 3, and this relationship was only weakly mediated by suboptimal parenting practices.

In summary, the evidence in favour of psychosocial mechanisms is, at best, inconsistent. On the one hand, it should not be surprising that individual mediators fail to fully (or even substantially) account for intergenerational continuities in antisocial behaviour because the association between parent and offspring antisocial behaviour is likely to be multiply determined and any one risk mechanism is unlikely to account for large portions of variance. Moreover, cohort effects may explain why psychosocial factors that link parent and offspring antisocial behaviour across one generation do not explain continuities in antisocial behaviour across subsequent generations. On the other hand, this implies that researchers should move towards testing cumulative risk models rather than models in which individual risk mechanisms are presumed to be the most salient (Rutter, 1979; Sameroff, Bartko, Baldwin, Baldwin, & Seifer, 1998). Moreover, the observed pattern of findings is consistent with the possibility that intergenerational continuities in antisocial behaviour are moderated by characteristics of the child or the family and that psychosocial factors might account for individual differences in offspring antisocial behaviour in certain families, but not others. These hypotheses are elaborated later in this chapter.

Biological models

Results from twin and adoption studies have shown that antisocial behaviour is moderately to highly heritable (Hicks, Krueger, Iacono, McGue, & Patrick, 2004; Moffitt, 2005; Rhee & Waldman, 2002). More recently, molecular geneticists have begun using linkage and association studies to identify specific genetic variants that are associated with antisocial behaviour in humans. The bulk of this work has implicated monoamine oxidase A (MAOA) variants, serotonin (5-HT) gene variants, and catechol O-methyltransferase (COMT) variants as being associated with aggressive and antisocial behaviour. Genetic studies are premised on the assumption that genetic variation underlies individual differences in neural function that, in turn, influence behaviour.

There have been two published genome-wide screens for genes associated with antisocial behaviour. Dick et al. (2004) conducted a genome-wide screen for genes influencing conduct disorder as reported retrospectively by a sample of adults selected for alcoholism. The strongest evidence of linkage was found to chromosomes 19 and 2. Genes in the region of chromosome 2 that were associated with conduct disorder symptomatology have also been associated with alcohol dependence, suggesting that these genes may be involved in impulsive, under-controlled behaviours more generally (Dick et al., 2004). Similarly, Stallings et al. (2005) conducted a genome-wide scan for genes influencing substance use and conduct problems in a sample of adolescent males being treated for substance abuse and delinquency and found the strongest linkage to chromosome 9. They also reported linkage to chromosome 17 for individuals reporting conduct problems without comorbid substance use problems. However, with the exception of the serotonin transporter promoter polymorphism, genes on these chromosomes have not been linked to conduct problems (Stallings et al., 2005).

Other studies have looked for associations between specific gene variants and antisocial behaviour. For example, one study of a large Dutch pedigree identified several male members who were characterized by borderline mental retardation and exhibited high levels of aggressive, impulsive behaviour (Brunner, Nelen, Breakefield, Ropers, & van Oost, 1993). Subsequent work determined that this behaviour was associated with a point mutation in the MAOA structural gene (which is located on the X chromosome) that resulted in marked reductions in MAOA activity and correlated reductions in monoamine concentrations (Brunner et al., 1993). However, this mutation is very rare. More common are variable number tandem repeat (VNTR) polymorphisms in other regions of the MAOA gene, some of which are functional. For example, Sabol, Hu, and Hamer (1998) identified a 30-base-pair repeat polymorphism in the promoter region of the MAOA gene and showed that promoter alleles with 3.5 or 4 copies of the repeat were transcribed 2–10 times more efficiently than alleles with 3 or 5 copies.

While some studies have shown that the low activity MAOA promoter variant is associated with antisocial personality disorder (Jacob et al., 2005) and antisocial alcoholism (Samochowiec et al., 1999; Schmidt et al., 2000), other researchers have failed to replicate these associations (Caspi et al., 2002; Haberstick, Smolen, & Hewitt, 2006; Huizinga et al., 2006; Kim-Cohen et al., 2006; Koller, Bondy, Preuss, Bottlender, & Soyka, 2003; Lu, Lee, Ko, Chen, & Shih, 1999; Nilsson et al., 2006; Saito et al., 2002; Widom & Brzustowicz, 2006; Young et al., 2006). Still others have reported that the *high* activity variant was associated with pervasive aggressive behaviour in children (Beitchman, Mik, Ehtesham, Douglas, & Kennedy, 2004) and aggressive and impulsive behaviour in adult men (Manuck, Flory, Ferrell, Mann, & Muldoon, 2000).

A number of serotonin transporter (5-HTT) and receptor (5-HTR) gene variants have also been associated with antisocial behaviour. Heils et al. (1995) identified an insertion/deletion polymorphism in the promoter region of the serotonin transporter gene. Individuals who have the short form of the allele transcribe less efficiently than individuals who carry the long form of the allele (Lesch et al., 1996). The short form of the serotonin transporter polymorphism has been associated with aggressive behaviour in 9-year-old children (Haberstick et al., 2006), with hostility and novelty seeking in adolescent drug users (Gerra et al., 2005), with conduct disorder (Sakai et al., 2006), with violent offending in adult males (Liao, Hong, Shih, & Tsai, 2004; Retz, Retz-Junginger, Supprian, Thome, & Rösler, 2004), and with antisocial alcoholism (Hallikainen et al., 1999). Other researchers have not replicated these findings (Davidge et al., 2004), although Davidge et al. (2004) did report that the 5-HTT VNTR 10-repeat allele was less common and the 12-repeat allele more common among children with high levels of aggression compared with controls. Moreover, Zalsman et al. (2001) reported that the long form of the transporter polymorphism was associated with violence in a sample of adolescent suicide attempters.

Serotonin receptor 1B (HTR1B) variants have also been implicated in antisocial behaviour. One study showed that the HTR1B-861C allele was more common among antisocial alcoholics (Lappalainen et al., 1998), but this association has not been replicated (Davidge et al., 2004; Huang, Grailhe, Arango, Hen, & Man, 1999; Kranzler, Hernandez-Avila, & Gelernter, 2002) and another study reported that the HTR1B-861C allele was less frequent among alcoholics with comorbid conduct disorder (Soyka, Preuss, Koller, Zill, & Bondy, 2004). Because the HTR1B-G861C polymorphism involves a silent mutation, it is likely to be in linkage disequilibrium with the true functional variant. Potential functional candidates include HTR1B-G-261T, which is located in the 5′ flanking region of the gene and is in linkage disequilibrium with G861C (Kranzler et al., 2002; Sinha, Cloninger, & Parsian,

2003). However, the HTR1B-G-261T polymorphism is not associated with antisocial behaviour (Kranzler et al., 2002) or antisocial alcoholism (Sinha et al., 2003).

Finally, the 5-HT2A receptor variant G1438A has been associated with impulsivity (Nomura et al., 2006) and criminality (Berggard, Damberg, Longato-Stadler, Hallman, Oreland, & Garpenstrand, 2003). The 5-HT2A receptor variant T102C has also been associated with impulsive behaviour (Bjork, Moeller, Dougherty, Swann, Machado, & Hanis, 2002) and with antisocial alcoholism (Hwu & Chen, 2000). However, for both 5-HT2A receptor variants, null associations with impulsivity have also been reported (Kusumi, Suzuki, Sasaki, Kensuke, Sasaki, & Koyama, 2002; Tochigi et al., 2005).

The COMT gene is located on chromosome 22 and has a common methionine (Met) to valine (Val) substitution at codon 158. Homozygosity for the Met allele is associated with a three- to fourfold reduction in enzyme activity relative to Val homozygotes (Lachman, Papolos, Saito, Yu, Szumlanski, & Weinshilboum, 1996). As reviewed by Volavka, Bilder, and Nolan (2004), the Met allele has been associated with aggressive and antisocial behaviour in four out of five studies of schizophrenic patients. However, in a study of clinic-referred children with attention deficit hyperactivity disorder, children who were homozygous for the Val allele had significantly more symptoms of conduct disorder than children who were heterozygous or homozygous for the Met allele, particularly if they also had low birth weight (Thapar et al., 2005). This finding was not replicated by Sengupta et al. (2006).

In summary, although researchers have detected associations between antisocial behaviour and a number of genetic variants, the literature is characterized by weak associations and failures to replicate. In some cases, failures to replicate may arise because behaviours are measured in different ways across different studies (e.g., impulsivity is measured with Go–No-Go tasks in some studies and with personality inventories in others) and because studies vary in terms of whether they include clinical samples versus samples of healthy participants. In this regard, studies of the genetics of antisocial behaviour are no different from genetic studies of other psychiatric phenotypes (Kendler, 2005). Moreover, although the function of some of these variants has been established, others are non-functional variants that are likely to be in linkage disequilibrium with yet-to-be-identified functional candidates.

Animal models may provide important leads to plausible candidate genes. Indeed, much of the focus on current candidate genes has been informed by studies of transgenic mice that showed elevated levels of aggression when genes encoding MAOA (Cases et al., 1995), COMT (Gogos et al., 1998), and 5-HT1B (Saudou et al., 1994) were knocked out. It is also possible that focusing on endophenotypes (Gottesman & Gould, 2003) may yield more replicable gene-outcome associations, as endophenotypes (versus behavioural phenotypes) are thought to be closer to the effects of gene action. For example, Meyer-Lindenberg et al. (2006) showed that the low activity variant of the MAOA gene was associated with limbic volume reductions, amygdala hyper-responsivity during emotional arousal, and diminished reactivity of prefrontal regions. Findings such as these shed light on potential brain mechanisms that link genes to behaviour.

Biosocial models

What is notable about family studies of antisocial behaviour is that inter-generational continuities, while often statistically significant, are generally modest in magnitude (Rutter, 1998). Moreover, siblings raised in the same criminogenic environment often differ in their propensity for antisocial behaviour (Farrington et al., 2001). Models that propose to explain how risk for antisocial behaviour is transmitted from parents to children must be able to account for heterogeneity in sibling outcomes and intergenerational discontinuities as well as continuities in antisocial behaviour. Biosocial models provide a promising explanatory framework in this regard. Biosocial models propose that risk for psychopathology is elevated when biologically vulnerable children encounter psychosocial adversities (Raine, 2002). Both the biological diathesis and the environmental trigger are required to substantially increase a child's risk for psychopathology. If supported, these models would suggest two things. First, main effect associations between genes and behaviour are often weak because the environmental risk required to trigger the genetic diathesis is absent. Second, intergenerational continuities in (and sibling similarity for) antisocial behaviour are typically modest in magnitude because not all children inherit the relevant genetic risk factors.

High rates of assortative mating for antisocial behaviour (Galbaud du Fort, Bland, Newman, & Boothroyd, 1998; Krueger, Moffitt, Caspi, Bleske, & Silva, 1998) make it plausible that, in many families, children will inherit a "double whammy" of genetic and environmental risk factors. This is of great concern given the growing evidence from quantitative and molecular genetics studies that genetic and psychosocial risks jointly increase liability to antisocial behaviour in children. For example, using data from a twin study, Jaffee et al. (2005) showed that physical maltreatment increased risk for conduct problems and DSM-IV conduct disorder among children who were at high, but not low, genetic risk for conduct problems. Given that physical maltreatment is more common among families in which parents have histories of antisocial behaviour and that antisocial behaviour is moderately heritable (Jaffee, Caspi, Moffitt, & Taylor, 2004), such gene × environment interactions may be one mechanism by which risk for antisocial behaviour is transmitted across generations.

Perhaps the best-replicated finding of an interaction between genetic and environmental risks involves the MAOA promoter variant and early adverse experiences such as maltreatment. As reported in a recent meta-analysis (Kim-Cohen et al., 2006) and in subsequent reports, individuals who possess the low activity MAOA variant are at significantly increased risk for a range of antisocial outcomes (and other emotional problems) in childhood and adulthood when they have also been maltreated or otherwise victimized (Caspi et al., 2002; Foley, Eaves, Wormley, Silberg, Maes, & Riley, 2004; Kim-Cohen et al., 2006; Nilsson et al., 2006; Widom & Brzustowicz, 2006), but not if they have been unexposed to significant psychosocial risk. These findings replicate those from animal studies in which early rearing experiences (e.g., peer-rearing vs. maternal-rearing) are experimentally manipulated (Newman et al., 2005). There have also been failures to replicate the MAOA × maltreatment interaction (Haberstick et al., 2005; Huizinga et al., 2006), although one such study may not be considered a genuine replication effort because of its highly selected sample and lack of control group (Young et al., 2006). As reported by Kim-Cohen et al. (2006) in their meta-analysis of five studies reporting MAOA × maltreatment effects, the overall effect size difference in the magnitude of the association between maltreatment and antisocial behaviour in the low versus high activity MAOA groups was small ($r = .18$), but statistically significant. Moreover, knowledge of both genetic and environmental risk factors may increase predictive accuracy. For example, Caspi et al. (2002) reported that 85% of men in their sample who had the low activity MAOA genotype and had been severely maltreated developed some form of antisocial behaviour and Nilsson et al. (2006) reported that their biosocial model accounted for significantly more variation in criminal behaviour than a purely psychosocial model did.

In summary, efforts to detect the joint effects of genetic and environmental risk factors are new and replications of existing findings are needed. Nevertheless, studies of gene × environment interactions hold great promise for improving predictive accuracy and for explaining intergenerational continuities and discontinuities in antisocial behaviour.

Future directions

Intergenerational studies of antisocial behaviour face a number of challenges (Patterson, 1998; Rutter, 1998; Shaw, 2003). On the one hand, studies that rely on retrospective reports of parents' antisocial behaviour or official records of parental criminal convictions face problems of recall bias and under-detection of antisocial behaviour. On the other hand, studies in which researchers gather prospective data on parent and offspring antisocial behaviour are beset by different problems. Whereas the parent generation is likely to be close in age (e.g., a birth cohort), they are unlikely to have made the transition to parenthood at exactly the same time. Consequently, the offspring generation may range widely in age and even when researchers can administer behavioural measures that are valid across a broad age range (e.g., the Achenbach family of measures; Achenbach & Rescorla, 2001) the very youngest sample members are frequently excluded from analyses, making what are often already small sample sizes even smaller and diminishing the power to detect effects.

Researchers who study intergenerational relations in antisocial behaviour are also challenged by questions about measurement timing. Although some researchers have argued that studies of intergenerational continuities should concern relations between the development of particular behaviours (e.g., antisocial behaviour) in children and the development of those same characteristics in parents when they were a similar age (Cairns, Cairns, Xie, Leung, & Hearne, 1998), intergenerational continuities are relatively weak when antisocial behaviour is measured at approximately the same age in the parent and offspring generations (Cairns et al., 1998; Cohen, Kasen, Brook, & Hartmark, 1998; Serbin, Cooperman, Peters, Lehoux, Stack, & Schwartzman, 1998; Smith & Farrington, 2004). Relationships are similarly weak when antisocial behaviour is measured in adolescence in one generation and early childhood in the next generation (Cohen et al., 1998; Conger et al., 2003; Hops, Davis, Leve, & Sheeber, 2003; Huesmann, Eron, Lefkowitz, & Walder, 1984), although this is not always true (Ehrensaft et al., 2003). Adult antisocial behaviour may be the best predictor of offspring antisocial behaviour simply because it is a proximal influence on the child's environment and because continuity from childhood to adulthood antisocial behaviour in the parent generation, although strong, is usually not perfect (Rutter, 1998).

Finally, although biosocial models provide a promising framework to explain both continuity and discontinuity in antisocial behaviour across generations, more research is needed to explicate the pathways by which genetic variants moderate effects of the environment on behaviour (Caspi & Moffitt, 2006). For example, genetic variants in the hypothalamic-pituitary-adrenal (HPA) axis and the serotonin system may be "stress-sensitive", resulting in neurohormonal changes in the face of chronic stress that lead to dysregulation of the HPA axis and, ultimately, behavioural pathology (Barr et al., 2004). Genetic variants may also moderate effects of life stressors on neural endpoints (e.g., amygdala activation) that have downstream effects on behaviour (Canli et al., 2006; Hariri et al., 2002; Meyer-Lindenberg et al., 2006). The effort to jointly estimate effects of genes and environments and to link them to behaviour via neural mechanisms is new and exciting and will require collaborative exchanges among molecular geneticists, neuroscientists, and social scientists. Although the study of intergenerational continuities in antisocial behaviour faces many conceptual and methodological challenges, progress in this enterprise may help to break the cycle of violence that carries such a heavy cost to families and to society.

References

Achenbach, T. M., & Rescorla, L. A. (2001). *Manual for the ASEBA school-age forms and profiles*. Burlington, VT: University of Vermont, Research Center for Children, Youth, and Families.
Barr, C. S., Newman, T. K., Shannon, C., Parker, C., Dvoskin, R. L., Becker, M. L., et al. (2004). Rearing condition and rh5-HTTLPR interact to influence

limbic-hypothalamic-pituitary-adrenal axis response to stress in infant macaques. *Biological Psychiatry*, *55*, 733–738.

Beitchman, J., Mik, H., Ehtesham, S., Douglas, L., & Kennedy, J. (2004). MAOA and persistent, pervasive childhood aggression. *Molecular Psychiatry*, *9*, 546–547.

Berggard, C., Damberg, M., Longato-Stadler, E., Hallman, J., Oreland, L., & Garpenstrand, H. (2003). The serotonin 2A–1438 G/A receptor polymorphism in a group of Swedish male criminals. *Neuroscience Letters*, *347*, 196–198.

Bjork, J. M., Moeller, F. G., Dougherty, D. M., Swann, A. C., Machado, M. A., & Hanis, C. L. (2002). Serotonin 2A receptor T102C polymorphism and impaired impulse control. *American Journal of Medical Genetics (Neuropsychiatric Genetics)*, *114*, 336–339.

Brunner, H. G., Nelen, M., Breakefield, X. O., Ropers, H. H., & van Oost, B. A. (1993). Abnormal behavior associated with a point mutation in the structural gene for monoamine oxidase A. *Science*, *262*, 578–580.

Cairns, R. B., Cairns, B. D., Xie, H., Leung, M.-C., & Hearne, S. (1998). Paths across generations: Academic competence and aggressive behaviors in young mothers and their children. *Developmental Psychology*, *34*, 1162–1174.

Canli, T., Qiu, M., Omura, K., Congdon, E., Haas, B. W., Amin, Z., et al. (2006). Neural correlates of epigenesis. *Proceedings of the National Academy of Sciences*, *103*, 16033–16038.

Capaldi, D. M., & Patterson, G. R. (1991). Relation of parental transitions to boys' adjustment problems: I. A linear hypothesis. II. Mothers at risk for transitions and unskilled parenting. *Developmental Psychology*, *27*, 489–504.

Capaldi, D. M., Pears, K. C., Patterson, G. R., & Owen, L. D. (2003). Continuity of parenting practices across generations in an at-risk sample: A prospective comparison of direct and mediated associations. *Journal of Abnormal Child Psychology*, *31*, 127–142.

Cases, O., Seif, I., Grimsby, J., Gaspar, P., Chen, K., Pournin, S., et al. (1995). Aggressive behavior and altered amounts of brain serotonin and norepinephrine in mice lacking MAOA. *Science*, *268*, 1763–1766.

Caspi, A., & Elder, G. H. J. (1988). Emergent family patterns: The intergenerational construction of problem behaviour and relationships. In R. A. Hinde & J. Stevenson-Hinde (Eds.), *Relationships within families: Mutual influences* (pp. 218–240). Oxford: Clarendon Press.

Caspi, A., McClay, J., Moffitt, T. E., Mill, J., Martin, J., Craig, I. W., et al. (2002). Role of genotype in the cycle of violence in maltreated children. *Science*, *297*, 851–854.

Caspi, A., & Moffitt, T. E. (2006). Gene–environment interactions in psychiatry: Joining forces with neuroscience. *Nature Review Neuroscience*, *7*, 583–590.

Cohen, P., Kasen, S., Brook, J. S., & Hartmark, C. (1998). Behavior patterns of young children and their offspring: A two-generation study. *Developmental Psychology*, *34*, 1202–1208.

Conger, R. D., Neppl, T., Kim, K. J., & Scaramella, L. (2003). Angry and aggressive behaviors across three generations: A prospective, longitudinal study of parents and children. *Journal of Abnormal Child Psychology*, *31*, 143–160.

Davidge, K., Atkinson, L., Douglas, L., Lee, V., Shapiro, S., Kennedy, J., et al. (2004). Association of the serotonin transporter and 5HT1D β receptor genes with extreme, persistent and pervasive aggressive behaviour in children. *Psychiatric Genetics*, *14*, 143–146.

Dick, D. M., Edenberg, H. J., Hesselbrock, V., Kramer, J., Kuperman, S., Porjesz, B., et al. (2004). A genome-wide screen for genes influencing conduct disorder. *Molecular Psychiatry, 9,* 81–86.

Ehrensaft, M. K., Wasserman, G. A., Verdelli, L., Greenwald, S., Miller, L. S., & Davies, M. (2003). Maternal antisocial behavior, parenting practices, and behavior problems in boys at risk for antisocial behavior. *Journal of Child and Family Studies, 12,* 27–40.

Faraone, S. V., Biederman, J., Jetton, J. G., & Tsuang, M. T. (1997). Attention deficit disorder and conduct disorder: Longitudinal evidence for a familial subtype. *Psychological Medicine, 27,* 291–300.

Faraone, S. V., Biederman, J., & Monuteaux, M. C. (2000). Attention-deficit disorder and conduct disorder in girls: Evidence for a familial subtype. *Biological Psychiatry, 48,* 21–29.

Farrington, D. P., Jolliffe, D., Loeber, R., Stouthamer-Loeber, M., & Kalb, L. M. (2001). The concentration of offenders in families, and family criminality in the prediction of boys' delinquency. *Journal of Adolescence, 24,* 579–596.

Fergusson, D., Horwood, L. J., & Ridder, E. M. (2005). Show me the child at seven: The consequences of conduct problems in childhood for psychosocial functioning in adulthood. *Journal of Child Psychology and Psychiatry, 46,* 837–849.

Foley, D. L., Eaves, L. J., Wormley, B., Silberg, J. L., Maes, H. H., & Riley, B. (2004). Childhood adversity, monoamine oxidase A genotype, and risk for conduct disorder. *Archives of General Psychiatry, 61,* 744.

Frick, P. J., Lahey, B. B., Christ, M. G., & Green, S. (1991). History of childhood behavior problems in biological relatives of boys with attention deficit hyperactivity disorder and conduct disorder. *Journal of Clinical Child Psychology, 20,* 445–451.

Galbaud du Fort, G., Bland, R. C., Newman, S. C., & Boothroyd, L. J. (1998). Spouse similarity for lifetime psychiatric history in the general population. *Psychological Medicine, 28,* 789–803.

Gerra, G., Garofano, L., Castaldini, L., Rovetto, F., Zaimovic, A., Moi, G., et al. (2005). Serotonin transporter promoter polymorphism genotype is associated with temperament, personality traits and illegal drugs use among adolescents. *Journal of Neural Transmission, 112,* 1397–1410.

Gogos, J. A., Morgan, M., Luine, V., Santha, M., Ogawa, S., Pfaff, D., et al. (1998). Catechol-*O*-methyltransferase-deficient mice exhibit sexually dimorphic changes in catecholamine levels and behavior. *Proceedings of the National Academy of Sciences, 95,* 9991–9996.

Gottesman, I., & Gould, T. (2003). The endophenotype concept in psychiatry: Etymology and strategic intentions. *American Journal of Psychiatry, 160,* 636–645.

Haberstick, B. C., Lessem, J. M., Hopfer, C. J., Smolen, A., Ehringer, M. A., Timberlake, D., et al. (2005). Monoamine oxidase A (MAOA) and antisocial behaviors in the presence of childhood and adolescent maltreatment. *American Journal of Medical Genetics Part B (Neuropsychiatric Genetics), 135B,* 59–64.

Haberstick, B. C., Smolen, A., & Hewitt, J. K. (2006). Family-based association test of the 5HTTLPR and aggressive behavior in a general population sample of children. *Biological Psychiatry, 59,* 836–843.

Hallikainen, T., Saito, T., Lachman, H. M., Volavka, J., Pohjalainen, T., Ryynanen, O.-P., et al. (1999). Association between low activity serotonin transporter promoter genotype and early onset alcoholism with habitual impulsive violent behavior. *Molecular Psychiatry, 4,* 385–388.

Hariri, A. R., Mattay, V. S., Tessitore, A., Kolachana, B., Fera, F., Goldman, D., et al. (2002). Serotonin transporter genetic variation and the response of the human amygdala. *Science, 297*, 400–403.

Heils, A., Teufel, A., Petri, S., Seemann, M., Bengel, D., Balling, U., et al. (1995). Functional promoter and polyadenylation site mapping of the human serotonin (5-HT) transporter gene. *Journal of Neural Transmission, 102*, 247–254.

Hicks, B. M., Krueger, R. F., Iacono, W. G., McGue, M., & Patrick, C. J. (2004). Family transmission and heritability of externalizing disorders: A twin-family study. *Archives of General Psychiatry, 61*, 922–928.

Hops, H., Davis, B., Leve, C., & Sheeber, L. (2003). Cross-generational transmission of aggressive parent behavior: A prospective, mediational explanation. *Journal of Abnormal Child Psychology, 31*, 161–169.

Huang, Y., Grailhe, R., Arango, V., Hen, R., & Man, J. (1999). Relationship of psychopathology to the human serotonin 1B genotype and receptor binding kinetics in postmortem brain tissue. *Neuropsychopharmacology, 21*, 238–246.

Huesmann, L. R., Eron, L. D., Lefkowitz, M. M., & Walder, L. O. (1984). The stability of aggression over time and generations. *Developmental Psychology, 20*, 1120–1134.

Huizinga, D., Haberstick, B. C., Smolen, A., Menard, S., Young, S. E., Corley, R. P., et al. (2006). Childhood maltreatment, subsequent antisocial behavior, and the role of monoamine oxidase A genotype. *Biological Psychiatry, 60*, 677–683.

Hwu, H., & Chen, C. (2000). Association of 5HT2A receptor gene polymorphism and alcohol abuse with behavior problems. *American Journal of Medical Genetics (Neuropsychiatric Genetics), 96*, 797–800.

Jacob, C. P., Muller, J., Schmidt, M., Hohenberger, K., Gutknecht, L., Reif, A., et al. (2005). Cluster B personality disorders are associated with allelic variation of monoamine oxidase A activity. *Neuropsychopharmacology, 30*, 1711–1718.

Jaffee, S. R. (2002). Pathways to adversity in young adulthood among early child bearers. *Journal of Family Psychology, 16*, 38–49.

Jaffee, S. R., Belsky, J., Harrington, H., Caspi, A., & Moffitt, T. E. (2006). When parents have a history of conduct disorder: How is the care-giving environment affected? *Journal of Abnormal Psychology, 115*, 309–319.

Jaffee, S. R., Caspi, A., Moffitt, T. E., Dodge, K. A., Rutter, M., Taylor, A., et al. (2005). Nature × nurture: Genetic vulnerabilities interact with child maltreatment to promote conduct problems. *Development and Psychopathology, 17*, 67–84.

Jaffee, S. R., Caspi, A., Moffitt, T. E., & Taylor, A. (2004). Physical maltreatment victim to antisocial child: Evidence of an environmentally mediated process. *Journal of Abnormal Psychology, 113*, 44–55.

Kendler, K. S. (2005). "A gene for . . .": The nature of gene action in psychiatric disorders. *American Journal of Psychiatry, 162*, 1243–1252.

Kim-Cohen, J., Caspi, A., Taylor, A., Williams, B., Newcombe, R., Craig, I. W., et al. (2006). MAOA, maltreatment, and gene–environment interaction predicting children's mental health: New evidence and a meta-analysis. *Molecular Psychiatry, 11*, 903–913.

Koller, G., Bondy, U., Preuss, W., Bottlender, M., & Soyka, M. (2003). No association between a polymorphism in the promoter region of the MAOA gene with antisocial personality traits in alcoholics. *Alcohol and Alcoholism, 38*, 31–34.

Kranzler, H., Hernandez-Avila, C., & Gelernter, J. (2002). Polymorphism of the 5-HT1B receptor gene (HTR1B): Strong within-locus linkage disequilibrium without association to antisocial substance dependence. *Neuropsychopharmacology, 26,* 115–122.

Krueger, R. F., Moffitt, T. E., Caspi, A., Bleske, A., & Silva, P. A. (1998). Assortative mating for antisocial behavior: Developmental and methodological implications. *Behavior Genetics, 28,* 173–186.

Kusumi, I., Suzuki, K., Sasaki, Y., Kensuke, K., Sasaki, T., & Koyama, T. (2002). Serotonin 5-HT$_{2A}$ receptor gene polymorphism, 5-HT$_{2A}$ receptor function and personality traits in healthy subjects: A negative study. *Journal of Affective Disorders, 68,* 235–241.

Lachman, H. M., Papolos, D., Saito, T., Yu, Y. M., Szumlanski, C. L., & Weinshilboum, R. M. (1996). Human catechol-O-methyltransferase pharmacogenetics: Description of a functional polymorphism and its potential application to neuropsychiatric disorders. *Pharmacogenetics, 6,* 243–250.

Lahey, B. B., Piacentini, J. C., McBurnett, K., Stone, P., Hartdagen, S., & Hynd, G. (1988). Psychopathology in the parents of children with conduct disorder and hyperactivity. *Journal of the American Academy of Child and Adolescent Psychiatry, 27,* 163–170.

Lappalainen, J., Long, J., Eggert, M., Ozaki, N., Robin, R., Brown, G., et al. (1998). Linkage of antisocial alcoholism to the serotonin 5-HT1B receptor gene in 2 populations. *Archives of General Psychiatry, 55,* 989–994.

Lesch, K. P., Bengel, D., Heils, A., Sabol, S., Greenberg, B., Petri, S., et al. (1996). Association of anxiety-related traits with a polymorphism in the serotonin transporter gene regulatory region. *Science, 274,* 1527–1531.

Liao, D.-L., Hong, C.-J., Shih, H.-L., & Tsai, S.-J. (2004). Possible association between serotonin promoter region polymorphism and extremely violent crime in Chinese males. *Neuropsychobiology, 50,* 284–287.

Loeber, R., & Stouthamer-Loeber, M. (1986). Family factors as correlates and predictors of juvenile conduct problems and delinquency. In M. Tonry & N. Morris (Eds.), *Crime and justice: An annual review of research* (pp. 29–149). Chicago: University of Chicago Press.

Lu, R. B., Lee, J. F., Ko, H. C., Chen, K., & Shih, J. (1999). No association of the MAOA gene with antisocial personality disorder. *Molecular Psychiatry, 4,* S98.

Manuck, S. B., Flory, J. D., Ferrell, R. E., Mann, J. J., & Muldoon, M. F. (2000). A regulatory polymorphism of the monoamine oxidase-A gene may be associated with variability in aggression, impulsivity, and central nervous system serotonergic responsivity. *Psychiatry Research, 95,* 9–23.

Maughan, B., & Rutter, M. (2001). Antisocial children grown up. In J. Hill & B. Maughan (Eds.), *Conduct disorders in childhood and adolescence* (pp. 507–552). Cambridge, UK: Cambridge University Press.

Meyer-Lindenberg, A., Buckholtz, J. W., Kolachana, B., Hariri, A. R., Pezawas, L., Blasi, G., et al. (2006). Neural mechanisms of genetic risk for impulsivity and violence in humans. *Proceedings of the National Academy of Sciences, 103,* 6269–6274.

Moffitt, T. E. (2005). The new look of behavioral genetics in developmental psychopathology: Gene–environment interplay in antisocial behaviors. *Psychological Bulletin, 131,* 533–554.

Moffitt, T. E., Caspi, A., Harrington, H., & Milne, B. J. (2002). Males on the life-course-persistent and adolescence-limited antisocial pathways: Follow-up at age 26 years. *Development and Psychopathology, 14,* 179–207.

Moss, H. B., Baron, D. A., Hardie, T. L., & Vanyukov, M. M. (2001). Preadolescent children of substance-dependent fathers with antisocial personality disorder: Psychiatric disorders and problem behaviors. *American Journal on Addictions, 10*, 269–278.

Newman, T. K., Syagailo, Y. V., Barr, C. S., Wendland, J. R., Champoux, M., Graessle, M., et al. (2005). Monoamine oxidase A gene promoter variation and rearing experience influences aggressive behavior in rhesus monkeys. *Biological Psychiatry, 57*, 167–172.

Nilsson, K. W., Sjoberg, R. L., Damberg, M., Leppert, J., Ohrvik, J., Alm, P. O., et al. (2006). Role of monoamine oxidase A genotype and psychosocial factors in male adolescent criminal activity. *Biological Psychiatry, 59*, 121–127.

Nomura, M., Kusumi, I., Kaneko, M., Masui, T., Daiguji, M., Ueno, T., et al. (2006). Involvement of a polymorphism in the 5-HT2A receptor gene in impulsive behavior. *Psychopharmacology, 187*, 30–35.

Patterson, G. R. (1998). Continuities – A search for causal mechanisms: Comment on the special section. *Developmental Psychology, 34*, 1263–1268.

Raine, A. (2002). Biosocial studies of antisocial and violent behavior in children and adults: A review. *Journal of Abnormal Child Psychology, 30*, 311–326.

Retz, W., Retz-Junginger, P., Supprian, T., Thome, J., & Rösler, M. (2004). Association of serotonin transporter promoter gene polymorphism with violence: Relation with personality disorders, impulsivity, and childhood ADHD psychopathology. *Behavioral Sciences and the Law, 22*, 415–425.

Rhee, S. H., & Waldman, I. D. (2002). Genetic and environmental influences on antisocial behavior: A meta-analysis of twin and adoption studies. *Psychological Bulletin, 29*, 490–529.

Rutter, M. (1979). Protective factors in children's responses to stress and disadvantage. In M.W. Kent & J. E. Rolf (Eds.), *Primary prevention of psychopathology: Social competence in children* (pp. 49–74). Hanover, NH: University Press of New England.

Rutter, M. (1998). Some research considerations on intergenerational continuities and discontinuities: Comment on the special section. *Developmental Psychology, 34*, 1269–1273.

Sabol, S., Hu, S., & Hamer, D. (1998). A functional polymorphism in the monoamine oxidase A gene promoter. *Human Genetics, 103*, 273–279.

Saito, T., Lachman, H. M., Diaz, L., Hallikainen, T., Kauhanen, J., Salonen, J. T., et al. (2002). Analysis of monoamine oxidase A (MAOA) promoter polymorphism in Finnish male alcoholics. *Psychiatry Research, 109*, 113–119.

Sakai, J. T., Young, S. E., Stallings, M. C., Timberlake, D., Smolen, A., Stetler, G. A., et al. (2006) Case-control and within-family tests for an association between conduct disorder and 5HTTLPR. *American Journal of Medical Genetics Part B (Neuropsychiatric Genetics), 141B*, 825–832.

Sameroff, A. J., Bartko, W. T., Baldwin, A., Baldwin, C., & Seifer, R. (1998). Family and social influence on the development of child competence. In M. Lewis & C. Feiring (Eds.), *Families, risk, and competence* (pp. 161–185). Mahwah, NJ: Lawrence Erlbaum Associates, Inc.

Samochowiec, J., Lesch, K. P., Rottman, M., Smolka, M., Syagailo, Y. V., Okladnova, O., et al. (1999). Association of a regulatory polymorphism in the promoter region of the monoamine oxidase A gene with antisocial alcoholism. *Psychiatry Research, 86*, 67–72.

Saudou, F., Amara, D., Dierich, A., LeMeur, M., Ramboz, S., Segu, L., et al. (1994).

Enhanced aggressive behavior in mice lacking 5-HT1B receptor. *Science, 265,* 1875.

Schmidt, L. G., Sander, T., Kuhn, S., Smolka, M., Rommelspacher, H., Samochowiec, J., et al. (2000). Different allele distribution of a regulatory MAOA gene promoter polymorphism in antisocial and anxious-depressive alcoholics. *Journal of Neural Transmission, 107,* 681–689.

Sengupta, S. M., Grizenko, N., Schmitz, N., Schwartz, G., Ben Amor, L., Bellingham, J., et al. (2006). *COMT* Val[108/158] Met gene variant, birth weight, and conduct disorder in children with ADHD. *Journal of the American Academy of Child and Adolescent Psychiatry, 45,* 1363–1369.

Serbin, L. A., Cooperman, J. M., Peters, P. L., Lehoux, P. M., Stack, D. M., & Schwartzman, A. E. (1998). Intergenerational transfer of psychosocial risk in women with childhood histories of aggression, withdrawal, or aggression and withdrawal. *Developmental Psychology, 34,* 1246–1262.

Shaw, D. S. (2003). Advancing our understanding of intergenerational continuity in antisocial behavior. *Journal of Abnormal Child Psychology, 31,* 193–199.

Sinha, R., Cloninger, C. R., & Parsian, A. (2003). Linkage disequilibrium and haplotype analysis between serotonin receptor 1B gene variations and subtypes of alcoholism. *American Journal of Medical Genetics Part B (Neuropsychiatric Genetics), 121B,* 83–88.

Smith, C. A., & Farrington, D. P. (2004). Continuities in antisocial behavior and parenting across three generations. *Journal of Child Psychology and Psychiatry, 45,* 230–247.

Soyka, M., Preuss, W., Koller, G., Zill, P., & Bondy, B. (2004). Association of 5-HT1B receptor gene and antisocial behavior in alcoholism. *Journal of Neural Transmission, 111,* 101–109.

Stallings, M. C., Corley, R. P., Dennehey, B., Hewitt, J. K., Krauter, K. S., Lessem, J. M., et al. (2005). A genome-wide search for quantitative trait loci that influence antisocial drug dependence in adolescence. *Archives of General Psychiatry, 62,* 1042–1051.

Stewart, M. A., deBlois, C. S., & Cummings, C. (1980). Psychiatric disorder in the parents of hyperactive boys and those with conduct disorder. *Journal of Child Psychology and Psychiatry, 21,* 283–292.

Thapar, A., Langley, K., Fowler, T., Rice, F., Turic, D., Whittinger, N., et al. (2005). Catechol O-methyltransferase gene variant and birth weight predict early-onset antisocial behavior in children with attention deficit/hyperactivity disorder. *Archives of General Psychiatry, 62,* 1275–1278.

Thornberry, T. P., Freeman-Gallant, A., Lizotte, A. J., Krohn, M. D., & Smith, C. A. (2003). Linked lives: The intergenerational transmission of antisocial behavior. *Journal of Abnormal Child Psychology, 31,* 171–184.

Tochigi, M., Umekage, T., Kato, C., Marui, T., Otowa, T., Hibino, H., et al. (2005). Serotonin 2A receptor gene polymorphism and personality traits: No evidence for significant association. *Psychiatric Genetics, 15,* 67–69.

Verlaan, P., & Schwartzman, A. E. (2002). Mother's and father's parental adjustment: Links to externalising behaviour problems in sons and daughters. *International Journal of Behavioral Development, 26,* 214–224.

Verona, E., & Sachs-Ericsson, N. (2005). The intergenerational transmission of externalizing behaviors in adult participants: The mediating role of childhood abuse. *Journal of Consulting and Clinical Psychology, 73,* 1135–1145.

Volavka, J., Bilder, R., & Nolan, K. (2004). Catecholamines and aggression: The role of COMT and MAO polymorphisms. *Annals of the New York Academy of Sciences*, *1036*, 393–398.

Welsh, B. C. (2003). Economic costs and benefits of primary prevention of delinquency and later offending: A review of the research. In D. P. Farrington & J. W. Coid (Eds.), *Early prevention of adult antisocial behaviour* (pp. 318–355). Cambridge, UK: Cambridge University Press.

Widom, C. S., & Brzustowicz, L. M. (2006). MAOA and the "cycle of violence": Childhood abuse and neglect, MAOA genotype, and risk for violent and antisocial behavior. *Biological Psychiatry*, *60*, 684–689.

Wozniak, J., Biederman, J., Faraone, S. V., Blier, H., & Monuteaux, M. C. (2001). Heterogeneity of childhood conduct disorder: Further evidence of a subtype of conduct disorder linked to bipolar disorder. *Journal of Affective Disorders*, *64*, 121–131.

Young, S. E., Smolen, A., Hewitt, J. K., Haberstick, B. C., Stallings, M. C., Corley, R. P., et al. (2006). Interaction between MAO-A genotype and maltreatment in the risk for conduct disorder: Failure to confirm in adolescent patients. *American Journal of Psychiatry*, *163*, 1019–1025.

Zalsman, G., Frisch, A., Bromberg, M., Gelernter, J., Michaelovsky, E., Campino, A., et al. (2001). Family-based association study of serotonin transporter promoter in suicidal adolescents: No association with suicidality but possible role in violence traits. *American Journal of Medical Genetics (Neuropsychiatric Genetics)*, *105*, 239–245.

9 Policy implications of present knowledge on the development and prevention of physical aggression and violence

Marianne Junger, Lynette Feder, Sylvana M. Côté and Richard E. Tremblay

This chapter describes what we believe to be the best possible policy to prevent physical aggression and violent crime. To begin with, some basic facts about physical aggression are presented. These facts offer a framework for preventive policies and help us to understand the results of the preventive interventions that are presented. Subsequently, a series of policy options are reviewed, and these various options are discussed in terms of the experimental evidence supporting them.

The focus here is mainly on the prevention of physical aggression or violence. Physical aggression is defined as attacks and injurious behaviour. For an extended discussion of the concept of aggression, readers are referred to Tremblay (2000). Physical aggression is generally labelled as "violence" in the scientific as well as in the public debate, although violence usually refers to behaviour committed by adolescents or adults, and not by children. In this review, physical aggression and violence are assumed to refer to the same category of behaviour. Most instances of physical aggression form a part of antisocial behaviour, and become "violent crime" when committed by juveniles or adults. Therefore, relevant literature will be used that covers related concepts, such as antisocial behaviour, crime or violent crime, as these concepts usually explicitly include physical aggression. In these cases, the concept employed is the one that is actually used by the original authors. Finally, this review is restricted to physical aggression with a pre-pubertal onset, and thereby excludes, for example, domestic violence or child maltreatment, except as long-term outcomes of interventions.

The problem

Violence constitutes a major problem in our society and it represents a key issue in public opinion, making it a political priority for many politicians. Unfortunately, there are few cures, if any, for the problem.

Objective costs of violence

In many ways, violence represents a heavy burden to society. Violence is damaging for the victims who are affected. Interpersonal violence causes about 73,000 deaths, and 20–40 hospital visits for every death for the whole of Europe, including the Eastern European countries (WHO European Region, 2005a). Alcohol is involved in up to 40% of these cases. Males predominate among both perpetrators and victims, and are more likely to die violently than females. Large differences exist within Europe. The risk of a violent death in the low- and middle-income countries is 14 times that of high-income countries. Violence has long-term psychological, behavioural and health effects. Being a victim of interpersonal violence can have long-lasting medical, behavioural and psychological consequences (WHO European Region, 2005a).

There are costs not only for the victims of violence, but also for the perpetrators. Being a violent person has early and long-lasting negative effects (see later section on negative outcomes of physical aggression). These effects become apparent in several ways. A British study showed that societal costs are much higher for children with conduct disorders than for children without conduct disorders. Scott, Knapp, Henderson, and Maughan (2001) compared three groups of children: those without conduct problems, those with conduct problems and those with a conduct *disorder*, all diagnosed at the age of 10 years. They investigated what costs had been made for these children up to the moment they reached the age of 28. They found that for the children without conduct problems the costs made were £7423. For the children with conduct problems these costs were 3.5 times higher (£24,324) and for children with a conduct disorder they were 10 times higher (£70,019). These differences were the result of costs made in various fields. Most of the costs were those following the commitment of a crime and criminal justice costs, but children with conduct problems or conduct disorder created more costs in the educational system (remedial teaching, costs as a result of truancy); they had received welfare more often, and they were responsible for costs in the mental health as well as the physical health system (Scott et al., 2001). For the USA similar results have been reported (Foster, Jones, & the Conduct Problems Prevention Research Group, 2005).

The subjective concerns of public opinion

Violence, that is, fear of it, is in itself also a source of concern for society: 24–30% of EU citizens are afraid of becoming a victim of crime within the next year (European Commission – Directorate-General Press and Communication, 2003); this fear is slightly higher for property crime, with 29% of EU citizens estimating that they will become the victim of a property crime within the next year and 24% estimating that they will become the victim of a robbery or personal assault. These estimates vary a lot by country, with the risk of assault estimated at 5% by Austrian citizens and 42% by Greek respondents (Figure 9.1).

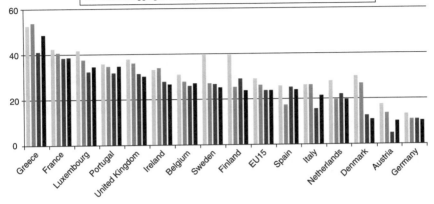

Figure 9.1 Do you fear being a victim of crime over the coming 12 months?

Source: European Commission – Directorate-General Press and Communication (2003, p. 9). © European Communities, 1995–2008.

Note: EU15, the 15 (future) new EU member countries.

Feelings of insecurity also vary between countries, with the Nordic countries feeling relatively safe and a number of Southern European countries feeling less safe. For example, in Denmark, 60% of citizens feel "very safe" in their neighbourhood. However, in Greece, only 27% feel very safe and 22% mentioned that they felt very unsafe in the neighbourhood they live in. Although it seems counter-intuitive, it has been documented relatively often that there is little relationship between the probability of becoming a victim of crime and feelings of insecurity (European Commission – Directorate-General Press and Communication, 2003).

Very often, the feelings of insecurity and estimations of the likelihood of being victimized are being interpreted as signs that citizens have a strong desire to be "tough on crime". That seems to be the way politicians interpret the wishes of their own population, in Europe as well as elsewhere. For example, 62% of EU citizens agree with the statement that "tougher sentences" would deter crime. However EU citizens seem to have more differentiation in their judgement. Overall, they are more likely to believe that young people can be deterred from committing crimes more by means of actively targeting them as subjects of *crime prevention programmes* (85%) than by means of tougher *sentencing policy* (62%) (European Commission – Directorate-General Press and Communication, 2003). More specifically EU citizens believe that young people are led into crime by poverty or unemployment (81%), and that they would commit less crime if they were taught better discipline (78%) or if they were better educated (67%) (European

Commission – Directorate-General Press and Communication, 2003). Interestingly, although opinions on prevention and reactions to crime vary widely per country, the support for prevention is universally high, usually more than 80%.

Lack of proper cure

After the fact, few reactions to violent crime, among adolescents and adults, seem to help to prevent it from happening again. Investing in more criminal justice seems a waste of time and money. Studies indicate that recidivism rates among those convicted to a prison sentence are usually around 75% (Wartna, Tollenaar, & Essers, 2005).

A recent meta-analysis looked at 111 studies that researched the association between type of sanction and recidivism (Smith, Goggin, & Gendreau, 2002). In total, 442,000 offenders were involved in these studies. The overall effect size was zero. The authors conclude that harsher sanctions had no deterrent effect on recidivism. These findings were consistent across subgroups of offenders, namely adult – youth, male – female and white – minority. Compared to community sanctions, a prison sentence produced a slight (3%) increase in recidivism. Furthermore, longer sentences were also associated with higher recidivism rates. Intermediate sanctions had no relationship with recidivism. This category included studies of intensive supervision, fines, boot camps, electronic monitoring, "Scared Straight", drug testing and restitution. No differential effects were found with respect to age group, gender and race. Smith et al. (2002) conclude that "getting tough on crime" by harsher punishment will not reduce recidivism, and this concerns all categories of offenders. These findings are very much the same as in older studies (Lipsey, 1992). Measures aiming at providing work after prison usually also found discouraging results with no notable effect on recidivism (Freeman, 1983; Terlouw, 1991; Van Dijk, 1994; Visher, Winterfield, & Coggeshall, 2006; Wilson & Herrnstein, 1985).

Some facts about physical aggression and violence that policy makers should know

The developmental course of physical aggression over a life course

In young children physical aggression can already be observed. From the age of 6 months on, mothers often report small incidents that can be described as physical aggression. According to mothers' reports, physical aggression becomes apparent in the first years of life and starts decreasing gradually from the age of 3 years on. Baillargeon, Tremblay, and Willms (1999) estimated that 70.1% of Canadian children (2–4 years old) display little physical aggression, 25.6% display some physical aggression and 3.5% relatively often show physical aggression (Baillargeon et al., 1999, 2002). These estimates will depend on the type of data that have been assembled and the choice of the cut-off score. The children in the "very often" category and their families will be one of the groups who might become the focus of preventive interventions.

Life-long stability of physical aggression

Aggressive behaviour is one of the most stable forms of behaviour (Caspi, 1993; Farrington, 1991; Fergusson, Horwood, & Lynskey, 1995; Herrnstein, 1995; Huesmann, Eron, Lefkowitz, & Walder, 1984; Loeber, 1991; Olweus, 1979; Verhulst & Van der Ende, 1992; Zumkley, 1994). A meta-analysis reported stability coefficients of .70–.80 over 1–5 years and of .60–.70 for 6–15 years (Olweus, 1979). Even among very young children a relatively high stability was reported, with stability coefficients of .73–.77 for the age group of 2–5 years (Shaw, Gilliom, & Giovannelli, 2000; Van Aken, Junger, Verhoeven, Van Aken, & Dekovic, 2007b), .73 for 17–23 months and .56 for 17–35 months. Age is important, because studies on antisocial behaviour show that the earlier children display antisocial behaviour, the more likely it is that they will continue to be antisocial in the future (Caspi & Silva, 1995; Huesmann et al., 1984; Moffitt, 1993; Nagin & Farrington, 1992; Olweus, 1979; Patterson & Yoerger, 1993).

Intergenerational stability of physical aggression

There is considerable intergenerational continuity in physical aggression. When parents have a history of violence and crime, the likelihood that their children will show the same behaviour is relatively high (Glueck & Glueck, 1950; Huesmann et al., 1984; Robins, 1966; Tremblay et al., 2004). This inter-generational transmission has been found in a sample of mothers who were relatively young. Serbin, Cooperman, Peters, Lehoux, Stack, and Schwartz-man (1998) found that aggressive behaviour and depressive symptoms in girls measured during primary school were predictive of aggressive behaviour and non-responsive behaviour of their children when these children were between the ages of 5 and 13 years old. This was remarkable, as there was a period of about 20 years between the measures of the mothers and their children.

Negative outcomes of physical aggression

Conduct disorders and aggressive behaviour are predictive of many types of negative outcomes. Aggressive children have a higher chance of having psy-chiatric problems in adulthood, such as depression, addiction, personality disorders (Matthys, 2003), substance abuse and smoking during pregnancy (Elliott, 1993; Kodl & Wakschlag, 2004), health problems (Bardone, Moffitt, Caspi, Dickson, Stanton, & Silva, 1998; Laub & Vaillant, 2000), a lower level of cognitive functioning (Huesmann, Eron, & Warnick Yarmel, 1987) and a higher likelihood of becoming a victim of crime (Shepherd & Farrington,

1995). Furthermore, they have a lower likelihood of graduating from school and a higher likelihood of becoming unemployed (Kokko & Pulkkinen, 2000; Robins, 1966).

Some basic facts and rules about interventions

Regarding interventions, there are a number of general rules. Below, four rules are discussed: the importance of adequate evaluation, early interventions generate more benefits than later interventions, the utmost importance of treatment fidelity and the absence of substantive guidelines.

Rule 1: The importance of adequate evaluation

It is of importance to stress the significance of adequate evaluations. Many authors have emphasized that randomized controlled trials (RCT) are the best way to test an intervention (Biglan, Mrazek, Carnine, & Flay, 2003; Leeuw, 2005). Of course, concluding that an intervention works and can be applied in the community requires more than one RCT. Several trials, including one within the community, may be needed. Many interventions are found to have no effects, and some have harmful effects. A well-known example is the drug-prevention programme "DARE" that was offered to children at school. This project was very popular in the USA. Over 15,000 law enforcement officers are active in delivery of DARE (Cunningham & Baker, 2003). Its goal was to provide information about drugs, to teach refusal skills and increase self-esteem. Several studies showed that DARE had no effect on drug use (Gottfredson, Wilson, & Nakaja, 1998; Lynam et al., 1999). The only reason for its popularity is probably its high feel-good factor (Lynam et al., 1999).

Another feel-good programme in the USA is "Scared Straight". This programme brings delinquent and at-risk youth into high-security prisons to be intimidated by long-term inmates. The goal is to deter future delinquent behaviour by exposing them to the scary nature of imprisonment. Television documentaries described the programme and claimed that it was very effective, with success rates of 80–90%. Perhaps because of the massive media coverage it received, the programme has been implemented in Norway, the United Kingdom and Canada as well. However, research could never confirm the positive media enthusiasm. A recent meta-analysis shows that none of the nine randomized evaluations showed any positive effect of the programme. On the contrary, the probability of recidivism among delinquents who participated in the Scared Straight programme is 1.6–1.7 times higher than for delinquents who did not participate in the programme (Petrosino, Turpin-Petrosino, & Buehler, 2002). Finally, many group programmes for adolescents have harmful effects (Dishion, McCord, & Poulin, 1999). Because of the potential harmful effects, one could easily defend the notion that it is unethical to expose youths to inadequately tested interventions.

Some authors warned against the dangers of pseudoscience. Research characterized by relatively poor designs and a small number of significant findings in a myriad of non-significant findings can be used to "sell" an intervention to the public (Gorman, 2003; Littell, 2006). Overall, it is important to maintain high standards in conducting evaluation studies.

Rule 2: Early interventions generate more benefits than later interventions

It seems logical that prevention is better than a possibly effective intervention to correct the occurrence of physical aggression after it becomes a persistent form of behaviour. It makes more sense to intervene with a preventive programme early in life than to provide an intervention later in life. Recent research has emphasized the importance of the early years in the healthy development of children (Shonkoff & Meisels, 2000). "The earlier the better" seems a wise guideline for policy makers. But do the facts support this rule? An economic analysis of interventions, based on an analysis of the investments that were made in relation to the outcomes (Carneiro & Heckman, 2003), concluded that the most effective way to allocate recourses, given the expected outcomes, is by investing a lot in the first years of life (up to 5 years old) and that interventions later in life produce increasingly less benefits. Investments early on produce much higher benefits than investments later (Carneiro & Heckman, 2003). Accordingly, based on the available evaluation studies, it becomes clear that the earlier one intervenes or invests in children, the better the likely outcomes for the child.

A problem is that actual policies usually differ from this ideal situation and generally invest more in older children, as problems tend to become more visible.

Rule 3: The utmost importance of treatment fidelity

It seems self-evident but it is crucially important to implement policies or interventions exactly as they were designed to be. The quality of implementation has been described as treatment fidelity or treatment integrity. A number of studies have shown that treatment fidelity is a predictor of success (Bellg et al., 2004; Miller & Binder, 2002).

A related issue is the quality of the professional executing the intervention. Olds et al. (2002) studied the differences between professional nurses and paraprofessionals delivering the "Nurse Family Partnership programme". They found that professional nurses achieved better results and that they were more responsive than paraprofessionals when making home visits to teenage mothers.

Rule 4: The absence of substantive guidelines

There are no universal rules other than rules 1, 2 and 3. There have been many overviews and meta-analyses of interventions (Barlow & Parsons, 2005;

Durlak, 1997; Durlak & Wells, 1997a, 1997b; Farrington & Welsh, 2005; Tremblay & Japel, 2003). Several attempted to find general and hopefully simple guidelines to guide policy. For instance, is it possible to advise home visits, because home visits would always result in benefits for children? This seems not to be the case. Similarly, some studies reported that, as a general rule, interventions should be broad and intensive, combining working with children, their family and their school (Battistich, 2001; Blok, Fukkink, Gebhardt, & Leseman, 2005; DiClemente, Hansen, & Ponton, 1996; Durlak, 1997; Greenberg, Domitrovich, & Bumbarger, 2001; Mulvey, Arthur, & Reppuci, 1993; National Institute on Drug Abuse, 2004; Schweinhart, 2004; Sherman, Gottfredson, MacKenzie, Eck, Reuter, & Bushway, 1997; Thornberry, Huizinga, & Loeber, 1995; Tremblay & Craig, 1995; Wasserman & Miller, 1998; Weissberg & Bell, 1997; Yoshikawa, 1994; Zigler, Taussig, & Black, 1992). Without doubt, there are interventions that are relatively broad and intensive and have been successful. However, having a broad and intensive programme in itself is no guarantee for success. For example, the "Infant Health and Development programme" was modelled according to the well-known and successful "Abecedarian project", and directed at families with infants that were born prematurely (born before 37 or fewer weeks gestation) and at low birth weight (2500 grams or less). It was a very expensive programme but it had no positive impact on children (Aos, Lieb, Mayfield, Miller, & Pennucci, 2004; Farran, 2000). Another example of an intensive and broad intervention with results that have not been convincing is Multi-System Therapy (MST). After successful first evaluation (Borduin et al., 1995), replications were not showing many benefits (Littell, Popa, & Forsythe, 2005). Furthermore, some home visiting programmes are effective but others are not (Kendrick et al., 2000; Sweet & Appelbaum, 2004). The same goes for preschool programmes. One programme may be called "preschool" but may be very different in content from other preschool programmes. Some preschool programmes have been effective in reducing problem behaviour and improve outcomes, but some have not (Clarke & Campbell, 1998; Nelson, Westhues, & MacLeod, 2003).

Are expensive interventions better than cheaper ones? A recent analysis by Aos et al. (2004) investigated the costs/benefits of interventions to reduce conduct problems and criminal behaviour. Their findings show that it cannot be concluded that cheap interventions produce bad results and expensive interventions produce better results. Some expensive interventions produced poor results, and some relatively cheap therapeutic interventions, such as Parent–Child Interaction Therapy (PCIT), produce good results. Similarly, a meta-analysis on attachment interventions concluded that "less is more". Effective interventions do not have to be broad. "The most effective interventions used a moderate number of sessions and a clear-cut behavioural focus in families with, as well as without, multiple problems." (Bakermans-Kranenburg, IJzendoorn, & Juffer, 2003, p. 195).

In conclusion, when selecting a specific programme it seems advisable to follow the four rules outlined above, to implement the programme exactly as it should be in order to attain good treatment fidelity and to use professionals who are highly qualified and train them well. Finally, it is difficult, at least at this moment, to distil general guidelines for effectiveness in terms of general and only roughly specified guidelines. At this moment the best policy is to consider which specific programmes are available, what the evaluation results were and whether there was a long-term impact on its participants.

Which policies are advisable?

Numerous factors influenced by multiple policies affect the healthy development of children. In general, public health policies affect children and their families. This section discusses seven types of interventions. To evaluate these options, the discussion is limited to experimental interventions that were evaluated by well-designed studies.

Intervention 1: Screen mothers

Screening issues have been reported to hinder the effective implementation of interventions. We suggest that screening issues should not be exaggerated. Tremblay et al. (2004) investigated which factors predicted whether a child would become a chronically aggressive child at the age of 4. They found that the best predictors were: having a sibling (odds ratio = 4); a low income (odds ratio = 2.6); a young mother (19 or younger at age of first birth; odds ratio = 3.1); antisocial behaviour of mother (odds ratio = 3.1); and smoking of mother during pregnancy (odds ratio = 2.2). Also important were: a dysfunctional family (odds ratio = 2.2) and coercive discipline practices (odds ratio = 2.3). The combination of being young and antisocial together elevated the risk of having a chronically aggressive child by a factor of 10.9. These findings emphasize the possibility of early screening. Most of these characteristics are known at pregnancy. It is therefore often unnecessary to wait for problems to occur. Women whose children are likely to be chronically aggressive can be identified during pregnancy. Further, these characteristics of mothers are not very difficult to measure. A complicated screening instrument seems unnecessary.

Intervention 2: Increase income

Having sufficient income constitutes the fundament of family life and the upbringing of children. Even in our Western societies some children grow up in poverty. Recent estimations state that 9.2% of the European population (EU states) live in absolute poverty (less than $20 a day) (Morrisson & Murtiny, 2004). Countries with low relative poverty[1] rates for children are mostly Nordic countries, with rates varying between 2.5% for Sweden and

5.2% for Denmark. Most European levels are at moderate levels, which range from 5.9% for the Czech Republic to 15.4% for Poland. The highest levels of poverty are found in the UK, namely 19.8%, and Italy, with 20.5% (UNICEF Innocenti Research Centre, 2000). Poverty is associated with poor outcomes in the fields of health, cognitive achievement and social behaviour (Adler et al., 1994; Costello, Compton, Keeler, & Angold, 2003; Morris, Gennetian, & Duncan, 2005; Rutter, Giller, & Hagell, 1998). Obviously, it is difficult to interpret this relationship in terms of causality. However, some experimental studies are available which investigated the effects of earning supplements on cognitive and social emotional outcomes in children.

Recently, a study presented findings on aggregated data from 13 employment-based welfare programmes in the USA and Canada. Participants were randomly assigned to programme groups or to "treatment as usual" groups. Two main approaches were tested: earning supplements and mandatory employment services. The study's goal was to determine what the impact was of these new services on the programme children in comparison with children of parents who were not in these programmes. In total 15,779 children (2–9 years old at the time of randomization) were assessed in this study with the aggregated data (Morris et al., 2005). Generally, the programmes boosted the income of the families by $800 to $2200 per year (which is about 5–12% of a standard deviation). One programme, the federal Earned Income Credit, provided nearly $4000 per year. Child outcomes that were studied included school achievement, externalizing and internalizing behaviour and health (Morris, 2002). The outcomes describing social behaviour included positive behaviour in the classroom, social skills and externalizing behaviour (including a few questions on physical aggression), internalizing behaviour[2] and self-reported delinquency (including fighting; see Huston et al., 2003). No specific information on physical aggression was presented. The findings can be summarized as follows (Morris, 2002; Morris et al., 2005).

First, children benefited from the programme only if it included parental employment in combination with earning supplements. Second, there were benefits for children's cognitive achievement and smaller improvements in social behaviour, including reductions in undesirable behaviours, such as externalizing behaviour and delinquency. It appeared that the cognitive benefits were relatively small, with effects sizes of, at most, .15 after 2–3 years of follow-up. After 4–5 years of follow-up these benefits became non-significant. The effects of the programmes on positive and externalizing behaviour were mainly neutral, but some positive effects for the experimental groups were found in four out of five programmes (Morris, 2002). Third, it appeared that the cognitive benefits were largely found in the younger children and not in the older children at the moment the programme started. Fourth, generally, no health effects were found for the programme children. Fifth, the authors report that in two programmes the effects on adolescents were to some extent harmful, especially on substance abuse. As mentioned above, no information is available for physical aggression. Information from the mothers as well as self-reports from the adolescents reported that they drank and smoked more. An Australian study supports the possible negative effects of more parental absence on the child's delinquent behaviours (Alexander, Baxter, Hughes, & Renda, 2005). It should be noted that in contradiction with this negative impact the results from a third programme, "New Hope", are positive for adolescents. Among other things, New Hope parents express more confidence in raising their adolescents than controls. Finally, in some cases, such as in the New Hope programme, the beneficial effects, both social and cognitive, seemed to be stronger for boys and less for girls. It seems also slightly more positive for African-Americans than for white children.

Little became known about why there were small improvements in cognitive achievement, slight improvements in social behaviour and small decreases in externalizing behaviour. Parenting behaviour was hardly affected by the programmes but one option mentioned was that programme parents made larger use of centre-based childcare and that this fact might explain these positive findings (Morris et al., 2005). Therefore, investigating the impact of childcare is important; this is done in a later section on Intervention 6.

Overall, the authors conclude that the fears of some – that sending mothers to work might affect their children negatively – were not supported. However, the positive results that were reported were relatively small and many comparisons were not differentiating the programme children and the control children (Morris et al., 2005). The present authors conclude that, on that basis, it is difficult to advise earning supplements as a policy measure in order to prevent physical aggression.[3]

Intervention 3: Increase access to existing services

Apart from raising the income of high-risk families, another relatively easy policy option might be to ameliorate access to existing services. A few randomized experiments have tried this option with mixed results. For example, the main goal of the home visiting programme "Comprehensive Child Development" was to help people solve their problems by helping them find their way in the existing services. The total costs were $240 million (over 5 years). Unfortunately, no positive effects of the programme could be demonstrated (St. Pierre & Layzer, 1999). One possible explanation was that the quality of the existing services, which were not known, might be insufficient.

Another example of a similar approach is Sure Start Local Programmes (SSLPs), which is in service at the moment in the UK (Melhuish et al., 2005). The main goal of SSLPs is to promote the functioning of children and families by improving services provided in the local programme areas. What makes it different from most interventions described in this essay is that it is *area based*, targeting *all* children under 4 and their families in particular areas. This means that services within an SSLP area are universally available and this approach limits stigmatization that may arise from specific individuals/families being targeted. Another characteristic is that, as a result of their local autonomy, SSLPs do not have a prescribed curriculum or specific set of services. Instead, each SSLP has extensive local autonomy concerning how it organizes its mission to improve and create services as needed, without a specification of how services are to be changed. SSLPs were advised that services should be evidence based and they were directed to sources of information on evidence-based interventions (Melhuish et al., 2005). SSLPs were situated in areas identified as having high levels of deprivation.

A recent detailed study assessed the early impact of SSLPs on child and family functioning. The study assessed 12,000 9-month-old and 3000 3-year-old children in 150 SSLP communities and a further 2800 (1500 9-month-olds and 1300 36-month-olds) in 50 comparison communities in 2003 and 2004. Thus allocation of communities to the experimental or control group was not randomized, and both groups were not similar on some variables.

The findings were slightly disappointing (Melhuish et al., 2005). Overall, not many significant effects were detected and they were usually small in magnitude. However, some positive but also some negative effects were described. On the positive side, older mothers of babies of 36 months reported less negative parenting and their children reported less problem behaviour, and this seemed to be the effect of SSLPs. But for teenage mothers the opposite seemed to be the case. Their children showed less verbal ability, less social competence and more behavioural problems. Overall, it seemed that the relatively well-to-do families within these disadvantaged neighbourhoods profited more from SSLPs, while the most disadvantaged families experienced harmful effects.

What is important is the possible explanation for these findings. The authors suggest several reasons (Melhuish et al., 2005):

- In practice, even though services are available for everybody, the less disadvantaged make more use of them than the most disadvantaged.
- Receiving home services, from home visitors who are not especially well trained, may not always be a source of support and satisfaction but of strain for the most disadvantaged families. Unless the home visitors are carefully selected and trained, they may not be able to achieve positive outcomes with problematic families. It is interesting to note that the Nurse Family Partnership was able to reach most of the very disadvantaged families and get good results with teenage mothers. This programme was very careful in the selection and training of the home visitors (Olds et al., 2002) and obtained good results with the most disadvantaged mothers.
- Working with less disadvantaged families may be easier and more gratifying than working with the most disadvantaged families.

It is important, according to the evaluation, to take into account not only the positive but also the negative impact. Although there are fewer very disadvantaged families and a greater number of less disadvantaged, in terms of the costs to society the most disadvantaged families may have a stronger impact on society.

It is concluded that a policy that had a single goal to increase access to existing services would have too little positive impact, would not have an impact for the most disadvantaged families and would therefore not be advisable.

Intervention 4: Promote the physical health of the mother and the child

In general it is clear that there are many links between the physical health of the mother and many types of outcomes in her child, among which are the cognitive functioning, social behaviour and health of the child, as measured by injury and hospitalization (Chapman & Scott, 2001; Serbin & Karp, 2003). More specifically, the health-related behaviour of the mother, whether she smokes, drinks or uses other substances such as cocaine, was linked in many studies to childhood outcomes. This is well known for extreme subpopulations, such as women who are severe substance abusers. Their children appear to be relatively severely impaired in terms of motor development, language development, cognitive development and playing skills, and they showed many signs of attention deficit hyperactivity disorder (ADHD; Budden, 1999). In large samples of the general population, relationships also have been assessed between alcohol, tobacco, cannabis use and stress, and developmental outcome for children (Huizing & Mulder, 2006; Linnet et al., 2003). This also occurs with behavioural outcomes such as ADHD, externalizing behaviour and physical aggression (Linnet et al., 2003; Sood et al., 2001). However, these findings are difficult to interpret, as the number of confounders is large and it is difficult in non-experimental studies to control all of them (Huizing & Mulder, 2006). Animal studies, however, corroborate the findings for humans and provide support for a link between substance abuse, generally, and negative cognitive and behavioural outcomes (Huizing & Mulder, 2006).

Interventions to improve health and child outcomes for women with an alcohol or drug problem during pregnancy have not been found to be very successful in terms of outcomes of the children (Doggett, Burrett, & Osborn, 2005). In contrast, programmes aimed more specifically at having women who smoke during pregnancy quit smoking do sometimes have positive effects. A recent study showed that a significant number of women quit smoking (Vries, Bakker, Mullen, & van Breukelen, 2006). In addition, smoking cessation interventions reduced low birth weight, preterm birth, and there was a 33 g increase in mean birth weight. Long-term effects on child outcomes of these experiments have not been reported up to now and the present authors could not trace a link with physical aggression as an outcome.

An RCT that improved mother's diet, by adding very-long-chain n-3 polyunsaturated fatty acids (PUFAs; cod liver oil) to her diet, has also been shown to improve IQ in children, but again no information on social behaviour was reported (Helland et al., 2003).

Child health: Improved diet

Malnutrition is, obviously, a major concern for children worldwide, especially in the developing countries. Malnutrition in the industrialized nations is less likely to result from insufficient food but rather from unhealthy diets, and specific deficiencies are still relatively common (Lambert et al., 2004; UNICEF, 2006). For example, globally, 2.2 billion people (38% of the world's population) live in areas with iodine deficiency (International Council for the Control of Iodine Deficiency Disorders, 2005). For Europe, it is estimated that 11% of the population are suffering from subclinical iodine deficiency disorders (WHO European Region, 2005b). Furthermore, 7.2% of the children have an iron deficiency (Male, Persson, Freeman, Guerra, Van 't Hof, & Haschke, 2001). These data illustrate that the nutritional status of Western countries is still a matter of concern (Lambert et al., 2004).[4]

It is also likely that children, including those in industrialized countries, come into contact with neuro-toxic metals such as lead or mercury, which can negatively affect their health, their cognitive and social development (Hubbs-Tait, Nation, Krebs, & Bellinger, 2005).

In the field of nutrition, various aspects of a child's physical health have been related to cognitive performance. Small for gestational age, no breast-feeding, iron and iodine deficiencies and protein-energy malnutrition are generally related to poorer IQ and cognitive achievement and sometimes ADHD-like symptoms (Grantham-McGregor, Fernald, & Sethuraman, 1999a, 1999b). However, poor nutrition is hardly ever an isolated factor and children growing up in poor circumstances are confronted with many other risk factors, such as poverty, maternal stress, dangerous living conditions and the presence of toxins such as lead, and are relatively more likely to be malnourished. In epidemiological studies, controlling for all relevant factors has generally proven difficult (Grantham-McGregor et al., 1999a, 1999b; Schmidt & Georgieff, 2006).

There have been a number of well-designed experimental studies investigating the relationship between dietary supplements and cognitive performance in children. Several studies showed that improved nutrition of mother (in pregnancy) and child improved IQ scores and other cognitive outcomes of children. This was the case when cod liver oil or iron was added to the mother's diet (Friel, Aziz, Andrews, Harding, Courage, & Adams, 2003; Grantham-McGregor et al., 1999b; Helland, Sith, Saarem, Saugstad, & Drevon, 2003; Hubbs-Tait et al., 2005; Zimmermann, Connolly, Bozo, Bridson, Rohner, & Grimci, 2006). Similarly vitamin–mineral supplements improve cognitive functioning. Often this is the case primarily for children who are not well nourished. For these children, dietary supplements have been shown to have a positive effect mainly on non-verbal IQ scores (Bellisle, 2004; Schoenthaler, Amos, Eysenck, Peritz, & Yudkin, 1991) or other measures of cognitive development (Grantham-McGregor, Walker, & Chang, 2000).

Only one study specifically investigated the relationship between malnutrition in the prenatal stage and antisocial behaviour in adult life. This study examined children born in The Netherlands during the hunger winter and compared them with children born earlier and later. It was found that prenatal exposure to famine did not affect children's cognitive capacities. Furthermore, when focusing the study on those children conceived during famine there appeared to be a higher risk for schizophrenia and, interestingly, the research team also found higher risk for antisocial personality. Neugebauer, Hoek, and Susser (1999) investigated a cohort of Dutch men born in large urban areas in 1944–1946. They were classified by the degree and timing of their prenatal exposure to nutritional deficiency. Antisocial personality disorder (ASPD) was assessed when these men were given psychiatric examinations for military induction at age 18 years ($N = 100,543$). The results showed that men exposed to severe maternal nutritional deficiency during the first and/or second trimesters of pregnancy exhibited increased risk for ASPD (adjusted odds ratio: 2.5). Third-trimester exposure to severe nutritional deficiency and prenatal exposure to moderate nutritional deficiency were not associated with risk for ASPD. These findings suggest that severe nutritional insults to the developing brain *in utero* may be capable of increasing the risk for antisocial behaviours in offspring (Neugebauer et al., 1999).

Apart from the previously mentioned study, the recent literature on nutrition and experimental supplementation studies is that outcome measures of social behaviour are often not included: the review by Grantham-McGregor et al. (2000) hardly mentions outcomes on social behaviour. Correlational studies do suggest links between nutritional status and social behaviour. Some of these elements, such as iron, have also been related to the child's temperament. Lower levels of neonatal haemoglobin and serum iron were found to be related to higher levels of negative emotionality, to lower levels of alertness and to lower soothability (Wachs, Pollitt, Cueto, Jacoby, & Creed-Kanashiro, 2005). These temperament characteristics are correlates of externalizing behaviour in young children (Van Aken, Junger, Verhoeven, Van Aken, & Dekovic, 2007a).

Interestingly, one iron supplementation study investigated social outcomes and reported that children who received iron supplements were, at the age of 12 months, more likely to show positive affect, to interact socially or to check their caregivers' reactions. A smaller proportion of the children in the supplements group resisted giving up toys and they were more easily soothed when upset (Lozoff, De Andraca, Castillo, Smith, Walter, & Pino, 2003). These findings suggest a possible link between nutritional status and physical aggressive behaviour.

Sometimes, iron supplements for children without iron deficiencies do also help to improve cognitive performance, as well as social behaviour (Lozoff et al., 2003), in RCTs and in comparison with a control group that is comparable in terms of poverty and social background and without iron deficiencies.

Raine, Mellingen, Liu, Venables, and Mednick (2003) reported on an experiment that included 176 3-year-old poor children (on the isle of Mauritius) and combined several types of interventions. The children in the experimental group received good nutrition, increased exercise and an educational boost. Raine and his colleagues (2003) tested the subjects for conduct disorder when they reached 17 years of age and found that there was significantly less conduct disorder in the experimental group. At the age of 23, self-reported crime was reduced by 34%. There was a trend for registered crime to be statistically reduced to about a third of the levels of the control subjects. They also found that the positive outcomes were especially prevalent in the experimental subjects who had been malnourished at the start of the study. This is the only study with crime as an outcome, but it is difficult in this study to know what element in the interventions caused the reduction in crime.

Older children

A number of RCTs in correctional facilities have also demonstrated that vitamin and mineral supplements can lead to overall decreases of up to 47% in aggressive and/or violent incidences and less serious rule violations in the USA (Schoenthaler & Bier, 2000) as well as in the UK (Gesch, Hammond, Hampson, Eves, & Crowder, 2002). A recent study investigated whether these findings could be replicated with school children 6–12 years of age (Schoenthaler & Bier, 2000). This study randomly allocated 80 children with school-discipline problems to either an experimental or a placebo group. Children in the experimental group received low-dose[5] vitamin–mineral tablets over the course of 4 months. Their previous findings were replicated, with the authors reporting an identical reduction of 47% in the antisocial behaviour of school children in the experimental group. Additionally, they found a 13% reduction in violent behaviour for those taking the vitamin supplements. It is interesting to note that the overall reduction in antisocial behaviour was, to a large extent, due to the improved behaviour in the most problematic juveniles.

Mechanisms

Of course several mechanisms may explain the relationship between nutritional status and social and cognitive outcomes. Among these possible mechanisms we mention improved brain anatomy or function and the functional isolation hypothesis (Grantham-McGregor et al., 1999a, 1999b):

1   Raine et al. (2003) suggested that, to explain their findings (see above), the link may be via better brain functioning leading to better IQ. However, preschool experiments leading to improved IQ did not always lead to improved behaviour, as was explained by Clarke and Campbell (1998).
2   It is also possible that children who are physically unhealthy do not

explore their environment as actively as healthy children do. Thereby they are under-stimulated and this leads to, among other things, lower cognitive achievement. This explanation seems applicable more strongly to the nutrition–cognition link than to an eventual nutrition–social behaviour link (Grantham-McGregor et al., 1999a, 1999b).

Obviously, none of the authors mentioned above believe that nutrition is the sole causal factor of violence, nor will it be the unique solution. However, as with income, one should remember that humans have biological and material needs that obviously constitute the basis of our social and mental lives. These needs should not be forgotten in sensible policies for children. Furthermore, it should be stressed that nutrition in young children is intimately related to social characteristics and the educational background of mothers, as indicators of their capacity to socialize their child. For example, a randomized experiment helping mothers to become more sensitive to reasons underlying the crying of their infants showed, among other things, that the feeding habits of mothers improved (Black, Siegel, Abel, & Bentley, 2001).

Intervention 5: The Nurse Family Partnership

The Nurse Family Partnership is a home visiting programme that was found to be relatively effective. It is important to note, as mentioned previously, that not all home visiting programmes are successful (Kendrick et al., 2000; Sweet & Appelbaum, 2004). For example, the Comprehensive Child Development home visiting programme was developed to help people, by means of home visits, to find their way to other services in the community. This programme cost $240 million over 5 years, and no positive effect could be established (St. Pierre & Layzer, 1999).

The Nurse Family Partnership targets first-time, low-income mothers. It consists of intensive and comprehensive home visitation by nurses. During pregnancy, the nurse will visit weekly for the first 4 weeks, then bi-weekly until the baby is born. After the baby is born visits are weekly for 6 weeks, then visits are bi-weekly until the child is 21 months old. Visits then become monthly with graduation at the child's second birthday. The primary mode of service delivery is home visitation, but the programme mothers use a variety of other health and human services in order to achieve its positive effects. The programme's goals were very broad: to improve the physical and mental health of the mother and her baby.

The programme was very thoroughly evaluated. Randomized trials were conducted with three different populations: Elmira, New York, 1977; Memphis, Tennessee, 1987; and Denver, Colorado, 1994. All three trials targeted first-time, low-income mothers. Many outcomes have been reported already. Follow-up research continues today, studying the long-term outcomes for mothers and children in the three trials.[6]

Many positive effects have been reported, in many different fields. For example, there were improvements in women's prenatal health, with reductions in prenatal cigarette smoking and in prenatal hypertensive disorders (Olds, Henderson, Kitzman, Eckenrode, Cole, & Tatelbaum, 1999). There were also reductions in children's healthcare encounters for injuries (Olds, Henderson, & Kitzman, 1994). Also, the researchers reported fewer unintended subsequent pregnancies and increases in intervals between first and second births. Furthermore, father involvement and women's employment improved, and there were reductions in families' use of welfare and food stamps. Children's school readiness also progressed: there were improvements in language, cognition and behavioural regulation (Olds et al., 1999). Most important in this essay, a 15-year follow-up of the Elmira trial reported that adolescents born to women who received nurse visits, in comparison with those in the comparison groups, had 61% fewer arrests, 72% fewer convictions and spent 98% fewer days in jail. In addition, they had fewer lifetime sex partners (0.92 vs. 2.48; $p = .003$), they smoked fewer cigarettes per day (1.50 vs. 2.50; $p = .10$) and spent fewer days consuming alcohol in the last 6 months (1.09 vs. 2.49; $p = .03$) (Olds et al., 1998a).

An important conclusion is that a successful intervention such as the Nurse Family Partnership generates a broad range of positive effects in the fields of social behaviour, cognitive functioning, health-related behaviour and economic outcomes. Most reviews seem to assume that this programme will also reduce physical aggression. Although this seems plausible it has not been explicitly reported (Olds et al., 1998b).

A recent meta-analysis of the cost-effectiveness of interventions aiming to reduce antisocial and criminal behaviour showed that the Nurse Family Partnership cost $9118 per child, but that the benefits were estimated to be $26,298 per child (Aos et al., 2004, p. 115).

Intervention 6: Childcare

Childcare is a culturally sensitive issue. Should children, especially infants and very young children, stay with their mother or can they be placed in childcare? What are the positive or possibly negative outcomes of childcare? Almost all studies have shown that generally childcare has a positive impact on the cognitive outcomes of children (Lowe Vandell & Wolfe, 2000; NICHD Early Child Care Research Network, 2002, 2004). Childcare of better quality leads to better cognitive outcomes (Belsky, 2003; Lowe Vandell & Wolfe, 2000).

The effects of childcare on social and emotional development are less clear. Some studies have suggested that childcare has a long-term somewhat negative impact on attachment security and social behaviour (Belsky, 2003; NICHD Early Child Care Research Network, 2004). This is especially true for children spending many hours per week in childcare but irrespective of quality of care (NICHD Early Child Care Research Network, 2004). However, these negative effects are not very strong (Belsky, 2003; Lowe Vandell & Wolfe, 2000).

On the other hand some positive outcomes have been reported as well. In fact Borge, Rutter, Côté, and Tremblay (2004) found that physical aggression was significantly more common in children from high-risk families looked after by their own parents than among children from high-risk families spending time in childcare. In low-risk families (84%), childcare had no impact on the level of physical aggression. Other longitudinal studies also reported positive impacts of high quality childcare. Again, the beneficial effects were most pronounced for children from high-risk backgrounds (Peisner-Feinberg et al., 2001). For example, a Swedish research study found that age of entry in childcare was related to social competence as well as school achievement (Andersson, 1992). The earlier children entered childcare (often before 1), the better the children performed on both outcomes at the age of 13. Of course, Swedish childcare is of high quality. Andersson's (1992) study shows that high quality care can be profitable for both the child's cognitive as well as his social and emotional development. It should be noted that most of the findings on the social-emotional aspects of childcare are based on correlational information. As far as we know, no experimental study as yet has investigated long-term social behavioural outcomes.

All in all, a policy that aims to promote child development would implement high quality childcare, especially for high-risk children, and would evaluate the results in an RCT. The potential benefits of childcare for children of ethnic minority groups in Europe are high. These children often have difficulties learning the main country's language and often start school with cognitive deficits. For these problems, childcare may be very beneficial. However, as mentioned above, the social implications have not been experimentally established. Only experimental designs will be able to produce adequate answers.

Intervention 7: The Perry-preschool programme

As is the case for home visiting programmes, not all preschool interventions have had an impact on social behaviour (Clarke & Campbell, 1998; Wilson, Lipsey, & Derzon, 2003). Most have been able to raise cognitive achievement, but only one has been shown to have long-term effects on many child outcomes, including social behaviour, and that is the Perry-preschool programme (Schweinhart, 2004; Schweinhart, Barnes, & Weikart, 1993). The participants were 3–4-year-old children of low IQ parents from African-American origin. The children followed the High/Scope curriculum for 2.5 hours a day, 5 days per week. Home visits were also performed on a weekly basis. As was the case for the Nurse Family Partnership, many positive child outcomes were reported in various areas. At the age of 40, the children of the programme performed much better in many ways than the control children. Fewer of the programme children dropped out school (33% versus 51%) or experienced grade retention (21% versus 41%). They also had a higher likelihood of getting a school degree (71% versus 54%). In terms of their economic position the programme children fared better. They more often had a job

(76% versus 62%), they earned more (more than $20,000: 29% versus 7%), had been dependent on welfare less often (59% versus 80%) and were more often the owner of their homes (37% versus 28%). Their mental health seemed to be better, they more often had a good relationship with their families (75% versus 64%) and fewer used sleeping pills or tranquillizers (17% versus 43%) or drugs such as marijuana or hashish (48% versus 71%) or heroin (0% versus 9%). Finally, in terms of involvement in crime, it appeared that the programme children were arrested less often (five arrests or more ever: 36% versus 55%) and were less often arrested for violent crimes (32% versus 48%). For various crime indicators they scored better than the control children (Figure 9.2).

The findings of the Perry-preschool programme have been criticized; although many comparisons favoured the programme group, on other comparisons the programme and the control groups did not differ significantly (Locurto, 1991). It should be noted, however, that a replication study confirmed the findings of the first study. Again the programme group fared much

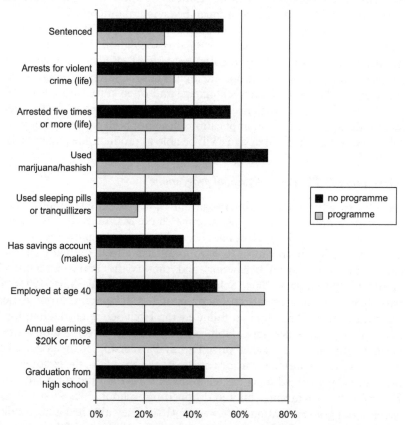

Figure 9.2 The Perry-preschool study: Summary of findings at the age of 40.
Source: Schweinhart (2003).

better in many ways; more specifically, the programme group had lower crime rates in comparison with the control group (Schweinhart & Weikart, 1997)

It is important to note that several preschool programmes were successful in terms of promoting the cognitive achievements of their participants but that they did not have the broad set of outcomes that the Perry-preschool programme obtained (Clarke & Campbell, 1998; Schweinhart, 2004). For example, a more directive programme with a strong cognitive orientation, such as the Abecedarian project, had fewer cross-over effects and did not have a long-term impact on social behaviour, crime or physical aggression.

The question is how these long-term outcomes of the Perry-preschool programme can be explained. The developers of the High/Scope curriculum that was applied in the Perry-preschool programme proposed that their specific method was the key to the programme's success. The High/Scope curriculum was based on the principles outlined by Piaget, who stated that children are active learners and need key experiences for their development. Moreover, there was a strong temporal structure in the planning of activities. Within this structure the children learned according to a "plan-do-review sequence": (1) *children express intentions*, (2) *children generate experiences*, and (3) *they reflect on their accomplishments* (Schweinhart et al., 1993). This "plan-do-review sequence" is a process that can be used in all situations throughout life. It can be hypothesized that this is one method by which individuals are to exercise self-control in their life. The authors speculate that this sequence might, in the end, be responsible for the long-term outcomes of their project (Schweinhart, 2004).

Clarke and Campbell (1998) analysed the outcomes of various preschool programmes, some of which reduced crime while others did not, and investigated what seemed to be essential in order to reduce crime. They state that, first, a childcare/preschool component seems to be necessary. Second, all the preschool projects that had an impact on crime included home visits, therefore it is plausible that the home visits were essential for the success. Third, it is unlikely that cognitive gains or improved school performance are necessary components for interventions in order to achieve reductions in crime. Several programmes that led to IQ gains and improved school achievement did not improve social behaviour (such as the Abecedarian project mentioned above). On the contrary, it may be counterproductive to only stress cognitive achievements at the cost of attention for social relationships. This may frustrate children, especially if they are in a school environment that is better than average (as was the case with the Abecedarian children), and therefore contrasts with their own improved but still limited cognitive possibilities (Clarke & Campbell, 1998). Clarke and Campbell (1998) conclude that improving academic skills to the exclusion of other goals may actually be detrimental to children. All in all, besides developing cognitive skills, children need to learn to take initiatives, to like school and to solve conflicts with other children. These findings support the findings of research that demonstrated the importance of social and emotional development of children and the link between cognitive achievement and emotional growth (Raver, 2002).

Finally, from the point of view of social policy, centre-based care has the advantage that it reaches (pre)school children from families that may be difficult to reach directly, because of cultural gaps and practical problems such as language difficulties, as is the case in Europe.

Several studies investigated the cost-effectiveness of the Perry-preschool programme (Schweinhart, 2003; Schweinhart et al., 1993). Overall, the costs of the programme per child were $14,716 and the total benefits were estimated to be at least $105,284, making it a rather "profitable" investment. An analysis by Rolnick (2003) showed that an investment in the Perry-preschool programme had a return on investment of 16% (after adjustment for inflation). In comparison, an investment in the same period on the US Stock Exchange had a return on investment rate of 7%.[7]

Discussion and conclusion: Towards an integrated family policy to prevent physical aggression

Why should governments intervene and promote the Nurse Family Partnership, provide high quality childcare and organize the Perry-preschool programme at a national level? Several reasons can be put forward. First, as mentioned previously, crime is a concern of virtually everybody in society. Second, children involved in physical aggression will become problematic citizens and become less productive members of society. They will be unemployed more often, pay fewer taxes, have unhealthy life styles and accordingly, become ill. Given the burden for society coupled with the unhappy prospects for aggressive individuals themselves, the government as the representative of the general public, has an important stake in healthy child development. In the end, several studies showed that it is an economically sound investment. What tips can we give to policy makers?

How should an integrated policy aiming at reducing physical violent behaviour be organized? It is beyond the scope of this chapter to reorganise the entire social policies of European nations. There are, however, a few tips that provide guidelines in thinking about new ways to help our children to develop better, and, more specifically, to become socialized, non-physically violent individuals.

Before presenting policy guidelines, it is necessary to note that the programmes described above were all found to reduce antisocial behaviour and crime. Only one programme explicitly reported a reduction in violent behaviour, namely the Perry-preschool programme. To the extent that various forms of antisocial behaviour and crime tend to be correlated relatively strongly it might be expected that a general reduction in crime implicates a reduction in violence. A methodological complication is that, because violent behaviour occurs less frequently than property crime, effects might be more difficult to demonstrate and to reach statistical significance. In the end, the question of whether prevention programmes, which have an impact on crime generally, affect violent behaviour as well, although plausible, needs to be proven empirically.

Finally, it is important to emphasize that some objectives are important in themselves and do not need to be pursued only because they reduce physical aggression. Fighting poverty and promoting health are such objectives. They constitute major and valuable objectives in themselves. They do not need to be pursued only for the sake of combating physical aggression.

This review has investigated what is known about effective interventions to prevent physical aggression and violence. This led to our proposing four rules on implementing an intervention: (1) the importance of rigorous (preferably experimental) evaluation; (2) seek to prevent rather than to intervene and do it early in a child's life rather than later; (3) pay attention to treatment fidelity when implementing programmes and, with that, the need for quality professionals who are thoroughly trained; and (4) there is an absence of substantive guidelines and recommendations of specific prevention programmes. With this in mind, we examined eight possible prevention strategies that have been rigorously evaluated.

Intervention 1: Screen mothers

It was argued that many potent risk factors, such as being antisocial, having little education and being young at the time of the first pregnancy, are known during pregnancy and allow early screening in a relatively easy way.

Intervention 2: Increase income

Experiments that made jobs and income supplements available to mothers of young children who were on welfare proved to be beneficial to children, but the benefits were very small. While there were gains in the cognitive development of children, these gains were not maintained after 4–5 years. Some studies have shown that children improved in terms of social behaviour. Overall, however, the findings are not very convincing that increasing income for a mother on welfare will lead to significant positive and long-lasting outcomes for the child.

Even as we note what the research indicates on increasing income, we want to be clear that improving the living conditions of the poor may be a worthy goal in and of itself. Duncan and Magnuson (2004), based on findings from their experimental studies (as discussed in Intervention 2) that income supplements have a small and short-term cognitive and social benefit for young children, formulated a reasonable policy option. They argue that maternal leave should be reimbursed at 100% for the first 6 months and that mothers should not work more than 30 hours a week for the following 6 months until the child is 1 year of age. Furthermore, they suggest that there should be generous child allowances for poor families that would continue until the child is 5 years of age. They stipulate that this would apply for a mother's first two children, with all additional children receiving no allowances.

An alternative option is based on the interpretation of the study done by Morris et al. (2005). Their research on income supplements led them to suggest that positive childhood outcomes were probably explained by the use of formal childcare. As a result, they argue that it would make sense to provide free childcare for young children from low-income families. Health care, childcare and (pre)school should then become available for these families at no additional costs. This would probably increase the use of these services for high-risk children without having to implement screening procedures to identify and treat high-risk families. While we are not recommending either policy, we do advocate for additional research on the effects that maternal leave and childcare have on the development of children.

Intervention 3: Increase access to existing services

Programmes that simply increased access to existing services consistently failed to show significant improvement in children's outcomes. In fact, in some cases and for high-risk groups adverse outcomes were reported (see Intervention 3, the Sure Start programmes). It is therefore clear that leading families towards existing services is not an advisable policy unless we can first be sure that these programmes are effective in having a positive impact on outcomes. This again establishes the need for rigorous research to evaluate programmes to ensure that they do not lead to unintentional harm.

Intervention 4: Promote the physical health of mother and child

Research shows that a mother's health is related to the cognitive outcomes in her child. In addition, some research finds a mother's health to be related to the social behaviour of her child. Additionally, the nutritional status of the child has consistently been found to relate to cognitive outcomes. Although only a few studies investigated social outcomes, the child's health also seems to be related to social behaviour. While much more research is needed to clarify the link between health and social behaviour, this line of enquiry offers a strong potential prevention programme.

Intervention 5: Home visiting

Most home visiting programmes have not been found to be successful, with the Nurse Family Partnership programme being one of the exceptions. It has not only produced significant results that have a positive impact on the mother and her child, but additionally has demonstrated beneficial effects on children's long-term outcomes across many different domains (including education, professional employment, social behaviour and criminal activity). While the data from this programme look very promising, we would caution that the Nurse Family Partnership has yet to be implemented and its results evaluated by those not connected to the programme, therefore we must also advise prudence until it is independently evaluated.

Intervention 6: Childcare

Large numbers of children make use of childcare. In European countries, these numbers are expected to continue to increase in the near future. Therefore, childcare provides a possible vehicle for reaching and assisting a significant number of children. Survey research led most researchers to agree that childcare demonstrates a positive impact on children's cognitive achievement, but they disagree whether there are positive effects on social behaviour. Studies taking into account the background of mothers reported that children from high-risk backgrounds were less physically aggressive when they were in childcare than when they stayed with their mothers. These findings suggest that policies desiring to promote positive child development should consider implementing high quality childcare, focused especially on high-risk children.

Intervention 7: Preschool

As was the case with home visiting, not all preschool programmes are effective, and some that have been found to be effective in improving cognition do not show positive results on social behavioural outcomes. An exception was the Perry-preschool programme, which did show long-term effects. Again, given the number of women who work and must rely on childcare or preschool programmes, this would seem to be a fertile avenue for increased research as, if found effective, it could be a vehicle for reaching a large number of children.

Intervention 8: Improve parenting skills

Our literature review did not reveal many parent effectiveness training programmes for parents of young children. The best possibility to improve parenting for young children was found in the Parent–Child Interaction Therapy programme. This programme is a therapy form that is indicated either when parents have parenting problems or abuse their children or, alternatively, when their child's behaviour is above the clinical range. In group format this programme may be applied more easily in a preventive way for families that are not yet problematic.

Though we have been critical of a number of preventive programmes, we strongly support policies that reduce violence. Our review indicates that they constitute a good strategy for the healthy development of children. They also carry with them the possibility of having an impact upon a broad range of social illnesses. As noted earlier, interventions found to be effective in reducing violence have also been found to have a positive impact on a number of other outcomes, including improved social relations, health behaviours and educational level and income. A recent meta-analysis of the cost-effectiveness of interventions aiming to reduce antisocial and criminal behaviour showed that the Perry-preschool programme, the Nurse Family Partnership and Parent–Child Interaction Therapy were cost-effective programmes (Aos et al., 2004, p. 115). Additionally, as physical aggression can be easily observed and measured, even in small children, it is fairly easy to target and reach the populations in need. We therefore argue that reducing violence is a good starting point in developing an effective and holistic integrated social policy.

Finally, it must be stressed that any social policy chosen would be more than the sum of the interventions that were reviewed. It would need to become an integrated system of care in order to improve the health and development of mothers and children. Within this system there must be special attention paid to verify whether chosen programmes constitute the best options for reducing aggressive and violent behaviour. However, it is important to emphasize that some objectives are important in and of themselves and therefore do not need to be pursued only because they may reduce physical aggression. So, for instance, we would argue that fighting poverty and promoting health amongst children are two such objectives.

With that in mind, we continue to recommend that policy makers seek out rigorous research to help formulate their preventive policies so as to implement the most effective programmes. Just as importantly, those attached to these programmes must commit to allowing rigorous research methods to ensure that their programmes are delivering on their promised benefits.

Notes

1 Usually relative poverty is defined as 50% of the median income in a country (UNICEF Innocenti Research Centre, 2000).
2 Both externalizing and internalizing behaviour are usually measured with the Child Behavior Checklist.
3 Obviously, other considerations, such as social justice, may play a role and lead to the support of earning supplements.
4 The World Health Organization publishes data on micro nutrition deficiencies at http://indorgs.virginia.edu/iccidd/mi/cidds.html
5 It contained 50% of the US recommended daily allowance (RDA).
6 See www.nursefamilypartnership.org
7 See: http://www.fightcrime.org/reports/CostBenefit.pdf

References

Adler, N. E., Boyce, T., Chesney, M. A., Cohen, S., Folkman, S., Kahn, R. L., et al. (1994). Socioeconomic status and health. The challenge of the gradient. *American Psychologist, 49*(1), 15–24.
Alexander, M., Baxter, J., Hughes, J., & Renda, J. (2005). *Evaluation of the impact of*

activity requirements for parenting payment customers on their children aged 13–15 years. The final report to the Department of Employment and Workplace Relations. Melbourne, Australia: Australian Institute of Family Studies.

Andersson, B.-E. (1992). Effects of day-care on cognitive and socioemotional competence of thirteen-year-old Swedish schoolchildren. *Child Development, 63,* 20–36.

Aos, S., Lieb, R., Mayfield, J., Miller, M., & Pennucci, A. (2004). *Benefits and costs of prevention and early intervention programs for youth* (No. 04-07-3901). Washington, DC: Washington State Institute for Public Policy.

Baillargeon, R. H., Tremblay, R. E., & Willms, D. J. (1999). *The prevalence of physical aggression in Canadian children: A multi-group latent class analysis of data from the first collection cycle (1994–1995) of the National Longitudinal Survey of Children and Youth (NLSCY).* Quebec, Canada: Applied Research Branch of Strategic Policy.

Baillargeon, R. H., Tremblay, R. E., Zoccolillo, M., Boivin, M., Pérusse, D., Japel, C., et al. (2002). *Intraindividual change in behaviour from 17 to 29 months in Québec Longitudinal Study of Child Development (QLSCD 1998–2002) – from birth to 29 months. Vol. 2, no. 7* (Collection Health and Wellness). Quebec, Canada: Institut de la Statistique du Quebec.

Bakermans-Kranenburg, M., IJzendoorn, M. v., & Juffer, F. (2003). Less is more: Meta-analysis of sensitivity and attachment interventions in early childhood. *Psychological Bulletin, 129,* 195–215.

Bardone, A. M., Moffitt, T. E., Caspi, A., Dickson, N., Stanton, W. R., & Silva, P. A. (1998). Adult physical health outcomes of adolescent girls with conduct disorder, depression, and anxiety. *Journal of the American Academy of Child and Adolescent Psychiatry, 37,* 594–601.

Barlow, J., & Parsons, J. (2005). Preventing emotional and behavioural problems: The effectiveness of parenting programmes with children less than 3 years of age. *Child Care, Health and Development, 31,* 33–43.

Battistich, V. (2001). Invited commentary on "preventing mental disorders in school-aged children: Current state of the field". *Prevention and Treatment, 4.*

Bellg, A. J., Borrelli, B., Resnick, B., Hecht, J., Minicucci, D. S., Ory, M., et al. (2004). Treatment fidelity workgroup of the NIH Behavior Change Consortium, US. *Health Psychology, 23,* 443–451.

Bellisle, F. (2004). Effects of diet on behaviour and cognition in children. *British Journal of Nutrition, 92,* S227–S232.

Belsky, J. (2003, 3/21/2005). The impact of child care on young children (0–2). *Encyclopedia on Early Childhood Development,* from http://www.excellence-earlychildhood.ca/documents/BelskyANGxp.pdf

Biglan, A., Mrazek, P. J., Carnine, D., & Flay, B. R. (2003). The integration of research and practice in the prevention of youth problem behaviors. *American Psychologist, 58,* 433–440.

Black, M. M., Siegel, E. H., Abel, Y., & Bentley, M. E. (2001). Home and videotape intervention delays early complementary feeding among adolescent mothers. *Pediatrics, 107,* E67.

Blok, H., Fukkink, R., Gebhardt, E., & Leseman, P. (2005). The relevance of delivery mode and other programme characteristics for the effectiveness of early childhood intervention. *International Journal of Behavioral Development, 29,* 48–57.

Borduin, C. M., Mann, B. J., Cone, L. T., Henggeler, S. W., Fucci, B. R., Blaske, D. M., et al. (1995). Multisystemic treatment of serious juvenile offenders: Long-term prevention of criminality and violence. *Journal of Consulting and Clinical Psychology*, *63*, 569–578.

Borge, A. I., Rutter, M., Côté, S., & Tremblay, R. E. (2004). Early childcare and physical aggression: Differentiating social selection and social causation. *Journal of Child Psychology and Psychiatry*, *45*, 367–376.

Budden, S. S. (1999). Intrauterine exposure to drugs and alcohol: How do the children fare? *Medscape General Medicine*, *1*(1), from http://www.medscape.com/home

Carneiro, P., & Heckman, J. J. (2003). *Human capital policy* (No. IZA DP No. 821). Bonn, Germany: Institute for the Study of Labor.

Caspi, A. (1993). Why maladaptive behaviors persist: Sources of continuity and change across the life course. In D. C. Funder, R. D. Parke, C. Tomlinson-Keasey, & K. Widaman (Eds.), *Studying lives through time* (pp. 343–376). Washington, DC: American Psychological Association (APA).

Caspi, A., & Silva, P. A. (1995). Temperamental qualities at age three predict personality traits in young adulthood: Longitudinal evidence from a birth cohort. *Child Development*, *66*(2), 486–498.

Chapman, D. A., & Scott, K. G. (2001). Intergenerational risk factors and child development. *Developmental Review*, *21*, 305–325.

Clarke, S. H., & Campbell, F. A. (1998). Can intervention early prevent crime later? The Abecedarian project compared with other programs. *Early Childhood Research Quarterly*, *13*, 319–343.

Costello, E. J., Compton, S. N., Keeler, G., & Angold, A. (2003). Relationships between poverty and psychopathology. A natural experiment. *Journal of The American Medical Association*, *290*, 2023–2029.

Cunningham, A., & Baker, L. (2003). Children who live with violence: Best evidence to inform better practice. Retrieved May 12, 2006, from http://ww4.psepc-sppcc.gc.ca/en/library/publications/children/violence/children_who_live_with_violence/background.html

DiClemente, R. J., Hansen, W. B., & Ponton, L. E. (1996). *Handbook of adolescent health risk behavior*. New York: Plenum Press.

Dishion, T. J., McCord, J., & Poulin, F. (1999). When interventions harm: Peer groups and problem behavior. *American Psychologist*, *54*, 755–764.

Doggett, C., Burrett, S., & Osborn, D. A. (2005). Home visits during pregnancy and after birth for women with an alcohol or drug problem. *The Cochrane Database of Systematic Reviews*, Art. No.: CD004456. DOI: 004410.001002/14651858.CD14004456.pub14651852.

Duncan, G. J., & Magnuson, K. (2004). Individual and parent-based strategies for promoting human capital and positive behavior. In P. L. Chase-Lansdale, K. Kiernan, & R. Friedman (Eds.), *Human development across lives and generations: The potential for change*. Cambridge: Cambridge University Press.

Durlak, J. A. (1997). *Successful prevention programs for children and adolescents*. New York: Plenum Press.

Durlak, J. A., & Wells, A. M. (1997a). Primary prevention mental health programs for children and adolescents: A meta-analytic review. *American Journal of Community Psychology*, *25*, 115–152.

Durlak, J. A., & Wells, A. M. (1997b). Primary prevention mental health programs: The future is exciting. *American Journal of Community Psychology*, *25*, 233–243.

Elliott, D. S. (1993). Health-enhancing and health-compromising lifestyles. In S. G. Millstein, A. C. Petersen, & E. O. Nightingale (Eds.), *Promoting the health of* adolescents. *New directions for the twenty-first century* (pp. 119–145). New York: Oxford University Press.

European Commission – Directorate-General Press and Communication (2003). *Results of Eurobarometer 58.0 (Autumn 2002). Analysis of public attitudes to insecurity, fear of crime and crime prevention.* Brussels, Belgium: European Commission.

Farran, D. (2000). Another decade of interventions for children who are of low income or disabled: What we know now. In J. P. Shonkoff & S. J. Meisels (Eds.), *Handbook of early childhood intervention* (2nd ed., pp. 510–549). New York: Cambridge University Press.

Farrington, D. P. (1991). Childhood aggression and adult violence: Early precursors and later-life outcomes. In D. J. Pepler & K. H. Rubin (Eds.), *The development and treatment of childhood aggression*. Hillsdale, NJ: Lawrence Erlbaum Associates, Inc.

Farrington, D. P., & Welsh, B. C. (2005). Randomized experiments in criminology: What have we learned in the last two decades? *Journal of Experimental Criminology*, *1*, 9–38.

Fergusson, D. M., Horwood, L. J., & Lynskey, M. T. (1995). The stability of disruptive childhood behaviors. *Journal of Abnormal Child Psychology*, *23*(3), 379–396.

Foster, E. M., Jones, D. E., & the Conduct Problems Prevention Research Group (2005). The high costs of aggression: Public expenditures resulting from conduct disorder. *American Journal of Public Health*, *95*, 1767–1772.

Freeman, R. B. (1983). Crime and unemployment. In J. Q. Wilson (Ed.), *Crime and public policy* (pp. 89–106). San Francisco, CA: Institue for Contemporary Studies.

Friel, J. K., Aziz, K., Andrews, W. L., Harding, S. V., Courage, M. L., & Adams, R. J. (2003). A double-masked, randomized control trial of iron supplementation in early infancy in healthy term breast-fed infants. *Journal of Pediatrics*, *143*, 582–586.

Gesch, C. B., Hammond, S. M., Hampson, S. E., Eves, A., & Crowder, M. J. (2002). Influence of supplementary vitamins, minerals and essential fatty acids on the antisocial behaviour of young adult prisoners: Randomised, placebo-controlled trial. *British Journal of Psychiatry*, *181*, 22–28.

Glueck, S., & Glueck, E. (1950). *Unraveling juvenile delinquency*. New York: The Commonwealth Fund, Oxford University Press.

Gorman, D. M. (2003). Prevention programs and scientific nonsense, *Policy Review*, *117*, 65–75.

Gottfredson, D. C., Wilson, D. B., & Nakaja, S. S. (1998). School-based crime prevention. In L. W. Sherman, D. Gottfredson, D. MacKinsey, J. Eck, P. Reuter, & S. Bushway (Eds.), *Preventing crime: What works, what doesn't, what's promising* (pp. 56–64). Washington DC: US Department of Justice.

Grantham-McGregor, S. M., Fernald, L. C., & Sethuraman, K. (1999a). Effects of health and nutrition on cognitive and behavioural development in children in the first three years of life. Part 1: Low birthweight, breastfeeding, and protein-energy malnutrition. *Food and Nutrition Bulletin*, *20*(1), 53–75.

Grantham-McGregor, S. M., Fernald, L. C., & Sethuraman, K. (1999b). Effects of health and nutrition on cognitive and behavioural development in children in the first three years of life. Part 2: Infections and micronutrient deficiencies: Iodine, iron, and zinc. *Food and Nutrition Bulletin*, *20*(1), 76–99.

Grantham-McGregor, S. M., Walker, S. P., & Chang, S. (2000b). Nutritional deficiencies and later behavioural development. *Proceedings of the Nutrition Society*, *59*, 47–54.

Greenberg, M. T., Domitrovich, C., & Bumbarger, B. (2001). The prevention of mental disorders in school-aged children: Current state of the field. *Prevention and Treatment*, 2004, from http://journals.apa.org/prevention/volume4/pre0040001a.html

Helland, I. B., Smith, L., Saarem, K., Saugstad, O. D., & Drevon, C. A. (2003). Maternal supplementation with very-long-chain n-3 fatty acids during pregnancy and lactation augments children's IQ at 4 years of age. *Pediatrics, 111*, e39–e44.

Herrnstein, R. J. (1995). *Criminogenic traits*. San Francisco, CA: ICS.

Hubbs-Tait, L., Nation, J. R., Krebs, N. F., & Bellinger, D. C. (2005). Neurotoxicants, micronutrients, and social environments. Individual and combined effects on children's development. *Psychological Science in the Public Interest, 6*(3), 57–121.

Huesmann, L. R., Eron, L. D., Lefkowitz, M. M., & Walder, L. O. (1984). Stability of aggression over time and generations. *Developmental Psychology, 20*, 1120–1134.

Huesmann, L. R., Eron, L. D., & Warnick Yarmel, P. (1987). Intellectual functioning and aggression. *Journal of Personality and Social Psychology, 52*(1), 232–240.

Huizing, A. C., & Mulder, E. J. H. (2006). Maternal smoking, drinking or cannabis use during pregnancy and neurobehavioral and cognitive functioning in human offspring. *Neuroscience and Biobehavioral Reviews, 30*, 24–41.

Huston, A. C., Miller, C., Richburg-Hayes, L., Duncan, G. J., Eldred, C. A., Weisner, T. S., et al. (2003). *New hope for families and children: Five-year results of a program to reduce poverty and reform welfare*. New York: MRDC.

International Council for the Control of Iodine Deficiency Disorders (2005). *Iodine deficiency disorder (IDD)*. Ottawa, Canada: World Health Oganization European Region.

Kendrick, D., Elkan, R., Hewitt, M., Dewey, M., Blair, M., Robinson, J., et al. (2000). Does home visiting improve parenting and the quality of the home environment? A systematic review and meta analysis. *Archives of Disease in Childhood, 82*, 443–451.

Kodl, M. M., & Wakschlag, L. S. (2004). Does a childhood history of externalizing problems predict smoking during pregnancy? *Addictive Behaviors, 29*, 273–279.

Kokko, K., & Pulkkinen, L. (2000). Aggression in childhood and long-term unemployment in adulthood: A cycle of maladaptation and some protective factors. *Developmental Psychology, 36*, 463–472.

Lambert, J., Agostoni, C., Elmadfa, I., Hulshof, K., Krause, E., Livingstone, B., et al. (2004). Dietary intake and nutritional status of children and adolescents in Europe. Nutrition in children and adolescents in Europe: What is the scientific basis? Proceedings of a workshop held on 14–16 May 2003, Rome, Italy. *British Journal of Nutrition, 92*(Suppl. 2), S147–S211.

Laub, J. H., & Vaillant, G. E. (2000). Delinquency and mortality: A 50-year follow-up study of 1,000 delinquent and nondelinquent boys. *American Journal of Psychiatry, 157*, 96–102.

Leeuw, F. L. (2005). Trends and developments in program evaluation in general and criminal justice programs in particular. *European Journal on Criminal Policy and Research, 11*, 233–258.

Linnet, K. M., Dalsgaard, S., Obel, C., Wisborg, K., Henriksen, T. B., Rodriguez, A., et al. (2003). Maternal lifestyle factors in pregnancy risk of attention deficit hyperactivity disorder and associated behaviors: Review of the current evidence. *American Journal of Psychiatry, 160*, 1028–1040.

Lipsey, M. W. (1992). Juvenile delinquency treatment: A meta-analytic inquiry into

555

the variability of effects. In T. D. Cook (Ed.), *Meta-analysis for explanation: A case book* (pp. 83–127). New York: Russell Sage Foundation.

Littell, J. H. (2006). The case for multisystemic therapy: Evidence or orthodoxy? *Children and Youth Services Review, 28*(4), 458.

Littell, J. H., Popa, M., & Forsythe, B. (2005). *Multisystemic therapy for social, emotional, and behavior problems in youth age 10–17.* Cochrane Library, Issue 3. Chichester, UK: John Wiley & Sons, Ltd.

Locurto, C. (1991). Beyond IQ in preschool programs? *Intelligence, 15*(3), 295.

Loeber, R. (1991). Questions and advances in the study of developmental pathways. In D. Cicchetti & S. L. Toth (Eds.), *Models and integrations* (Vol. 3, pp. 97–116). Pittsburgh: University of Pittsburgh, Western Psychiatric Institute and Clinic.

Lowe Vandell, D., & Wolfe, B. (2000). *Child care quality: Does it matter and does it need to be improved?* (No. 78). Wisconsin-Madison: Institute for Research on Poverty.

Lozoff, B., De Andraca, I., Castillo, M., Smith, J. B., Walter, T., & Pino, P. (2003). Behavioral and developmental effects of preventing iron-deficiency anemia in healthy full-term infants. *Pediatrics, 113*, 846–854.

Lynam, D. R., Milich, R., Zimmerman, R., Novak, S. P., Logan, T. K., Martin, C., et al. (1999). Project DARE: No effects at 10-year follow-up. *Journal of Consulting and Clinical Psychology, 67*, 590–593.

Male, C., Persson, L. Å., Freeman, V., Guerra, A., Van't Hof, M. A., & Haschke, F. (2001). Prevalence of iron deficiency in 12-mo-old infants from 11 European areas and influence of dietary factors on iron status (Euro-Growth Study). *Acta Paediatrica, 90*, 492–498.

Matthys, W. (2003). Oppositioneel-opstandige en antisociale gedragsstoornissen. In A. J. M. Bonnet-Breusers, R. A. Hirasing, K. Hoppenbrouwers, H. B. H. Rensen, & M. M. Wagenaar-Fischer (Eds.), *Praktijkboek jeugdgezondheidszorg (v3.2-1–v3.2-26)* (Vol. V3.2-1–V3.2-26). Amsterdam: Elsevier.

Melhuish, E., Belsky, J., Leyland, A., Anning, A., Hall, S. D., Tunstill, J., et al. (2005). *Early impact of Sure Start local programmes on children and families. Research information* (No. 13). Birkbeck, UK: Institute for the Study of Children, Families and Social Issues.

Miller, S. J., & Binder, J. L. (2002). The effects of manual-based training on treatment fidelity and outcome: A review of the literature on adult individual psychotherapy. *Psychotherapy: Theory/Research/Practice/Training, 39*(2), 184.

Moffitt, T. E. (1993). Adolescence-limited and life-course-persistent antisocial behavior: A developmental taxonomy. *Psychological Review, 100*, 674–701.

Morris, P. A. (2002). The effects of welfare reform policies on children. *Social Policy Report, XVI*(1), 1–18.

Morris, P. A., Gennetian, L. A., & Duncan, G. J. (2005). Effects of welfare and employment policies on young children: New findings on policy experiments conducted in the early 1990s. *Social Policy Report, XIX*(2), 3–18.

Morrisson, C., & Murtiny, F. (2004). *History and prospects of inequality among Europeans.* Paris, France: Centre de Recherche en Économie et Statistique (CREST).

Mulvey, E. P., Arthur, M. W., & Reppuci, N. D. (1993). The prevention and treatment of juvenile delinquency: A review of the research. *Clinical Psychology Review, 13*, 133–167.

Nagin, D. S., & Farrington, D. P. (1992). The stability of criminal potential from childhood to adulthood. *Criminology, 30*(2), 235–260.

National Institute on Drug Abuse (2004). *Lessons from prevention research. Science-based facts on drug abuse and addiction* (NIDA InfoFacts). Bethesda, MD: National Institutes of Health (NIH).

Nelson, G., Westhues, A., & MacLeod, J. (2003). A meta-analysis of longitudinal research on preschool prevention programs for children. *Prevention and Treatment, 6,* 1–32.

Neugebauer, R., Hoek, H. W., & Susser, E. (1999). Prenatal exposure to wartime famine and development of antisocial personality disorder in early adulthood. *Journal of the American Medical Association, 282,* 455–462.

NICHD Early Child Care Research Network (2002). Early child care and children's development prior to school entry: Results from the NICHD Study of Early Child Care. *American Educational Research Journal, 39,* 133–164.

NICHD Early Child Care Research Network (2004). Early child care and children's development in the primary grades: Follow-up results from the NICHD Study of Early Child Care. *American Educational Research Journal, 43,* 537–570.

Olds, D. L., Henderson, C. R. J., Cole, R., Eckenrode, J., Kitzman, H., Luckey, D., et al. (1998a). Long-term effects of nurse home visitation on children's criminal and antisocial behavior: 15-year follow-up of a randomized controlled trial. *Journal of the American Medical Association, 280*(14), 1238–1244.

Olds, D. L., Henderson, C. R. J., & Kitzman, H. (1994). Does prenatal and infancy nurse home visitation have enduring effects on qualities of parental caregiving and child health at 25 to 50 months of life? *Pediatrics, 93,* 89–98.

Olds, D. L., Henderson, C. R. J., Kitzman, H. J., Eckenrode, J. J., Cole, R. E., & Tatelbaum, R. C. (1999). Prenatal and infancy home visitation by nurses: Recent findings. A review of 20 years of research on a program that employs nurses as home visitors. *The Future of Children, 9,* 44–65.

Olds, D. L., Pettitt, L. M., Robinson, J., Henderson, C. J., Eckenrode, J., Kitzman, H., et al. (1998b). Reducing risks for antisocial behavior with a program of prenatal and early childhood home visitation. *Journal of Community Psychology, 26,* 65–83.

Olds, D. L., Robinson, J., O'Brien, R., Luckey, D. W., Pettitt, L. M., Henderson, C. R. J., et al. (2002). Home visiting by paraprofessionals and by nurses: A randomized, controlled trial. *Pediatrics, 110,* 486–496.

Olweus, D. (1979). Stability of aggressive reaction patterns in males: A review. *Psychological Bulletin, 86*(4), 852–875.

Patterson, G. R., & Yoerger, K. (1993). Developmental models for delinquent behavior. In Hodgins (Ed.), *Mental disorder and crime* (pp. 140–172). Newbury Park: Sage.

Peisner-Feinberg, E. S., Burchinal, M. R., Clifford, R. M., Culkin, M. L., Howes, C., Kagan, S. L., et al. (2001). The relation of preschool child-care quality to children's cognitive and social developmental trajectories through second grade. *Child Development, 72,* 1534–1553.

Petrosino, A., Turpin-Petrosino, C., & Buehler, J. (2002). "Scared Straight" and other juvenile awareness programs for preventing juvenile delinquency. *The Cochrane Database of Systematic Reviews, Issue 2,* Art. No.: CD002796. DOI: 10.1002/14651858.CD002796.

Raine, A., Mellingen, K., Liu, J., Venables, P., & Mednick, S. A. (2003). Effects of environmental enrichment at ages 3–5 years on schizotypal personality and antisocial behavior at ages 17 and 23 years. *American Journal of Psychiatry, 160*(9), 1627–1635.

Raver, C. C. (2002). Emotions matter: Making the case for the role of young children's emotional development for early school readiness. *Social Policy Report, XVI*(1), 3–18.

Robins, L. N. (1966). *Deviant children grown up*. Baltimore: Williams & Wilkins.

Rolnick, A. (2003). *Investments in children prevent crime and save money* (Fight crime: Invest in kids: 3). A research brief, Washington, DC (www.fightcrime.org).

Rutter, M., Giller, H., & Hagell, A. (1998). *Antisocial behavior by young people*. Cambridge, UK: Cambridge University Press.

Schmidt, A. T., & Georgieff, M. K. (2006). Early nutritional deficiencies in brain development: Implications for psychopathology. In D. Cicchetti & D. J. Cohen (Eds.), *Developmental psychopathology* (2nd ed., Vol. 2, pp. 259–291). Hoboken, NJ: John Wiley & Sons, Inc.

Schoenthaler, S. J., Amos, S. P., Eysenck, H. J., Peritz, E., & Yudkin, J. (1991). Controlled trial of vitamin–mineral supplementation: Effects of intelligence and performance. *Personality and Individual Differences, 12*(4), 351–362.

Schoenthaler, S. J., & Bier, I. D. (2000). The effect of vitamin–mineral supplementation on juvenile delinquency among American schoolchildren: A randomized, double-blind placebo-controlled trial. *Journal of Alternative and Complementary Medicine, 6,* 7–17.

Schweinhart, L. J. (2003, April). *Benefits, costs, and explanation of the High/Scope Perry-preschool program*. Paper presented at the Meeting of the Society for Research in Child Development, Tampa, FL, USA.

Schweinhart, L. J. (2004). *The High/Scope Perry-preschool study through age 40: Summary, conclusions, and frequently asked questions* (monograph). Ypsilanti, MI: High/Scope Educational Research Foundation.

Schweinhart, L. J., Barnes, H. V., & Weikart, D. P. (1993). *Significant benefits. The High/Scope Perry-preschool study through age 27* (Monograph No. 10). Ypsilanti, MI: High/Scope Press.

Schweinhart, L. J., & Weikart, D. P. (1997). The High/Scope Perry-preschool curriculum comparison study through age 23. *Early Childhood Research Quarterly, 12,* 117–143.

Scott, S., Knapp, M., Henderson, J., & Maughan, B. (2001). Financial cost of social exclusion: Follow up study of antisocial children into adulthood. *British Medical Journal, 323,* 191–196.

Serbin, L. A., Cooperman, J. M., Peters, P. L., Lehoux, P. M., Stack, D. M., & Schwartzman, A. E. (1998). Intergenerational transfer of psychosocial risk in women with childhood histories of aggression, withdrawal, or aggression and withdrawal. *Developmental Psychology, 34,* 1246–1262.

Serbin, L. A., & Karp, J. (2003). Intergenerational studies of parenting and the transfer of risk from parent to child. *Current Directions in Psychological Science, 12,* 138–142.

Shaw, D. S., Gilliom, M., & Giovannelli, J. (2000). Aggressive behavior disorders. In C. H. Zeanah, Jr. (Ed.), *Handbook of infant mental health* (2nd ed., pp. 397–411). New York: Guilford Press.

Shepherd, J., & Farrington, D. P. (1995). Preventing crime and violence. *British Medical Journal, 321,* 271–272.

Sherman, L. W., Gottfredson, D. C., MacKenzie, D., Eck, J., Reuter, P., & Bushway, S. (1997). *Preventing crime: What works, what doesn't, what's promising. A report to the United States Congress, prepared for the National Institute of Justice*. College

214   *Junger et al.*

Park, MD: University of Maryland, Department of Criminology and Criminal Justice.

Shonkoff, J. P., & Meisels, S. J. (Eds.). (2000). *Handbook of early childhood intervention* (2nd ed.). New York: Cambridge University Press.

Smith, P., Goggin, C., & Gendreau, P. (2002). *The effects of prison sentences and intermediate sanctions on recidivism: General effects and individual differences* (User Report 2002–01). Ottawa, Canada: Solicitor General Canada.

Sood, B., Delaney-Black, V., Covington, C., Nordstrom-Klee, B., Ager, J., Templin, T., et al. (2001). Prenatal alcohol exposure and childhood behavior at age 6 to 7 years: I. Dose-response effect. *Pediatrics, 108*, e34.

St. Pierre, R. G., & Layzer, J. I. (1999). Using home visits for multiple purposes: The comprehensive child development program. *The Future of Children, 9*, 134.

Sweet, M. A., & Appelbaum, M. L. (2004). Is home visiting an effective strategy? A meta-analytic review of home visiting programs for families with young children. *Child Development, 75*, 1435–1456.

Terlouw, G.-J. (1991). *Criminaliteits preventie onder allochtonen; evaluatie van een project voor Marokkaanse jongeren* (Vol. 109). Arnhem: Gouda Quint.

Thornberry, T. P., Huizinga, D., & Loeber, R. (1995). The prevention of serious delinquency and violence. In J. C. Howell, B. Krisberg, D. Hawkins, & J. J. Wilson (Eds.), *Sourcebook on serious, violent, and chronic juvenile offenders* (pp. 213–237). Thousand Oaks, CA: Sage.

Tremblay, R. E. (2000). The development of aggressive behavior during childhood: What have we learned in the past century? *International Journal of Behavioral Development, 24*, 129–141.

Tremblay, R. E., & Craig, W. M. (1995). Developmental crime prevention. In M. Tonry & D. P. Farrington (Eds.), *Building a safer society. Strategic approaches to crime prevention* (Vol. 19, pp. 151–236). Chicago: University of Chicago Press.

Tremblay, R. E., & Japel, C. (2003). Prevention during pregnancy, infancy and the preschool years. In D. P. Farrington & J. W. Coid (Eds.), *Early prevention of adult antisocial behaviour* (pp. 205–242). Cambridge, UK: Cambridge University Press.

Tremblay, R. E., Nagin, D. S., Séguin, J. R., Zoccolillo, M., Zelazo, P. D., Boivin, M., et al. (2004). Physical aggression during early childhood: Trajectories and predictors. *Pediatrics, 114*, 43–50.

UNICEF (2006). *Progress for children. A report card on nutrition* (No. 4, May 2006). New York: UNICEF Strategic Information Section, Division of Policy and Planning.

UNICEF Innocenti Research Centre (2000). *A league table of child poverty in rich nations* (Innocenti Report Card No. 1, June 2000). Florence, Italy: Innocenti Research Centre.

Van Aken, C., Junger, M., Verhoeven, M., Van Aken, M. A. G., & Dekovic, M. (2007a). Externalizing behaviors and minor unintentional injuries in toddlers: Common risk factors? *Journal of Pediatric Psychology, 32*, 230–244.

Van Aken, C., Junger, M., Verhoeven, M., Van Aken, M. A. G., & Dekovic, M. (2007b). Parental personality, parenting and toddlers: Externalizing behaviors. *European Journal of Personality, 21*(8), 993–1015.

Van Dijk, J. J. M. (1994). Security first. *Tijdschrift voor Criminologie, 36*, 19–24.

Verhulst, F. C., & Van der Ende, J. (1992). Six-year stability of parent-reported problem behavior in an epidemiological sample. *Journal of Abnormal Child Psychology, 20*(6), 595–610.

Visher, C. A., Winterfield, L., & Coggeshall, M. (2006). Systematic review of non-custodial employment programs: Impact on recidivism rates of ex-offenders. *The Campbell Collaboration Reviews of Intervention and Policy Evaluations (C2-RIPE)* (Vol. February 2006). Philadelphia, PA: Campbell Collaboration.

Vries, H. d., Bakker, M., Mullen, P. D., & van Breukelen, G. (2006). The effects of smoking cessation counseling by midwives on Dutch pregnant women and their partners. *Patient Education and Counseling 63*(1–2), 177–187.

Wachs, T. D., Pollitt, E., Cueto, S., Jacoby, E., & Creed-Kanashiro, H. (2005). Relation of neonatal iron status to individual variability in neonatal temperament. *Developmental Psychobiology, 46*, 141–153.

Wartna, B. S. J., Tollenaar, N., & Essers, A. A. M. (2005). *Door na de gevangenis: Een cijfermatig overzicht van de strafrechtelijke recidive onder ex-gedetineerden* (Vol. 228). Den Haag, The Netherlands: Boom.

Wasserman, G. A., & Miller, L. S. (1998). The prevention of serious and violent juvenile offending. In R. Loeber & D. Farrington (Eds.), *Serious and violent juvenile offenders* (pp. 197–248). Thousand Oaks, CA: Sage.

Weissberg, R. P., & Bell, D. N. (1997). A meta-analytic review of primary prevention programs for children and adolescents: Contributions and caveats. *American Journal of Community Psychology, 25*, 207–214.

WHO European Region (2005a). *Injuries and violence in Europe. Why they matter and what can be done.* Copenhagen, Denmark: World Health Oganization European Region.

WHO European Region (2005b). *Nutrition and food security. Micronutrient deficiencies.* Copenhagen, Denmark: World Health Oganization European Region.

Wilson, J. Q., & Herrnstein, R. (1985). *Crime and human nature.* New York: Simon and Schuster.

Wilson, S. J., Lipsey, M. W., & Derzon, J. H. (2003). The effects of school-based intervention programs on aggressive behavior: A meta-analysis. *Journal of Consulting and Clinical Psychology, 71*, 136–149.

Yoshikawa, H. (1994). Prevention as cumulative protection: Effects of early family support and education on chronic delinquency and its risks. *Psychological Bulletin, 115*, 28–54.

Zigler, E., Taussig, C., & Black, K. (1992). Early childhood prevention. A promising preventative for juvenile delinquency. *American Psychologist, 47*, 997–1006.

Zimmermann, M. B., Connolly, K., Bozo, M., Bridson, J., Rohner, F., & Grimci, L. (2006). Iodine supplementation improves cognition in iodine-deficient school-children in Albania: A randomized, controlled, double-blind study. *American Journal of Clinical Nutrition, 83*(1), 108–114.

Zumkley, H. (1994). The stability of aggressive behavior: A meta-analysis. *German Journal of Psychology, 18*, 273–281.

10 From child development to human development[1]

Jacques van der Gaag

Early child development (ECD) and human development (HD) are closely linked. Early child development refers to the combination of physical, mental, and social development in the early years of life – those dimensions that are commonly addressed by integrated programmes of ECD. These programmes include interventions to improve the nutrition, health, cognitive development, and social interaction of children in the early years (Myers, 1992; Young, 1997).

Human development refers to similar dimensions – education, health (including nutrition), social development, and growth – but at the scale of a nation. The multidimensional framework for HD used in this chapter is a variant of one first proposed by the United Nations Development Programme in 1990. (In)equality is included in the discussion, but an even broader concept of HD would include additional dimensions such as human rights (Sen, 1999).

Human development, broadly defined, is the overarching objective of most international and multinational development programmes. Because HD is so closely linked to ECD, investing in ECD is the natural starting point for these programmes and for the public policy that frames them.

Four critical "pathways" link ECD to HD. The first pathway runs through education. Interventions during the early years of a child have multiple benefits for subsequent investments in the child's education, ranging from on-time enrolment in elementary school to an increased probability of progressing to higher levels of education. The second pathway is through health. Like education, investments in health are an investment in human capital and have long-term benefits. The third pathway links the notion of improved social behaviour (as a result of being enrolled in an ECD programme) with the formation of social capital. This linkage is more speculative, but is suggested by some interesting research results. In the fourth pathway, ECD is linked to HD by the potential of ECD programmes to address inequality in society. And, ultimately, education, health, social capital, and equality are linked to economic growth and hence to HD.

All these linkages are discussed in this chapter, which concludes with suggestions for further research to close some of the gaps in knowledge identified. To provide context, the chapter opens with a brief history of development economics.

Development economics: A brief history

The history of development economics is well described in the *Handbook of Development Economics*, Volume 1 (Chenery & Srinivasan, 1989), which is recommended for serious readers. A key point to note in this chapter is that early approaches to development, which were characterized by mathematical planning models, have been replaced gradually by development models, which recognize that people are both the means and the ultimate cause of development. These more recent models underscore the importance of investing in (young) people as a central means to foster development.

The shift from planning models to people is illustrated by the salient contributions of four Nobel laureates in economics, all of whom were rewarded for their work on development. The first Nobel laureate in economics was Jan Tinbergen, who shared the prize in 1969 with Ragna Frisch. Tinbergen's influence on the field can still be felt around the world.

Tinbergen initially studied physics and, later, applied mathematical planning models to the economies of developing countries, mainly to determine optimal levels of investments. The planning, at least in concept, comprised three stages. First, at the macro level, a desired level of economic growth was chosen. Since labour was thought to be abundantly available, this desired growth rate determined the optimal level of overall investment. At the middle stage, the optimal distribution of this investment by region and by industry was determined, and, at the third stage, individual investments for projects were evaluated and allocated. Apart from the abundance of labour (to be recruited from rural areas), no people were included in these planning models.

It would be unfair to Tinbergen (who entered or, rather, invented the field of development economics because of concern for the living conditions of the world's poor) to suggest that people were forgotten in the development process. On the contrary, people were seen as an important production factor. Consequently, education was an important element in these models. Investments in education needed to be planned, as were investments in roads or in machines. Indeed, skilled labour (the result of such investments) could also be allocated by region or industry and, if needed, even imported.

Omitted from these early models, however, was the (economic) behaviour of people. In 1979, the Nobel Prize for economics was awarded to T. W. Schultz (and W. A. Lewis). Schultz's major contribution to the field was in showing that the behaviour of people in developing countries is, like the people in developed countries, that of a rational *homo economicus*, reacting to incentives and opportunities. He stressed the importance of investing in human capital (skills and knowledge) to increase productivity (especially in agriculture) and entrepreneurship.

A third Nobel laureate (in 1993), R. W. Fogel, emphasized the importance of "people development" in yet another way. Taking a historical view, Fogel underscores the importance of the contribution of technological change to physiological improvements. He concludes that the "technophysio" evolution (as termed by him) accounts for about half of British economic growth over the past two centuries. He states: "Much of this gain was due to the improvement in human thermodynamic efficiency. The rate of converting human energy input into work output appears to have increased by about 50% since 1790" (Fogel, 2000, pp. 78–79). Fogel is also one of the few economists who have recognized the importance of long-term health effects from deprivation during early childhood.

A. Sen, who received the Nobel Prize in 1998, also recognized the central role of investing in people. The resulting higher income, from higher productivity, reduces poverty and increases economic well-being. However, Sen also underscores better health, higher education levels, and improved nutrition as separate goals that, in addition to higher income, represent non-monetary aspects of the quality of life (i.e., of "human development") that are valuable in and of themselves. In his book *Development as Freedom* (Sen, 1999), he extends this concept to emphasize that individual freedom is the ultimate goal of economic life. In this treatise, Sen uses a very broad definition of freedom, which includes freedom from hunger, disease, ignorance, all forms of deprivation, poverty, as well as political and economic freedom and civil rights.

Linking ECD to HD: Four pathways

Education

The first pathway from ECD to HD is through education. The importance of ECD for subsequent educational performance, and the role of education in economic and human development, are well known and supported by extensive scientific evidence accumulated from neurophysics, paediatrics, the medical sciences, child development, education, sociology, and economics. Ample evidence documents the importance of the early months and years in life for a child's physical, mental, and social development (Cynader & Frost, 1999; McCain & Mustard, 1999; Myers, 1992; Young, 1997). The rapid development of the brain during the early months and years is crucial, and newborns who receive proper care and stimulation will be readier to enter school on time and to learn.

Children participating in ECD programmes receive psychosocial stimulation, nutritional supplementation, and health care, and their parents receive training in effective childcare. Children who have participated in these programmes show higher intelligence quotients and improvements in practical reasoning, eye and hand coordination, hearing and speech, and reading readiness (Myers, 1992). Grade repetition and dropout rates are lower, performance at school is higher, and the probability that a child will progress to higher levels of education increases (Barnett, 1995, 1998; Grantham-McGregor, Walker, Chang, & Powell, 1997; Karoly et al., 1998; Schweinhart, Barnes, & Weikart, 1993).

Over the long term, these children benefit from earlier schooling, better schooling, and more schooling, making them more productive and more "successful" as adults. Being well educated is the best predictor of "success" as an adult, regardless of how success is defined. The definition of success, as a better job and higher income in the market-place or increased and improved production at home (e.g., childcare, nutritional practices, family health), can differ from case to case, but higher education is always associated with greater well-being, broadly defined (Haveman & Wolfe, 1984; Psacharopoulos, 1994).

The public benefits of education are also well known. For society, they include greater ability to adopt new technologies, better functioning of democratic processes, lower fertility rates, and lower crime rates (Carnoy, 1992; Rutter, Giller, & Hagell, 1998). As firmly established in the economic literature on development, education is also important for economic growth (Barro, 1997).

The education pathway clearly demonstrates that the link between ECD and HD is straightforward, as abundantly documented by scientific evidence. Increased investments in ECD programmes can be fully justified, and usually are, based on this evidence alone (Van der Gaag & Tan, 1998). Good education is a goal in itself and fosters economic prosperity, yet three additional pathways deserve at least the same attention as education.

Health

For many decades, the leading development agencies, including the World Health Organization, the United Nations Children's Fund (UNICEF), and the World Bank, have emphasized the importance of providing good nutrition, immunization, and other basic health care services for young children. The health benefits of these services are immediately evident (Bundy, 1997; Pan American Health Organization, 1998; Stephenson, Latham, Adams, Kinoti, & Pertet, 1993) and the cost-effectiveness of interventions to improve these services are well established (Horton, 1999). Despite this knowledge, shamefully millions of children in developing countries still die before they have lived 1 year, and those who survive suffer from a myriad of easily preventable diseases.

ECD programmes can make a dramatic difference. They are associated with decreased morbidity and mortality among children, fewer cases of malnutrition and stunting, improved personal hygiene and health care, and fewer instances of child abuse.

Less well known are the strong links between trauma in the early years of life (e.g., from malnutrition, even *in utero*, and infectious diseases) and an individual's health as an adult. Recent studies show that the links between health and nutrition in the early years of life and one's health status as an adult are much more numerous and stronger than previously known. The range of adult health outcomes now known to be associated with growth *in utero* and early life development, or lack of, include blood pressure, respiratory function, and schizophrenia. Childhood social and educational factors also are strongly associated with physical and mental health outcomes in adult life (Wadsworth & Kuh, 1997).

Scientific evidence of these links is also available in relation to the crucial period of brain development *in utero* and shortly after birth (Barker, 1998; Ravelli, 1999). Infant malnutrition has been associated with diabetes and reduced stature as an adult. Infection early in life has been related to the development of chronic bronchitis, acute appendicitis, asthma, Parkinson's disease, and multiple sclerosis in adulthood. And, low birth weight has been correlated with subsequent increased blood pressure, chronic pulmonary disease, cardiovascular disease, coronary heart disease, and stroke. Thus, although an investment in basic health and nutritional services for young children can be justified by immediate health and anthropometric outcomes for children, the linkage to their health status as adults heightens the importance of the interventions, which are standard components of integrated ECD programmes.

The linkage to adult health status is also significant for HD efforts. Evidence indicates that the association between adult health status and economic well-being is at least as strong as the association between education and economic well-being (Hertzman, 1999; Smith, 1999). Adults with better health, higher life expectancy, and better weight and height measures tend to have higher productivity, less absenteeism from work, and higher incomes than their less fortunate counterparts.

However, the causality in the relationship between health status and economic well-being remains in question. Does good health lead to higher productivity (income) or does a higher income enable one to buy better health? Both relationships – health as cause and as effect – have been proved true. Where it is possible to establish that good or poor health came first, a subsequent economic effect can be determined (e.g., the reduced earning power of an adult stunted by malnutrition as a child) (Bundy, 1997; Thomas & Strauss, 1997). The converse – higher income leading to better health – also is well documented (Acheson, 1998). Clearly, better health results in higher income in many instances, but additional research is needed to further unravel the dual relationship.

To establish a definitive link between health and the HD of a nation, the health-and-income nexus must be aggregated across individuals, for populations. Recent studies demonstrate this link. Like education, the health status of a population is related to the economic growth of that population (Barro, 1997; Pritchett & Summers, 1996; World Health Organization, 1998). Key examples in Africa are the economic (growth-reducing) effects of malaria and the epidemic of acquired immuno-deficiency syndrome (AIDS; Bloom & Sachs, 1998).

Surprisingly, most of the studies of health and economic growth are recent, and additional research is needed to understand more fully the many ways in which the health of a population, which is a good in itself, can influence the wealth of a nation. But, the fact that the link is very important is no longer debatable. Like education, the health pathway from ECD to HD is clear. If increasing the wealth of a nation is an overall objective, beginning with the health of a newborn is a logical first step.

Social capital

The "social" benefits of ECD programmes are less well defined than the health and education benefits but they still exist. Many studies of the effects of ECD programmes note the change in children's behaviour (Kagitcibasi, 1996; Karoly et al., 1998). They are less aggressive and more cooperative, they behave better in groups, and they accept instructions (e.g., from parents) well. Overall the children have higher self-concepts and are more socially adjusted.

A few long-term (tracer) studies point to similar outcomes for the children's adult life: improved self-esteem, social competence, motivation, and acceptance of the culture's norms and values. In particular, evidence suggests that participation in ECD programmes leads to reduced criminal behaviour and less delinquency as an adult (Schweinhart et al., 1993; Yoshikawa, 1995; Zigler, Taussig, & Black, 1992).

The link between improved social behaviour and the formation and maintenance of "social capital" has yet to be established. Social capital includes many distinct social phenomena. At the macro level, it refers to informal institutional arrangements, trust, ethnic social networks, non-legal market arrangements, and other related phenomena (Coleman, 1990; Putnam, 1993). At the individual level, it refers to a person's ability to draw upon social networks to better pursue his or her own interests, a phenomenon that usually involves reciprocal arrangements similar to the exchange of "IOU" slips when obtaining financial credit (Coleman, 1988, 1990; Lin, 1999).

Studies of the social benefits of ECD programmes suggest that the benefits will continue later in life. As the brain needs to be wired properly for academic learning, so it needs to be prepared suitably for social learning. If studies can truly establish the link between the social benefits of ECD programmes and improved skills of adults in creating and utilizing social capital, the link to HD can easily be made. To do so only requires that the benefits to social capital at the individual level be aggregated to society as a whole. Although social capital is an ill-defined concept that refers to many different social phenomena, this linkage has already been established firmly in the sociology and economic literature (Narayan, 1997; Woolcock, 1999). Much empirical evidence has been acquired recently, and although it does not directly make the link between children and adults, as suggested above, it is convincing and growing.

Interest in the link between culture, or values, and economic performance is increasing. Recent studies suggest that "values" is an important concept for explaining differences in the growth of nations (Fukuyama, 1995). If researchers determine that ECD programmes can instil values that are reflected subsequently in adult behaviour, the link between ECD and HD through the pathway of social capital may be even greater than suggested here.

Equality

The fourth pathway, "equality", refers to a "level playing field". It is inextricably linked to the previous three pathways. Equality may refer to a level playing field in education, health, or social capital. And, like education, health, and social capital, equality is a good in itself and contributes to the economic performance of a nation. If ECD programmes can be shown to contribute to achieving a more equal society, the link between ECD and HD, through the pathway of equality, can be easily established. In fact, ECD programmes can contribute greatly to a levelling of the playing field if they are well targeted (Barros & Mendonca, 1999). With a relatively small investment, ECD programmes can decrease the disadvantage of poor children, compared with their more fortunate counterparts, in nutritional status, cognitive and social development, and health. The benefits of greater equality begin right after birth.

For adults, equality in education and health leads to equality of opportunity; better education and health lead to higher income. Significantly, data show that countries with a more equitable distribution of income are also healthier (Deaton, 1999; Hertzman, 1999; Wilkinson, 1996). The evidence is undeniable, yet the reasons for the relationship are being debated. Nevertheless, the link between more equality of opportunity early in life and more equality in education, income, and health later in life appears to be strong, as does the aggregate link between greater equality in income and the health of society. And, again, the benefits begin with ECD.

Finally, numerous studies show that greater equality leads to higher sustainable growth (Aghion, Caroli, & Garcia-Pefialosa, 1999; Barro, 1997). The link between ECD and HD, through the pathway of equality, is complex but strong.

Early child development: Benefits and research needs

Table 10.1. summarizes the benefits of ECD – better education, improved health, increased social capital, and greater equality. All of these outcomes are of value themselves, and the benefits are immediately tangible at the time of intervention (i.e., in a child's early years). ECD programmes are most often justified by the immediate benefits to a child's social and cognitive development and health and nutritional status. Yet, as discussed above, these outcomes have positive, long-term consequences for the children as they mature into adults and for their nations as a whole. Except for the pathway

Table 10.1 Benefits of early child development

Benefits of ECD	Pathways linking ECD to HD			
	Education	Health	Social capital	Equality
For children (immediate)	Higher intelligence, improved practical reasoning, eye and hand coordination, hearing and speech; reading readiness; improved school performance; less grade repetition and dropout; increased schooling	Less morbidity, mortality, malnutrition, stunting, child abuse; better hygiene and health care	Higher self-concept: more socially adjusted; less aggressive; more cooperative; better behaviour in groups; increased acceptance of instructions	Reduced disadvantages of poverty; improved nutritional status, cognitive and social development, and health
For adults (long term)	Higher productivity; increased success (better jobs, higher incomes); improved childcare and family health; greater economic well-being	Improved height and weight; enhanced cognitive development; fewer infections and chronic diseases	Higher self-esteem; improved social competence, motivation, acceptance of norms and values; less delinquency and criminal behaviour	Equality of opportunity, education, health, and income
For society	Greater social cohesion; less poverty and crime; lower fertility rates; increased adoption of new technologies; improved democratic processes; higher economic growth	Higher productivity; less absenteeism; higher incomes	Improved utilization of social capital; enhanced social values	Reduced poverty and crime; better societal health; increased social justice; higher sustainable economic growth

Notes: ECD, Early child development; HD, human development.

of education, these long-term benefits are usually ignored by government officials and policy makers.

The link between ECD and HD through the pathway of education is clearly established and abundantly documented. New developments in health research, particularly those addressing the relationship between child health and adult health, also provide ample evidence of a link between ECD and HD. As additional research findings become available, the pathway of health is likely to become as significant to HD as is education. International organizations and governments may need to fundamentally rethink health care efforts worldwide and to direct a much larger share of health care budgets to the health care of children, especially in their early years. The aim will be not only to address children's immediate health problems, but also to reduce their future health risks as adults.

The pathway of social capital is currently less clear, but suggestive. The link between social behaviour as a child and as an adult needs to be confirmed, and the link between social behaviour and social capital is still weak. The literature on social capital is relatively young, but current evidence indicates that this pathway for ECD to HD will become as firmly established as the pathways of education and health.

The pathway of equality from ECD to HD is undeniable and, as noted, is linked to the other three pathways. The finding that income equality is related to the health of society is a recent and surprising one, which reinforces the importance of ECD and suggests far-reaching policy implications.

Education, health, social capital, and equality are all important contributors to economic growth. Together with economic growth, they constitute the mutually reinforcing elements of a comprehensive framework for HD, as depicted in Figure 10.1. This framework could be expanded easily, for example, to include gender issues or poverty (as it relates to equality).

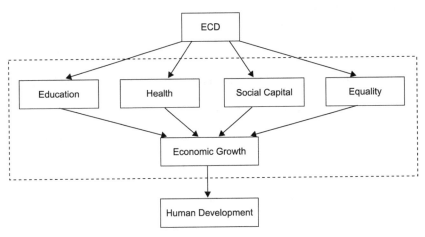

Figure 10.1 A comprehensive framework for human development.

Well-executed and well-targeted ECD programmes are initiators of HD. They stimulate improvements in education, health, social capital, and equality that have both immediate and long-term benefits for the children participating in the programmes. Investments in ECD programmes are in many ways investments in the future of a nation.

Acknowledgement

The author thanks Wendy Janssens for excellent research assistance during the preparation of this chapter.

Note

1 This chapter has been previously published as: Van der Gaag, J. (2002). From child development to human development. In M. E. Young (Ed.), *From early child development to human development* (pp. 63–78). Washington, DC: World Bank Publications. © International Bank for Reconstruction and Development/The World Bank.

References

Acheson, D. (1998). *Independent inquiry into inequalities in health: Report*. London: The Stationery Office.

Aghion, P., Caroli, E., & Garcia-Pefialosa, C. (1999). Inequality and economic growth: The perspective of the new growth theories. *Journal of Economic Literature*, *37*, 1615–1660.

Barker, D. J. P. (1998). *Mothers, babies and health in later life*. Edinburgh: Churchill Livingstone.

Barnett, W. S. (1995). Long-term effects of early childhood programs on cognitive and school outcomes. *The Future of Children*, *5*(3), 25–50.

Barnett, W. S. (1998). Long-term cognitive and academic effects of early childhood education on children in poverty. *Preventive Medicine*, *27*, 204–207.

Barro, R. J. (1997). *Determinants of economic growth: A cross-country empirical study*. Cambridge, MA: MIT Press.

Barros, R. P. de, & Mendonca, R. (1999). *Costs and benefits of pre-school education in Brazil*. Rio de Janeiro: Institute of Applied Economic Research.

Bloom, D. E., & Sachs, J. D. (1998). Geography, demography, and economic growth in Africa, Harvard Institute for International Development. *Brookings Papers on Economic Activity*. Washington, DC: Brookings Institution.

Bundy, D. A. P. (1997). Health and early child development. In M. E. Young (Ed.), *Early child development: Investing in our children's future* (pp. 11–38). Amsterdam: Elsevier Science.

Carnoy, M. (1992). *The case for investing in basic education*. New York: United Nations Children's Fund.

Chenery, H., & Srinivasan, T. N. (1989). *Handbook of development economics, Volume 1*. New York: North Holland.

Coleman, J. (1988). Social capital in the creation of human capital. *American Journal of Sociology*, *94*, S95–S120.

Coleman, J. (1990). *Foundations of social theory.* Cambridge, MA: Harvard University Press.

Cynader, M. S., & Frost, B. (1999). Mechanisms of brain development: Neuronal sculpting by the physical and social environment. In D. P. Keating and C. Hertzman (Eds.), *Developmental health and the wealth of nations: Social, biological, and educational dynamics* (pp. 153–184). New York: Guilford Press.

Deaton, A. (1999). Inequalities in income and inequalities in health. *National Bureau of Economic Research Working Paper No. W7141.* New York: NBER.

Fogel, R. W. (2000). *The fourth great awakening.* Chicago: University of Chicago Press.

Fukuyama, E. (1995). *Trust: The social virtues and the creation of prosperity.* New York: Free Press.

Grantham-McGregor, S. M., Walker, S. P., Chang, S. M., & Powell, C. A. (1997). Effects of early childhood supplementation with and without stimulation on later development in stunted Jamaican children. *American Journal of Clinical Nutrition, 66,* 247–253.

Haveman, R. H., & Wolfe, B. L. (1984). Schooling and economic well-being: The role of nonmarket effects. *Journal of Human Resources, 19*(3), 377–407.

Hertzman, C. (1999). Population health and human development. In D. P. Keating and C. Hertzman (Eds.), *Developmental health and the wealth of nations: Social, biological, and educational dynamics* (pp. 21–40). New York: Guilford Press.

Horton, S. (1999). Economics of nutritional investments (draft). In R. D. Semba and M. W. Bloem (Eds.), *Nutrition and health in developing countries* (pp. 859–872). Totowa, NJ: Humana Press.

Kagitcibasi, C. (1996). *Family and human development across cultures: A view from the other side.* Mahwah, NJ: Lawrence Erlbaum Associates, Inc.

Karoly, L. A., Greenwood, P. W., Everingham, S. S., Hoube, J., Kilburn, M. R., Rydell, C. P., et al. (1998). *Investing in our children: What we know and don't know about the costs and benefits of early childhood interventions.* Washington, DC: RAND.

Lin, N. (1999). *Inequality in social capital: Evidence from urban China. Creation and returns of social capital in education and labor markets.* Center for Research in Experimental Economics and Political Decision Making/University of Amsterdam, Institute of Information and Computing Sciences (ICS)/University of Groningen and ICS/Utrecht University.

McCain, M. N., & Mustard, J. F. (1999). *Reversing the real brain drain: Early years study, Final report.* Toronto: Publications Ontario.

Myers, R. G. (1992). *The twelve who survive.* London: Routledge.

Narayan, D. (1997). *Voices of the poor: Poverty and social capital in Tanzania.* Washington, DC: World Bank.

Pan American Health Organization (1998). *Nutrition, health and child development: Research advances and policy recommendations,* Scientific Publication No. 566. Washington, DC: PAHO.

Pritchett, L., & Summers, L. H. (1996). Wealthier is healthier. *Journal of Human Resources, 31*(4), 841–868.

Psacharopoulos, G. (1994). Returns to investment in education: A global update. *World Development, 22*(9), 1325–1343.

Putnam, R. (1993). The prosperous community – social capital and economic growth. *The American Prospect, 356,* 4–9.

Ravelli, A. C. J. (1999). *Prenatal exposure to the Dutch famine and glucose tolerance and obesity at age 50*. Thela Thesis. Amsterdam: University of Amsterdam.

Rutter, M., Giller, H., & Hagell, A. (1998). *Antisocial behavior by young people*. Cambridge: Cambridge University Press.

Schweinhart, L. J., Barnes, H. V., & Weikart, D. P. (1993). *Significant benefits: The High/Scope Perry-preschool study through age 27*. Ypsilanti, MI: High/Scope Press.

Sen, A. (1999). *Development as freedom*. New York: Alfred A. Knopf.

Smith, J. P. (1999). Healthy bodies and thick wallets: The dual relation between health and economic status. *Journal of Economic Perspectives, 13*(2), 145–166.

Stephenson, L. S., Latham, M. C., Adams, E. J., Kinoti, S. N., & Pertet, A. (1993). Physical fitness, growth and appetite of Kenyan schoolboys with hookworm, *Trichuris trichiura* and *Ascaris lumbricoides*. Infections are improved four months after a single dose of albendazole. *Journal of Nutrition, 123*, 1036–1046.

Thomas, D., & Strauss, J. (1997). Health and wages: Evidence on men and women in urban Brazil. *Journal of Econometrics, 77*, 159–185.

Van der Gaag, J., & Tan, J.-P. (1998). *The benefits of early child development programs: An economic analysis*. Washington, DC: World Bank, Human Development Network.

Wadsworth, M. E., & Kuh, D. (1997). Childhood influences on adult health. *Paediatric and Perinatal Epidemiology, 11*, 2–20.

Wilkinson, R. G. (1996). *Unhealthy societies: The afflictions of inequality*. London: Routledge.

Woolcock, M. (1999). *Managing risk, shocks, and opportunity in developing economies: The role of social capital*. Washington, DC: World Bank, Development Research Group.

World Health Organization (1998). *Health, health policy, and economic outcomes. Health and development satellite*. Geneva: WHO.

Yoshikawa, H. (1995). Long-term effects of early childhood programs on social outcomes and delinquency. *The Future of Children, 5*(3), 51–75.

Young, M. E. (1997). *Early child development. Investing in our children's future*, International Congress Series No. 1137. Amsterdam: Elsevier Science.

Zigler, E., Taussig, C., & Black, K. (1992). Early childhood intervention: A promising preventative for juvenile delinquency. *American Psychologist, 47*(8), 997–1006.

11 Inconvenient truths: Behavioural research and social policy[1]

Anne C. Petersen

Why is social policy so seldom based on what we know from research? The goal of this chapter is to provide useful principles and approaches to increase the likelihood that research will result in positive policy implementation. We recognize that many researchers do not aim to influence policy; the rewards in the world of research do not generally require, and may even discourage, this orientation. But there are many researchers, especially those focused on youth, who would like to improve the lives of young people; doing so typically requires structural policy change. This chapter is directed at those researchers who are interested in influencing policy to achieve positive change among youth.

Introduction: Inconvenient truths

Where does the "inconvenient truth" come in? As former US Vice President and Presidential candidate Al Gore has demonstrated in his documentary film of that name, research results (specifically about global climate change) can be inconvenient when they contradict the position of a political regime. This chapter will identify some examples of "inconvenient truths" resulting from behavioural research. Conversely, research results can be used in ways not intended by the researchers, as with the way behavioural science results were used by many selectively repressive governments from the middle of the 20th century on, to enslave or less directly control subgroups of the population (Elkins, 2005; Richter & Dawes, 2008; Zimbardo, 2007). The "truths" of the underlying behavioural research are just as "inconvenient" when applied for negative or destructive purposes as is research that is ignored by repressive governments.

As background, it is important to recognize that research and policy may have similar goals, most notably to improve society. But each also has specific contexts, approaches, and goals that have likely diverged in wealthier countries. (Less wealthy countries are less likely to invest scarce resources in research, especially on behavioural issues. But when they choose to do so, for example with a research institute, they seem to be more likely to use the research results.) However, some (e.g., World Bank, 2007) have noted the importance of keeping politics out of the knowledge-generating process, to avoid biasing or even totally subverting the process. Stokes (1997) greatly advanced thinking on this topic with his important book *Pasteur's Quadrant* in which he clearly laid out the purpose of knowledge generation and articulated a strong rationale for "applied" and policy-relevant research. Research is primarily focused on discovering truth in basic phenomena (which Stokes noted also happens with "applied" research). Researchers are rewarded for making contributions that advance knowledge. Influencing policy is not necessarily a part of the rewards of research achievement. Policy makers, in contrast, function within a context that typically requires election with some degree of accountability to or popularity with the electorate. (This, of course, varies from country to country with few countries having direct representation as does the USA.) Policy makers in the United States have proven to be more interested in a powerful story than data, and more often use emotion than evidence to persuade. Power is the chief motivator among many policy makers; even those who base their actions primarily in principles need to pay attention to those who wield power.

Providing information to policy makers is a double-edged sword. Researchers cannot guarantee that the information will be used for good purposes. Abuse or misuse of research is always a possibility. For example, Richter and Dawes (2008) found massive suppression of research results about child development under *apartheid* in South Africa, especially results that contradicted the policy agenda of the country (for example, research finding strengths among black children). Zimbardo (2007) has used his life-long programme of research on human motivation and control of behaviour to document the possibility of evil in each of us and our institutions, requiring appropriate countervailing policies. He makes explicit links between research findings of the Stanford Prison Experiments and real life examples, such as the unethical behaviour at Abu Ghraib Prison. Can abuse or misuse of research be prevented? Not likely. The Zimbardo approach of making the implications explicit is helpful for those hoping to establish policies to protect humans from abuse, but the same implications can be and have been used by those interested in power and control of other humans. What is needed then are possible approaches for limiting the destructive use of research results, starting with recognizing the possible "dark sides".

In all of this, we are assuming the situation in which there is a clear outcome of research: the research is of the highest quality, with careful attention to validity and specifically generalizability of results, along with any limitations. This requires more extensive research than typically exists on most questions. The Zimbardo research mentioned above is an example of rigorous research grounded in theory, with elegant research designs and ample replication.

When research is of poorer quality, its implementation into social policy is less likely to be effective, thus limiting impact, for good or ill. Such research, however, reflects poorly on the entire research establishment. That indeed is an inconvenient truth!

A more typical situation, especially for social/behavioural research, is that of incompletely studied hypotheses. Because so many social/behavioural theories or even variables are highly contextual, it is nearly impossible to study a phenomenon in all contexts. Some have even argued that generalizability in this field is not an appropriate goal; rather the variations should be studied and understood. For example, some parental behaviour styles were found to be effective with young people from middle class populations in the USA (Baumrind, 1971). Research now has consistently shown that in most contexts authoritative parenting (i.e., parenting that is warm and responsive while still providing firm, consistent rules and standards for youth behaviour) has the most positive outcomes in general (Lamborn, Mounts, Steinberg, & Dornbusch, 1991; Steinberg, 2001) but effectiveness depends on some basic assumptions such as a general level of child safety and security. In contexts where young people cannot be safe and secure except with high levels of parental monitoring or even control, effective parental behaviour patterns look quite different (e.g., Ceballo & McLoyd, 2002; McLeod, Kruttschnitt, & Dornfeld, 1994).

The parenting example just given is one in which there is enough research to characterize the variations in contexts that require different behaviour. For many questions, there simply is not enough research to know what the recommended policy stance should be. Insufficient research does not always keep researchers from exaggerating or even presenting false claims from research (e.g., Martinson, Anderson, & deVries, 2005). Social/behavioural scientists are no different from other researchers in this regard. Indeed, we may be fortunate that there are not usually large financial gains to be had for most social/behavioural research. The field of drug discovery research, for example, is full of cases in which the research is incomplete in terms of generalizability (e.g., for whom is the drug effective or ineffective and in whom does it produce adverse results?). Yet, the prospect of significant financial gain typically propels a drug through the required clinical trial process as quickly as possible, with some likelihood that the desire for financial gain will cause owners of the drug to suppress adverse findings or perhaps even to fabricate data to increase a speedy introduction into markets with the most positive claims.

Underlying assumptions

To even engage the discussion of the relationship between research and social policy, it is essential to frame such a discussion. Several underlying assumptions are required. Most important is the assumption that both researchers and policy makers are seeking positive human development. The instances in which repressive governments controlled human behaviour, with death for those who refused to be controlled (for example, with the "Mau Mau Rebellion" documented by Elkins, 2005), were not seeking positive human development; their goals were rather greed, control of natural resources, and/

or positive human development for only a subgroup of people. (The latter goal is not one this author believes is achievable; no one achieves positive human development when any subgroup is suppressed.) To generalize about these examples in history, some people were regarded as less worthy, expendable, necessary "collateral damage" relative to pursuit of the primary goals. But this argument projects negative intent where it probably did not exist. What Zimbardo's research (e.g., 2007) makes clear is that human beings can persuade themselves that they are doing the right thing while in fact engaging in evil acts. Given this human capacity for evil, it is even more important that we approach policy with humility and clear intent. An advance analysis of possible unintended consequences, and especially of negative consequences, together with identification of approaches to minimize these consequences is also important. Petersen (2006) describes one such approach using systems thinking.

A second underlying assumption is that learning or perhaps knowledge (depending on the state of evidence) is valued. Again, totalitarian regimes do not seek "knowledge" except when it will serve the predefined goals. A country in which new and perhaps different evidence is not appreciated and supported is also one in which it is very difficult to conduct research. Even governments that cannot be considered totalitarian but tend toward control of information and people may ignore "inconvenient truths" from research results. (For example, the Bush administration in the USA denied the scientific findings on global climate change, and suppressed on federal agency websites many kinds of scientific findings reflecting "inconvenient truths" relative to political stances.) Most governments may have difficulty being totally open to new "truths" from research because it may require flexibility and perhaps changing positions, something most politicians avoid for fear of being considered quixotic or even inconsistent. It may be more difficult now to totally control information, with mass communication tools like the internet and the web.

A third important underlying assumption is related to the second and is especially difficult in all countries with democratic and especially populist governments. Research is based on a systematic scientific method and is quite rational. Politics, in contrast, is often highly emotional, with vivid cases achieving primacy over even strong data. Policy related to incarceration in the USA has had little relationship with the body of research on effective practices, whether for deterrence of future crime or rehabilitation (Barkow, 2005). A single vivid exceptional case of horrific criminal behaviour can be used to generate fear and mobilize votes on policy totally inconsistent with all overall evidence, as has been the case repeatedly in the USA. What is the motivation of the politicians? Is it simply winning the election if they can appear strong and tough and therefore attractive to voters who have been manipulated to be fearful? Or is it greed from those with financial interests in the prison system? It seems likely that all possible combinations of motivation have existed in the USA. Conventional wisdom in Washington, DC, the political centre of the

USA, is that manipulation of fear is the most predictable way to gain a positive vote, regardless of the underlying issue. In contrast, most people, even those who are highly intellectual and rational, are unlikely to vote solely on the basis of data. Research on the power of persuasive messages demonstrates that a strong story is essential (Hamilton, 2006). Supporting data can help but it cannot succeed alone. Thus the underlying assumption here is that both researchers and policy makers at least understand how the other group works, and respect each other enough to find common ground on the evidence/story continuum so that they are not working at cross-purposes. Most policy researchers have learned the communication principle above and will seek a compelling example to make the inferences from their data vivid to policy makers. While we have framed the assumption in terms of mutual respect, it is usually up to the scientists to learn to become effective communicators to policy makers.

Finally, while some policy may be international, most is local and some national. The assumption here is that policy will only work within a community that shares some common values. The aim is to attend to the generality or limitations of the argument and inferences. Because the author knows it best, most examples are drawn from the USA.

Similarly, this chapter rests on an important assumption about science, and especially scientists. Scientists must remain objective about their results. There have been cases in which researchers claimed to speak as scientists but without providing supporting data or evidence for the claims, as their true intent was advocacy (Petersen, 2006). Each of us has a right to speak out as citizens about issues of importance to us, but it is important to be clear when we are speaking about scientific data and when we are speaking from a position of ethics or belief. Speaking as scientists about matters of belief without support of scientific data only undermines the entire enterprise.

A few definitions are also important in this chapter. *Research* is intended to refer to normal science: theory-based hypothesis testing in which the results can lead to rejection of the hypothesis. *Policy research* can be of two types: research on existing policy or research designed to inform policy making; this chapter is primarily focused on the second type. *Policy* is defined by Webster's dictionary (1970) as "any governing principle, plan, or course of action". Policy is established in most democratic societies at many levels, from international to village, and by various sectors depending on their purview (e.g., water policy, health policy, etc.). While the focus here is primarily on public policy such as that made by government officials, it is important to note that policy is also established by non-governmental professional organizations for the conduct of their members or constituents (e.g., physicians, school systems, etc.). As already noted, policy may be wise and beneficial to most or cruel and benefiting few, with all possibilities in between. Policy is of interest to researchers because it can sustain changes achieved by effective programmes. This approach to policy requires consideration of *systems*, defined as structures, processes, or relationships.

Youth problem behaviour research and policy

Given all the issues already discussed, what is known about the status of youth policy and specifically what is the status of policy related to youth problem behaviour research? In general, most policy appears not to be aligned with research, although the situation is much better in some countries than others, depending on the national orientation toward fostering healthy development generally and having the national resources to support these approaches. In the United States, a recent federal report (Catalano, Berglund, Ryan, Lonczak, & Hawkins, 2004) reviewing positive youth development programmes concluded that "models of healthy development hold the key to both health promotion and health prevention of problem behaviors" (p. 101). This report cited evidence that policy makers, practitioners, and prevention scientists have all converged on this conclusion. They cite new evidence providing empirical demonstration that the same risk and protective factors that predict problem behaviours also predict positive outcomes.

Treatment programmes for problem behaviour are absent in many countries, except for incarceration and related punishments that typically include no rehabilitation. Recent research by Moffitt (1993) would suggest a different approach in any case, with her conclusion that only 5% of adolescent anti-social behaviour is likely to persist into adulthood, and that small groups must be treated before adulthood and preferably earlier in childhood to help those young people to achieve different outcomes. To our knowledge, no policy has yet been implemented that would target highly aggressive pre-schoolers and their families for special interventions likely to change the course of development.

The preferred approach, except for the small group of youth just mentioned, is to foster positive development for youth (e.g., Larson, 2000; Lerner, 2005). Pittman, Diversi, and Ferber (2002) identified some framing questions for 21st century policy at the community or country level to "help adolescents become adults who are problem free, fully prepared, and fully engaged in their communities" (Pittman et al., 2002, p. 149). The questions "create the framework from which specific policies and decisions can be discussed by policy makers and the public" (p. 151).

- What are the desired *outcomes and goals?* The community or country might wish to focus on improved school graduation rates, or improved health status on a variety of indicators. More common are efforts to reduce some problem such as teen smoking or pregnancy.
- What are the *inputs* at play? Inputs refer to existing services for basic needs, supports, and opportunities needed for healthy development.
- What are the *settings* involved? Depending on the specific issue being addressed, there will be some context or setting in which a programme takes place – such as a school, a youth organization, or the broader community.

- Who are the *actors?* These might be youth themselves, families, teachers, businesses, youth workers, or any combination of these and others.
- What is the *time frame?* This gets at the timing, duration, and intensity of any efforts.
- Who is the *target group?* Will the effort focus on all youth or selected subgroups?
- What are the expected *youth roles?* Youth may be recipients or active participants, depending on cultural values about appropriate roles.

Pittman and colleagues (2002) also identify a set of important principles that have resulted from global youth research (e.g., Brown, Larson, & Saraswathi, 2002; Larson, 2002; Larson, Brown, & Mortimer, 2003; McCall & Groark, 2000; Saraswathi & Larson, 2002; Shanahan, 2000; Shanahan, Mortimer, & Kruger, 2002; Youniss, Bales, Christmas-Best, Diversi, McLaughlin, & Silbereisen, 2002). The four principles are:

1. Social policy has to focus on positive outcomes and non-academic outcomes as clearly as it focuses on negative outcomes and academic success.
2. Social policy should be firmly connected to older and younger populations.
3. Social policy should reach across a range of settings and systems, providing a full range of services, supports, and opportunities.
4. Social policy should prominently feature the voices and actions of young people themselves as agents of positive change.

These principles result from research concluding that working with young people where they are has the best chance of achieving sustainable results. They are whole people not just students, and therefore need policy that recognizes their wholeness. Similarly, they have histories in childhood and will become adults. They interact with others older and younger in many settings on a continuing basis. Therefore, programmes need to recognize the temporal and contextual embeddedness of youth development. Finally, youth are capable of being powerful positive agents of change, for themselves and their communities. Their positive development will be most sustainable if they are guided but not led, and appreciated for the strengths, ideas, and especially the energy they have.

Global youth policy

The foregoing references and examples are largely drawn from research by US and European researchers. The recent report from the World Bank (2007) titled *World Bank Development Report 2007* is an outstanding and clearly-written summary of knowledge from youth programme and policy innovations around the world, and is largely consistent with the conclusions from research. Most remarkably, this report on development from one of the foremost multinational development agencies is focused on youth as the central strategy. The World Bank report for 2007 takes the perspective that youth must be a focus of development policy because "young people will greatly influence the future of their nations" (p. 2). The report is framed around five important youth transitions that have the biggest long-term impacts on how human capital is kept safe, developed, and deployed: (1) continuing to learn, (2) starting to work, (3) developing a healthful lifestyle, (4) beginning a family, and (5) exercising citizenship. This framework permits application to every society, despite different timing of the transitions. In general, youth is defined as the standard 12–24 years of age but the report explicitly recognizes that in many societies the transitions may occur earlier or later than this age range.

The World Bank report also focuses explicitly on effective youth policy, using a "youth lens" (Figure 11.1). Three strategic directions are identified: (1) opportunities (including the usual education and health foci but also includes less common but equally important components of working life and giving youth a voice), (2) capabilities (including developing youth capabilities to choose well among opportunities by recognizing youth as decision-making agents and by helping to ensure that they are informed, resourced, and judicious), and (3) second chances (recognizing that many young people have already experienced bad luck or bad choices but still have many years left to benefit from opportunities if they can get "back on track").

The report gathers urgency from the recognition of two current trends: that more young people are receiving a primary education and are ready to benefit from further education; and that lower fertility rates in many countries provide the opportunity for youth to enter the workforce without as many non-working dependents. It also explicitly recognizes research demonstrating that making labour more productive is the best way to reduce poverty. The challenges to productivity include capitalizing on increased

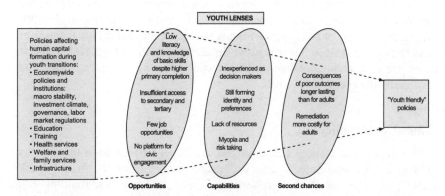

Figure 11.1 Youth lenses. From World Bank (2007), © International Bank for Reconstruction and Development/The World Bank.

education levels (including improving the quality of primary education and improving both the availability and quality of secondary and higher education) and severe threats to health (such as HIV/AIDS). Research demonstrates the economic importance of addressing these challenges, as well as their importance for quality of life.

Youth demographics vary across nations and generally demonstrate a relationship in which more children and youth in a population correlate with low national or per capita income. Nonetheless, many low-income nations can capitalize on being "young" by increasing human capital and productivity of youth. Of the 1.5 billion people globally between the ages of 12 and 24 years, 1.3 billion are in developing countries, which is the most ever in history. Dramatic declines in fertility rates are projected to plateau within the next decade or so in rapidly growing economies such as China and Chile. A predominance of the young is projected to continue for up to 40 years in other countries, such as most of the countries in sub-Saharan Africa. Large numbers of young people are a drain on a nation if they remain uneducated and unemployed for long periods, wasting human resources. If a nation sees this human resource as an opportunity to build human capital, youth can become a significant engine for economic development. For example, 40% of the higher growth in East Asia over Latin America in the period 1965–1990 is attributable to faster growth of its working age population and better policies for trade and human capital development of young people.

Powerful examples from various countries are given to demonstrate the role that youth policy can play in producing more positive outcomes for youth and the nation's economic development. For one example, Bell, Shantayanan, and Gersbach (2006) used an "overlapping-generations" model to estimate the effects of human capital investments in Africa. These researchers estimated that Kenya will not recover its 1990 levels of human capital and per capita income until 2030. A programme that invested in both post primary education and health of young adults would produce more dramatic gains (about a fourfold increase) than the educational subsidy alone.

Public policy can make an enormous difference in the opportunities of youth, especially when markets do not work. In terms of the youth transition related to learning, policy can make it possible for youth to attend school and also to increase the quality of that education, both of which are crucial factors in human capital development and future economic gains of nations. As for starting a productive work life, policy can reduce the periods of work inactivity – which not only mean wasted human resource but also create scars that are most powerful for the most disadvantaged – and can correct for information failures that lead to disincentives for work entry and for employment of youth. While youth are generally healthier than their older counterparts, they make choices that may compromise their future health. Building the capacity to make wise decisions is, therefore, extremely important. For this, young people need both information and capacity to make and act on wise decisions. Similarly, beginning a family requires both good nutrition and reproductive health services, as well as the capacity to make wise decisions about these. Becoming a citizen is intimately linked to identity development, and requires understanding of both rights and responsibilities. Being an effective citizen requires basic skills, information, and opportunities to participate. Beginning to participate while still young provides an excellent way to produce better programmes and policy and to develop the skills of younger people to be effective citizens.

The *World Bank Development Report 2007* concludes with an excellent summary chapter on all policy goals, directions, actions, and programmes. Examples are provided of every aspect but the chapter notes, however, that too few promising programmes are evaluated. This would seem to be an opportunity for university researchers to partner with donors (e.g., foundations) to build systematic feedback into programmes and to produce evaluation research on whether the promises of the programmes were realized. Youth can play a useful role in providing feedback about programme effectiveness and making assessments of whether progress was made.

While this report is to be applauded for recognizing the central importance of youth to development globally, it seems to suggest that both youth development and development generally can be achieved with "top-down" approaches. There is reason to question whether a singular focus on such approaches will be effective, with the primary one being the importance of individual and community engagement in development efforts. The present author has argued (Petersen, 2007) that *people* are the primary drivers of development, not money, citing the many development failures among the top-down efforts compared with the success of efforts that engage people, such as micro lending among others (e.g., Easterly, 2006). In most countries, enabling infrastructure including supportive policies is necessary for effective development outcomes. But they are not likely to be sufficient. To achieve the significant changes required for national advancement as for individual development, the affected individuals must be engaged.

Bottom-up approaches for positive youth development

There are many good examples of positive youth development programmes around the world, documented by the Fall 2006 *Newsletter* of the International Society for Behavioral Development (Barber & Weichold, 2006). A US example is that of Lerner and colleagues who have developed a 4-H programme of positive youth development (Lerner, Almerigi, Theokas, & Lerner, 2005a; Lerner et al., 2005b) that produced highly promising early results. An excellent global study is that of Verma and colleagues on street children in developing countries (Verma, 2008).

An example that is especially comprehensive, grounded in theory, and matches the principles discussed by Pittman and colleagues (2002) is that of Bogenschneider (1996). She proposed a theory for positive youth development, planned a programmatic approach embedded in community, and influenced policy at the state level to implement the ideas.

Bogenschneider's (1996) ecological risk/protective theoretical framework combines two major perspectives: the epidemiological risk-focused model (e.g., Hawkins, 1995; Hawkins, Catalano, & Miller, 1992) and the resiliency or protective process approach (Garmezy, 1983; Rutter, 1987; Werner, 1992). Bogenschneider integrates these two approaches with the ecological theory of human development (Bronfenbrenner, 1979) to bring in all the important contexts for youth, and developmental contextualism (Lerner, 1995) to include the dynamic relationship over time between these contexts and developing youth.

Central to her framework is simultaneously strengthening resiliency in youth and protective factors in their environments while also reducing risks in the youth and their community. Since protective factors are only needed in the face of risks, the model affords consideration of all, with application as needed. She argues that her framework better permits understanding of human development and generates principles that guide the design, delivery, and evaluation of prevention programmes. She and her university-based team have partnered with 22 communities in the US state of Wisconsin to help them create communities empowered to nurture the healthy development of youth.

In describing how to use this framework for building prevention programmes, policies, and community capacity, Bogenschneider (1996) identifies twelve principles that are also recommended by other prevention scholars:

1. Identify the real issues facing local youth (by collecting data and engaging community discussions).
2. Establish well-defined goals that target the risk and protective processes associated with the identified youth issue or problem.
3. Be comprehensive in addressing both risk and protective processes in several levels of the human ecology (because problem behaviours have no single cause, but many).
4. Collaborate with stakeholders in the community or neighbourhood (to engage local ownership and existing services).
5. Educate coalition members on current theory and research on adolescent development, prevention programming, and community process (using local data).
6. Tailor the plan to the community, reducing risks that exist locally and building protective processes that do not exist (use assessments of needs, assets, and capacities).
7. Involve the target audience (i.e., youth) in programme design, planning, and implementation.
8. Be sensitive to cultural, ethnic, and other forms of diversity in the neighbourhood or community (and engage that diversity in the coalition and the support staff).

9. Intervene early and continuously (to engage when change is most possible and to sustain new healthier patterns).
10. Select developmentally appropriate prevention strategies (in terms of timing, type, and focus of programmes).
11. Anticipate how changes in one part of the system may affect changes in the system or other settings (use the whole system to reinforce positive change and consider possible unintended side effects, and minimize them in advance or limit adverse effects by watching for them during the programme).
12. Evaluate effectiveness by monitoring changes in risk and protective processes (over time and in multiple settings).

The Wisconsin Youth Futures coalitions were established in communities ranging from small rural communities to large inner-city neighbourhoods. Coalitions consisted of 30–35 individuals, including judges, school leadership and teachers, law enforcement officials, local government officials, leaders of parent/teacher associations, business leaders, representatives of community service clubs, parents, and young people. The focus was on specific youth problems such as drug and alcohol use, prejudice and intolerance, and youth violence. Community members and the university team collected data from youth to identify risks and opportunities. In five or six meetings, coalition members learned about youth development, and established priorities. Then the coalition assessed community resources and support for youth and then identified plans to address gaps. Members developed a comprehensive, multi-dimensional plan to be implemented by the university team and local volunteers.

While comprehensive results of this programme have been difficult to obtain, the Wisconsin Youth Futures team has been able to verify that the programme has some results of the predicted sort, and there have been many policy impacts. For example, more community support from the local coalitions seemed to produce lower adolescent alcohol use (Mills & Bogenschneider, 2001). Youth Futures coalitions used the data from their youth to identify gaps and needs, in the youth and their community, so as to avoid redundant efforts and focus services at the local level on areas of need. Seventeen of the coalitions gave highest priority to alcohol and other drug use among youth. They generated more than 30 local policies to reduce adolescent alcohol use. For example, local coalitions were able to better align local policies and practices with their intentions to support good behaviour as well as to discourage or punish bad behaviour. In one community, both teens and those who provide alcohol to minors must appear before the judge, a change from only requiring the teen to appear, so that there is better tracking and it is not only young people who are required to be responsible. Many other examples could be cited with the area of alcohol use. Youth Futures coalitions generated many other policy changes as well, including some at the state level.

Thus the Wisconsin Youth Futures community coalitions appear to provide an effective and efficient way to create better environments for youth, by using community research to provide valuable information on youth needs and gaps in services, and to come together to create solutions that make a difference. Sustainability in these efforts will be of interest going into the future. And youth behaviour outcomes, both constructive engagement in their lives as well as reduced problem behaviour, will be important to track.

Summary

The local approach for policy influence used in this example is desirable for many reasons. First, young people and their families live in communities. This is the proximal environment that can enable or constrain development. While nations or other levels of government can also adversely affect youth development and should not be ignored, the local level needs to be at least a focus of policy influence. Second, the community policy level is more likely to reflect the demographics as well as the other assets and deficits of the people living there. Research has demonstrated that "one size does not fit all" – policy prescriptions need to work for the people, and preferably have emerged bottom up from the people. From a research perspective, local variations will provide valuable information about the extent of diversity in assets, needs, desires, and so forth.

Cost is likely to be a very important consideration to policy makers. Community-based work is likely to be provided by volunteers and be less expensive than top-down work, but we do not yet have cost information on the programme described here. Other studies have examined costs in youth programmes (e.g., Aos, Phipps, Barnowski, & Leib, 2001). The single most important variable increasing costs is the extent to which professionally trained staff are required for effective implementation.

Will this approach work around the world? The Kellogg Foundation Latin America/Caribbean Program "Promoting Regional Development" (2007) uses a similar approach, developing community coalitions committed to working on behalf of young people. Diverse communities are engaging and supporting youth in the poorest regions of Latin America and the Caribbean: north-eastern Brazil, the high Andes (Peru, Bolivia, and part of Ecuador), and a region including most of Central America, southern Mexico, and the island of Haiti and the Dominican Republic. These efforts have already produced many persuasive examples of effectiveness. Again, more definitive results will hopefully emerge from evaluation information.

Conclusions

After decades of neglect, and worse, by many communities and nations there are now promising approaches to address youth problem behaviour through community coalitions that focus on fostering positive youth development and reducing risks through attention to both young people and their environments. Programmes addressing local conditions and needs are most likely to engage the proximal factors needed for young people to grow and thrive. Young people are born with the potential to be effective adults but in too many situations they are discouraged or even prevented from reaching their potential. Programmes such as Wisconsin Youth Futures hold promise of truly fostering positive youth development and reducing youth problems.

At the same time, the research-based wisdom demonstrated in the *World Bank Development Report 2007* is to be applauded as well. Recognition of transitions in youth development, and how these might provide opportunities for national efforts that recognize cultural variations in their youth as well as variations in available infrastructure, provides a strong framework for effective programmes.

Combining the two approaches – top down and bottom up – would seem the most powerful of all approaches. Local empowerment and development of youth is certainly necessary and is likely to be sufficient for successful adulthood unless the nation thwarts the development of youth and their communities. Outmigration of motivated youth with sufficient capacity is a likely outcome of national constriction of development opportunities, but bottom-up development efforts from the community combined with top-down national supports and incentives are likely to provide a winning combination for successful national development with a highly effective next generation.

Note

1 An earlier version of this chapter was presented by the author at the Workshop "Development of Behavior Problems: State of Knowledge and Policy Implications", on 8/9 June 2006, Utrecht, The Netherlands.

References

Aos, S., Phipps, P., Barnowski, R., & Leib, R. (2001). *The comparative costs and benefits of programs to reduce crime. Version 4.0*. Olympia, WA: Washington State Institute for Public Policy.

Barber, B. L., & Weichold, K. (2006). Introduction to research on interventions targeting the promotion of positive development, *ISSBD Newsletter* (Number 2, Serial No. 50). www.issbd.org/resources/files/ISSBD050_online.pdf.

Barkow, R. E. (2005). Federalism and the politics of sentencing. *Columbia Law Review, 105*.

Baumrind, D. (1971). Current patterns of parental authority. *Developmental Psychology Monographs, 4*(2), 1–103.

Bell, C., Shantayanan, D., & Gersbach, H. (2006). The long-run economic costs of AIDS: A model with an application to South Africa. *World Bank Economic Review, 20*(1), 55–89.

Bogenschneider, K. (1996). An ecological risk/protective theory for building prevention programs, policies, and community capacity to support youth. *Family Relations*, *45*, 127–138.

Bronfenbrenner, U. (1979). *The ecology of human development*. Cambridge, MA: Harvard University Press.

Brown, B. B., Larson, R. W., & Saraswathi, T. S. (2002). *The world's youth: Adolescence in eight regions of the globe*. New York: Cambridge University Press.

Catalano, R. F., Berglund, M. L., Ryan, J. A. M., Lonczak, H. S., & Hawkins, J. D. (2004). Positive youth development in the Unites States: Research findings on evaluation of positive youth development programs. *Annals of the American Academy of Political and Social Science*, *591*(1), 98–124.

Ceballo, R., & McLoyd, V. C. (2002). Social support and parenting in poor, dangerous neighborhoods. *Child Development*, *73*, 1210–1321.

Easterly, W. R. (2006) *White man's burden: How the West has spent so much and accomplished so little*. New York: Penguin Press.

Elkins, C. (2005). *Imperial reckoning: The untold story of Britain's gulag in Kenya*. New York: Henry Holt & Co, Inc.

Garmezy, N. (1983). Stressors of childhood. In N. Garmezy & M. Rutter (Eds.), *Stress, coping, and development in children* (pp. 43–84). New York: McGraw-Hill.

Hamilton, J. T. (2006). *All the news that's fit to sell: How the market transforms information into news*. Princeton, NJ: Princeton University Press.

Hawkins, J. D. (1995, August). Controlling crime before it happens: Risk-focused prevention. *National Institute of Justice Journal*, pp. 10–18.

Hawkins, J. D., Catalano, R. F., & Miller, J. Y. (1992). Risk and protective factors for alcohol and other drug problems in adolescence and early adulthood: Implications for substance abuse prevention. *Psychological Bulletin*, *112*(1), 64–105.

Kellogg Foundation Latin America/Caribbean Program (2007). *Promoting Regional Development*. http://www.wkkf.org/default.aspx?tabid=75&CID=321&NID=618 Language ID=0

Lamborn, S. D., Mounts, N. S., Steinberg, L., & Dornbusch, S. M. (1991). Patterns of competence and adjustment among adolescents from authoritative, authoritarian, indulgent, and neglectful families. *Child Development*, *62*, 1049–1065.

Larson, R. W. (2000). Toward a psychology of positive youth development. *American Psychologist*, *55*, 170–183.

Larson, R. W. (2002). Globalization, societal change, and the new technologies: What they mean for the future of adolescence. *Journal of Research on Adolescence*, *12*(1), 1–30.

Larson, R., Brown, B., & Mortimer, J. (2003). *Adolescents' preparation for the future: A report from a study group on adolescence in the twenty first century*. New York: Blackwell Publishers.

Lerner, R. (1995). *America's youth in crisis: Challenges and options for programs and policies*. Thousand Oaks, CA: Sage.

Lerner, R. M. (2005, September). *Promoting positive youth development: Theoretical and empirical bases*. White paper prepared for a workshop on the science of adolescent health and development, National Research Council, Washington, DC.

Lerner, R. M., Almerigi, J. B., Theokas, C., & Lerner, J. V. (2005a). Positive youth development: A view of the issues. *Journal of Early Adolescence*, *25*(1), 10–16.

Lerner, R. M., Lerner, J. V., Almerigi, J. B., Theokas, C., Phelps, E., Gestsdottir, S., et al. (2005b). Positive youth development, participation in community youth development programs, and community contributions of fifth-grade adolescents:

Findings from the first wave of the 4-H Study of Positive Youth Development. *Journal of Early Adolescence, 25*(1), 17–71.

Martinson, B., Anderson, M., & deVries, R. (2005). Scientists behaving badly study. *Nature, 435*, 737–738.

McCall, R. B., & Groark, C. J. (2000). The future of child development research and public policy, *Child Development, 71*(1), 197–204.

McLeod, J. D., Kruttschnitt, C., & Dornfeld, M. (1994). Does parenting explain the effects of structural conditions on children's antisocial behavior? A comparison of blacks and whites. *Social Forces, 73*(2), 575–604.

Mills, J., & Bogenschneider, K. (2001). Can communities assess support for preventing adolescent alcohol and other drug use? Reliability and validity of a community assessment inventory. *Family Relations, 50*, 355–375.

Moffitt, T. E. (1993). Adolescence-limited and life-course-persistent antisocial behavior: A developmental taxonomy. *Psychological Bulletin, 100*(4), 674–701.

Petersen, A. C. (2006). Conducting policy-relevant developmental psychopathology research. *International Journal of Behavioral Development, 30*(1), 39–46.

Petersen, A. C. (2007). *Health and development in Africa: What are the engines for growth and change?* Invited lecture sponsored by the Alliance for the Earth Sciences, Engineering, and Development in Africa (AESEDA), The Pennsylvania State University. www.globalphilanthropyalliance.org/download/Anne_Petersen_AESEDA_4_07.ppt

Pittman, K., Diversi, M., & Ferber, T. (2002). Social policy supports for adolescence in the twenty-first century: Framing questions. *Journal of Research on Adolescence, 12*(1), 149–158.

Richter, L., & Dawes, A. (2008). South African psychological research on child development: A history of bias and neglect. In C. van Ommen & D. Painer (Eds.), *Interiors. A history of South African psychology* (pp. 286–323). Pretoria: University of South Africa Press.

Rutter, M. (1987). Psychosocial resilience and protective mechanisms. *American Journal of Orthopsychiatry, 57*, 316–331.

Saraswathi, T. S., & Larson, R. (2002). Adolescence in global perspective: An agenda for social policy. In B. B. Brown, R. W. Larson, & T. S. Saraswathi (Eds.), *The world's youth: Adolescence in eight regions of the globe* (pp. 344–362). New York: Cambridge University Press.

Shanahan, M. J. (2000). Pathways to adulthood in changing societies: Variability and mechanisms in life course perspective. *Annual Review of Sociology, 26*, 667–692.

Shanahan, M., Mortimer, J. T., & Kruger, H. (2002). Adolescence and adult work in the twenty-first century, *Journal of Research on Adolescence, 12*(1), 99–120.

Steinberg, L. (2001). We know some things: Adolescent–parent relationships in retrospect and prospect. *Journal of Research on Adolescence, 11*, 1–19.

Stokes, D. E. (1997). *Pasteur's quadrant: Basic science and technological innovation.* Washington, DC: Brookings Institution Press.

Verma, S. (2008). *Mapping typologies of risk and opportunity among street children in developing countries.* Invited Symposium, 2008 ISSBD Biennial Meeting, Wurzburg, Germany.

Webster's New Twentieth Century Dictionary of the English Language – Unabridged (2nd ed.) (1970). New York: World Publishing Company.

Werner, E. (1992). The children of Kauai: Resiliency and recovery in adolescence and adulthood. *Journal of Adolescent Health, 13*, 262–268.

World Bank (2007). *World Bank Development Report 2007*. http://go.worldbank.org/AR3D4L0E40.

Youniss, J., Bales, S., Christmas-Best, V., Diversi, M., McLaughlin, M., & Silbereisen, R. (2002). Youth civic engagement in the twenty-first century. *Journal of Research on Adolescence, 12*(1), 121–148.

Zimbardo, P. (2007) *Lucifer effect: Understanding how good people turn evil*. New York: Random House.

Author index

Subject index

For Product Safety Concerns and Information please contact our EU representative GPSR@taylorandfrancis.com Taylor & Francis Verlag GmbH, Kaufingerstraße 24, 80331 München, Germany